Critical Issues in the Early Development of Premature Infants

Critical Issues in the Early Development of Premature Infants

SIBYLLE K. ESCALONA

Yale University Press
New Haven and London

Designed by Sally Harris
and set in Times Roman type by
The Composing Room of Michigan.
Printed in the United States of America by
The Alpine Press, Inc., Stoughton, Mass.

Library of Congress Cataloging-in-Publication Data

Escalona, Sibylle K. (Sibylle Korsch), 1915–
Critical issues in the early development of premature infants.

Includes bibliographies.
1. Infants (Premature)—Development—Longitudinal studies. 2. Infants (Premature)—Family relationships—Longitudinal studies. 3. Infants (Premature)—Psychology—Longitudinal studies. 4. Child psychology—Longitudinal studies. I. Title. [DNLM: 1. Infant, Premature—growth & development. WS 410 E74c]
RJ250.3.E83 1987 618.92′01 87–6110
ISBN 0–300–03516–0 (alk. paper)

The paper in this book meets the guidelines for permanence and durability of the Committee on Production Guidelines for Book Longevity of the Council on Library Resources.

10 9 8 7 6 5 4 3 2 1

Contents

Figures

Tables

Appendixes

Acknowledgments

The research project upon which this book is based was made possible, in part, by USPHS grant HD01799; by the W. T. Grant Foundation; by the March of Dimes/Birth Defects Foundation; and by the Barbra Streisand Foundation.

So many different persons were involved in planning the study, in collecting and analyzing the data, and in thinking about the meaning of what was learned that an adequate acknowledgment of each individual is impossible. My heartfelt gratitude goes to each and every person who took an active role in the endeavor.

My friend and colleague Harvey H. Corman, M.D., played a major role during all phases of the work, from its inception in 1973 through a critical review of the manuscript in 1986. His unfailing support and his wisdom enabled me to overcome obstacles that at times seemed insurmountable. Bruce A. Grellong, Ph.D., assumed major responsibility for data collection and for the development and validation of assessment instruments. Ina Wallace, Ph.D., planned and executed the computer programs and statistical analyses. She also assumed responsibility for the follow-up studies. Among those who proved vital mainstays of the project were the following: Laurel Lardaro, Regina Ciambrone, Nancy Kaplan, and Lynn Myers. Evelyn Lipper, M.D., served as project pediatrician throughout. Last but not least, Herbert H. Vaughan, Director of the Rose F. Kennedy Center for Research in Mental Retardation and Human Development, initiated the entire venture.

PART I Setting the Stage

Chapter 1

What We Did and Why

The facts and ideas presented in this volume are based on a longitudinal study of 106 infants and their families. All of the infants were patients in a neonatal intensive care unit in a municipal hospital affiliated with a medical school. We became acquainted with the families soon after each baby's birth and conducted regular research sessions until the children had reached the age of 40 months.

The larger research program which made this study possible was a collaborative venture under the auspices of the Rose F. Kennedy Center for Research in Mental Retardation and Human Development of the Albert Einstein College of Medicine, Yeshiva University, New York. Neuroscientists, neonatologists, pediatricians, and developmental psychologists jointly studied this group of high-risk infants in order to learn more about the interactions between biologic and environmental factors that lead to diverse developmental outcomes. Other publications have reported on neurological and medical aspects of this issue, such as the assessment of neurobehavioral status in neonates (Kurtzberg 1979) and precursors of developmental deficits (Lipper et al. 1981; Wallace et al. 1982; Rose and Wallace 1985). For the developmental psychology unit, however, the opportunity to maintain regular contact with a group of low-birthweight infants and their families over some years offered challenges that went beyond the identification of impaired or deviant development.

We thought that a detailed description of the development and life experience of more than a hundred children would be of interest in its own right, the more so when accompanied by information about perinatal complications as well as about physical development and health status. Research on high-risk infant populations has typically focused on global variables such as birthweight or socioeconomic status and on selected outcome variables such as IQ or neuropathology at later ages. What we have come to know about the impact of childrearing practices and sociocultural characteristics upon social and cognitive development, in fact, is derived from the the study of normal child development. And, with some exceptions (Pavenstedt 1967), phenomenological accounts of child behavior in the context of ordinary life situations have dealt with middle-class children, so that our understanding of normal child development and the theories that support it are based largely on studies of middle-class children and their families. Yet even for them, systematic and comprehensive accounts of the behavioral events that—in context and sequence—constitute the life experience and development of very young children are not available.

For a small segment of the urban population we had an opportunity to fill this gap in information. As it happened, the composition of our research population seemed tailor-made for a more comprehensive study. The socioeconomic background of participating families covered the entire spectrum, from those who were grossly deprived to those who held professional or executive positions and lived in relative affluence. Also, the three dominant ethnic groups in our region, black, Hispanic, and Caucasian, were well represented. These circumstances invited a thorough examination of the developmental patterns that emerge under widely different conditions of childrearing, and the systematic description of the daily life and the development of this group thus became one of the aims of our study. Research procedures were therefore planned to focus as much on family functioning, the broader sociocultural and physical aspects of the child's environment, and childrearing practices as on each child's cognitive and psychosocial development.

Before we describe how we went about accomplishing this goal, it seems important to acquaint the reader with the assumptions, the theoretical frame of reference, and even the investigators' attitudes insofar as they guided our efforts. Objectivity—that is, the constraint of being factual and systematic—should not be confused with the absence of a point of view. The facts selected as relevant, the methods of ascertaining them, the organization of the data once they are collected, the very style in which material is presented—all reflect the basic orientation of the researchers.

Our perspective on issues in child development leans heavily on concepts that derive from the framework of psychoanalytic ego psychology. Piaget's theory of cognitive development also influences our thinking, especially as to the manner in which postulated structural changes in the mental apparatus are linked to observable changes in the scope and complexity of cognitive activity. A kinship to other developmental theories generally characterized by such terms as structural, dynamic, and holistic will become apparent. What these theories have in common is the assumption that transformations in behavior integration are in the general direction of increasing differentiation, increasing complexity, and increasingly hierarchical organization, and also that each major transformation results in the emergence of capacities not previously present. These changes are conceptualized as occurring on the psychological level: they refer to a succession of stable patterns of mental functioning. Thus the complex process of becoming a sentient, socially-related, thinking, problem-solving, and potentially creative individual cannot be understood by reduction to the physiological structures and processes upon which it rests. This statement in no way minimizes the importance of the biologic substratum. In the case of infants at biologic risk, such as our research population, the importance of central nervous system characteristics as determinants of behavior and development is highlighted simply because immaturity and deficits in brain functioning constitute the risk factor. In principle, the physiologic and specifically neural underpinnings of behavior and development are equally crucial in normal individuals. In what follows we shall describe some of the consequences of central nervous system deficits for the child's manner of responding to environmental circumstances and the resulting variations in cognitive and psychosocial development.

This broad sketch of where we fit in the spectrum of current thinking in child development is intended to convey the rationale for a research design that links such intrapersonal variables as impulse control to measures of ability such as IQ and that seeks to trace the roots of these developmental acquisitions to patterns of experience and behavior that were prominent in each child's life during the first few years. From the outset we knew that we could not possibly obtain a comprehensive picture of each child's significant experience, nor could we capture all the vital aspects of early personality development. Even intensive and sophisticated case studies fall short of such a goal. Much more is this so when data must be obtained during half-day-long sessions at intervals of six months or more. Much will be said about the shortcomings and limitations necessarily entailed by practical constraints as well as by the fact that there are many dimensions of developmental change for which adequate techniques of assessment do not exist. The reader will find the material we report to be far more modest and circumscribed than might be suggested by the generalizations we have offered. Nonetheless, some of the implications of our view will be mentioned briefly because they underlie the use to which data were put.

We regard the young organism as engaging with all aspects of the relevant environment and as shaping his own experience to some degree beginning on the first day of life. The readiness, or rather the necessity, to respond actively to the perceived environment derives from built-in properties of the organism which take the form of action impulses and later of felt needs, urges, wishes, interests, and goals. The biopsychic energies that compel behavior are difficult to define. Yet all psychological theories include the notion of some sort of energy or force to impel adaptation and development. Psychoanalysis, for example, postulates inborn instinctual drives and their derivatives; for Piaget the concept of an equilibrium between the child's adaptive repertoire and the actual adaptive challenge is a key notion; and instrumental learning theories assume an inherent tendency to arousal in the service of satisfaction or relief from tension. In the absence of a conceptually satisfying formulation concerning the energic components of behavior, it is nonetheless possible to discern the manifestations of forces and impulses at work.

What can be observed and studied are the ego functions that regulate and channel impulses and motivations. In fact, increasingly flexible and complex regulatory processes and mechanisms provide a key index of ego development. Increasing self-control and changing patterns of self-regulation are the basis of developmental progress in all spheres: cognition, affect, social transactions, and perceptual/motoric functions. If we and others refer to such regulatory controls as central, it is because the *same* structural and functional changes underlie development in each of these domains. By the same token, it is generally recognized that affect, perception, cognition, interpersonal relationships, and other spheres of functioning are highly interdependent and very closely interwoven during the early years of life.

A word is in order about how our results are organized and presented. We were confronted with a large mass of information about each child. In order to make sense of the material it was necessary to look at the same and related data in many different ways. A large number of calculations yielded an unconscionable number of tables which were similar to one another yet not redundant. Large portions of the data were of the kind that transforms what is essentially descriptive and qualitative information into numbers. Such numbers do not lend themselves to statistical reduction, although analysis of variance (ANOVA) and simple correlations were applicable to some of our data. The more interesting and important findings emerged only when the data were divided into subgroupings much too small to permit proper statistical evaluation. Thus our quantitative description was often limited to such devices as scattergrams and percentages.

It proved impossible to elucidate the findings and the relationships between them and to interpret results in the customary manner. That is, were we to document each assertion sufficiently to allow the reader to judge its validity, the tedium of inspecting innumerable tables would be intolerable and continuity of thought would be disrupted. Yet documentation is an indispensable requirement of empirical research. We have dealt with the problem by using graphic representations whenever possible so that the reader can observe important data trends with ease.

Another departure from the usual format came about because the effort to trace many facets of developmental change led us to devise numerous assessment instruments and to employ quasi-experimental methods drawn from other research projects. To have included a description of these procedures in the body of the text would have rendered the text nearly unreadable. Yet an explanation of the meaning of the scores, and of how they were obtained, is essential. The appendixes contain full descriptions of each research procedure. We thought it best to reproduce the manual and scoring blanks in the form actually used by the research staff. In consequence, there are instances (for example, achievement motivation) where the manual defines the variable and explains its relevance to our study. In others (for example, socioeconomic background) the rationale was self-evident but the interpretation and scoring of individual items required explication.

Last, we offer an introductory overview of the ground plan for the longitudinal study itself and for this book as well. We used our data to explore the sociocultural conditions that yielded sharply different life experiences for these children and further to trace the consequences of different patterns of experience for development during the first years of life. With a few exceptions, this report is limited to the period between 28 and 40 months of age. In different sections of this book the reader will find:

• An account of the objective background characteristics and diverse caretaking arrangements that differentiate socioeconomic groups.

• An account of selected patterns or aspects of experience that emerged as the combined result of biologic or other child characteristics and what the childrearing environment provided. Certain aspects of experience are massively different in the separate socioeconomic groups (as represented in our sample) and to some extent in different ethnic groups as well. Nearly all experience patterns were found in each of the social groups, although the groups differed from one another in the frequency with which each pattern was represented.

• For the sample as a whole, and for each of three subgroups, an analysis of the relationship between socioeconomic status (SES) and several developmental outcome measures will be described. Stable patterns of experience for each SES group and the associations between experience patterns (EP) and developmental outcome will be reported for the sample as a whole and also separately for each SES group.

The two primary measures of developmental progress were cognitive test scores and assessments of impulse control. In addition, neuropathology (as identified by pediatric/neurological examination)[1] and behavioral maladjustment (as determined by an assessment instrument for adjustment status) were regarded as outcome measures. That neurological illness and multiple soft neurological signs would occur with some frequency in a group of premature infants was to be expected. What we had not anticipated was that an appreciable number of these youngsters, although biologically sound, would develop fairly severe behavioral maladaptations at the ages of 2 and/or 3 years.

The relationships among environmental settings, experience patterns, cognitive development, and adjustment status are more clear-cut and easier to demonstrate within what, for want of a better term, we called the intact group: that is, those children in our research group who showed no neuropathology and no severe behavior difficulty. The relevant relationships are more difficult to trace among deviant children for the following reasons, among others: Deviant children respond atypically to many situations, and caretaking adults often modify their childrearing techniques in order to accommodate the special needs of the children. For these reasons our results are reported first for the intact group (part II) and then for the two deviant groups (part III).

Quantitative statements cannot reflect the infinite variety in the interplay of forces and conditions that may yet receive the same rating or score. More important, graphs and tables are remote from the meanings, the personal relationships, and the social ambience that, for each individual, constitute the unique family drama from which our numbers are derived. We therefore offer a number of vignettes of both intact and deviant children. We hope that these descriptions of individual children, presented as interludes, will convey to the reader our sense of the importance of early life experience and early development.

1. When appropriate, clinical neurological examination was supplemented by additional procedures and specialty consultations.

Chapter 2

How We Went About Achieving Our Goals

Recruitment and the Research Visit

During the year 1975/76 all families of patients in the neonatal intensive care unit were invited to participate in the follow-up study provided that the infants had a birthweight of less than 2500 grams and a gestational age of less than 36 weeks, or were small for gestational age by the Dubowitz criteria (Dubowitz 1970). In addition, we required that the mother be able to communicate reasonably well in English. The great majority of the mothers would have signed the consent form almost at once, but we asked that the matter first be discussed with the father or other important members of the family. Preliminary conversations were informal and took place over a period of several days. Although there was no remuneration, we did offer the family individualized and convenient medical supervision of the child as well as regular developmental evaluations and a full report of the results. Later, when parents and staff had come to know one another rather well, we learned that the parents and grandparents had responded primarily to the interest we showed in them as individuals and in their concerns about the baby.

While the babies were still inpatients, research activity was focused on medical and neurologic aspects. The follow-up study proper began when the children had reached the age of 7 months, corrected for prematurity. At that time and on each of the following visits the child was seen for extensive examination, and prolonged interviews were held with the mother and/or other family members. Visits were scheduled to take place at the following ages in months: 7, 15, 28, 34, and 40. The long hiatus between the 15- and 28-month visits was the unhappy consequence of a temporary funding crisis. A 22-month visit which had been planned for the entire group was limited to children for whom we felt special concern.

Demographic information was collected during the first few visits. These data were coded and later processed by computer. Many socioenvironmental variables were determined anew during each visit in order to monitor the changes taking place. These, as well as the interval history, were also coded and computer-stored separately for each visit. (For the socioenvironmental coding protocol, see Appendix A.)

We asked that for each visit the child be brought by the mother or whoever had primary responsibility for the baby's care. Fathers, grandparents, siblings, other relatives, and friends were welcome. Quite often, research visits became a family outing. Interviews with caretakers, most often the mother, were a leisurely affair, informal but not unstructured. Every effort was made to use our clinical skills in order to cover, as spontaneously as possible, the large number of topics and items required for coding and related to demographic and developmental issues. We knew from earlier experience and confirmed again that information offered in the course of a natural conversation in which the mother is an active participant is generally more accurate than are answers to direct questions. This is true even of concrete facts such as the size of the apartment. The mother and the others were encouraged to express their thoughts and feelings about anything at all, but only if and when it was they who initiated conversation on topics not directly related to the child. A good many of the mothers clearly valued the opportunity to speak their mind to an interested yet unintrusive listener. Precisely because the interviews often met a felt need, great care was taken to respect the informants' reserve and defensive attitudes. A clinically probing interview would have been inappropriate and unwise. In the research context and within the given time limitations it would have been impossible to offer therapeutic support. It was therefore important to prevent the development of a strong personal relationship, which all too readily comes to imply a promise of help with personal problems—a promise we would have been unable to keep. Interviews were cordial at all times, and with most families an easy, trusting, and mutually respectful relationship was established.

It is worth noting that it was possible to maintain such contact over some years with a population that is often described as less than cooperative. Most of our families were black or Hispanic, and most were poor. Such groups are said to break appointments readily and to dislike extensive verbal interchanges with professionals. The fact that of the 117 families[1] who came for the 7-month visit 104 were still with us at 40 months speaks for itself. Of the thirteen cases lost to the study two died, most moved to distant places, and two did not respond to invitations to return. As has been true with other programs serving similar populations, it required patience and flexibility to maintain reasonably regular schedules. Mothers overslept, "forgot," had more pressing appointments, or—as it was put to us—could not get themselves together. They might not make it until the third try. Transportation was provided, and we tried in every way to meet the family's convenience. It also helped a great deal that one staff member maintained liaison with our families and offered them some practical assistance. She telephoned mothers between visits, made a point of meeting them briefly when they had other appointments in the building, arranged for specialty consultations, and on request provided information about community resources. Many a time she helped a mother to fill out bewildering forms. Thus those families ill equipped to deal with the bureaucracy had a friend and resource at the project.

1. This includes nine children who suffered severe brain damage and were excluded from this research sample.

Over the years the research staff came to feel a good deal more than sympathy for our families. We learned to respect and admire the energy and determination needed to maintain a household, take care of children, live up to obligations to the extended family, and cope with illness, public agencies, and the threat and actuality of robbery, violence, and all the other hazards that beset the urban poor. By the same token, we had an unusual opportunity to realize the vitality, strength, and richness of human relationships and the capacity for sheer enjoyment shown by many of these families.

Research visits to project quarters lasted from three to six hours. Always they included developmental testing, a pediatric/neurological examination, a play interview (from 15 months onward), and the family interview. In addition, we administered a number of quasi-experimental procedures to obtain information on behavioral dimensions or on psychological functions that are of phase-specific relevance. For the age levels with which we are concerned in this book, these special procedures consisted of standardized techniques to assess the following areas: mother-child interaction, including response to separation from the mother, impulse control, concept formation, and perception of the self (precursors of body image). At the 34-month visit we added an assessment of achievement motivation as well as the Level of Aspiration test, which reflects response to success and failure. At the last visit the World Test was administered. It taps the ability to structure space in the service of mental representation as the child is asked to "build something" using realistic miniature toy props. The data obtained through these supplementary procedures were invaluable in that they provided a more complete and dynamic picture of each child's cognitive and psychosocial functioning. This information is used in the illustrative vignettes but not in the more formal quantitative analysis. All of the special procedures are described in the appendixes and, where appropriate, the scoring manual is reproduced.

Valuable information about child and family was also obtained as the youngster was fed, dressed, toileted, and observed at play during the time the mother spent closeted with the interviewer. Throughout such in-between periods other staff conversed with the attending family members about what was going on and especially about the degree to which the child's behavior was or was not similar to what was seen at home.

Standard Tests of Cognitive Development

The intellectual development of the children was monitored chiefly by means of serial administration of intelligence tests. At the ages of 7 and 15 months[2] we used the Bayley Scales of Mental Development (Bayley 1969), which yield a mental developmental index (MDI) very similar to the IQ. Beginning at 28 months, the

2. Through 15 months we calculated age with a correction for prematurity; thereafter chronological age was used.

Stanford-Binet Intelligence Test was given (Terman and Merrill 1973). For more than half of our subjects the lowest level of the Stanford (2.0 years) was beyond their reach or coincided with the most difficult items they could achieve. In these instances or when the number of items from the Stanford that were applicable was too small to yield a reasonable sample of cognitive competence, the Bayley Scales were administered once again. Forty children were given both tests. In this small sample the mental age scores resulting from the two instruments were in close agreement.

We are well aware of the limitations of the IQ and agree with much of the criticism that has been leveled at these scores when they are used as the sole measure of a child's ability. Intelligence in the broader meaning of the term—that is, cognitive, adaptive, problem-solving, and learning ability—is only partially tapped by standard tests. A child may well be sophisticated and innovative in social or other contexts, may even be precocious in some aspects of development, and yet may be ill prepared to deal with formboards, words, pictures, and other components of the test in the required manner. This is more likely to occur when the type of problem presented during the test is alien to the family culture in which the child lives. It is for this reason that we sought to supplement test findings by assessing additional realms of cognitive functioning insofar as this was possible to do during a single visit.

The well-known fact that intelligence tests are culture-bound is of special relevance to our research population, so many of whom came from poor black or Hispanic homes. The age norms that determine scores are based on representative samples of the entire U.S. population, which is predominantly white and middle class. These norms reflect the biologically given capacities of the organism as it matures, but they also reflect the result of such training, teaching, opportunity, and constraint as are generally provided for the majority of children in our society. For these and other reasons there can be little doubt that IQs are unfair in the sense that they may classify as dull some bright children who have had no opportunity to learn the requisite skills. Beyond this, the tests may fail to tap areas that have been cultivated in the child's milieu but are not representative of the majority. Inevitably, value judgments are imbedded in test composition and enter the evaluation of results.

From a broadly humanistic point of view, it may be no better to have a normal than a borderline IQ. Practically speaking, impoverished or delayed cognitive development in the areas included in standard tests is a serious handicap because success in school rests primarily on the variety of abilities measured by the tests. It is a familiar story to hear that poor children often enter kindergarten and first grade ill prepared to meet school demands. They may not be accustomed to concentrate on a learning task or to pay close enough attention to profit from a teacher's explanation. Even sitting still without speaking as the spirit moves them can be difficult—not necessarily because they are unable to concentrate and learn but because what is talked about and taught does not build on previous interests and practiced activities. Nor is the subject matter congruent with things in which persons in the home environment have shown an interest.

Minority populations, be they poor, non-white, or both, are also part of the larger society. They must participate in and adapt to the institutions of the dominant group. In a technological society, academic learning failure has profound consequences for material and vocational success. In a substantial number of poor children one can observe a malign sequence that begins with slow or retarded cognitive development during the preschool years and leads to insufficient academic progress and finally to a lack of fitness for skilled vocational careers. All the parents in our study, even the least educated and the least ambitious, were well aware of this. They wanted very much for their children to do well in school, to become good wage earners and good citizens or, at the very least, to be "smart" enough to stay out of trouble. Thus, both to the individuals concerned and to society at large, early cognitive development as measured by intelligence tests is an important issue.

After all the caveats about the IQ, something more positive needs to be said as well. We have found that in the case of very young children the IQ reflects more about overall development than is true at later ages. In the absence of conditions that prevent full and interested participation on the child's part, such as extreme shyness, fatigue, ill health, or unconquerable negativism, IQs do indicate progress, delay, or precocity in overall development. In our experience, a two- or three-year-old who performs markedly below age standards in the testing situation is extremely likely also to be immature in the realm of social interactions, in his affect manifestations, in his relative self-sufficiency, in his play, and in his capacity to cope with everyday problems. In terms of developmental theory, it makes good sense to find a greater correspondence between IQ scores and more broadly defined developmental status in children below the age of about 4 than in older children. While affective, social, perceptual, and cognitive development remain interdependent throughout life, they are inseparable in infancy and very closely interwoven in early childhood. Therefore the maturity of a set of cognitive functions is more likely to reflect the level of maturity in other areas of functioning in very young children than in somewhat older ones.

What has been said so far about the limitations and strengths of standard intelligence tests refers to children who fall behind in their cognitive and psychosocial development. Things are less clear at the other end of the range. At the time of this writing, American families tend to place a very high value on early achievement. Skills that formerly were not expected to appear until a somewhat later age, such as word, color, and form recognition, are taught in the nursery. Reading is felt to be a desirable skill at age 3 or 4. In general much of what used to be considered school learning has moved into informal as well as formal preschool education. Many of the toys and games used with very young children are similar to test items and can be thought of as training geared not only to later educational requirements but also to competent test taking.

Preschoolers do respond to such "cognitive enrichment" with accelerated (by previous standards) development of certain skills. Yet it has not been demonstrated that early readers become better readers or that the ability to recite numbers without comprehending what they denote leads to greater prowess in arithmetic. In the case of language acquisition it has long been known that among highly gifted individuals a fair proportion learned to speak relatively late. When precocity occurs spontaneously, it often heralds superior intellectual endowment, but this is a very different thing from precocious learning fostered by energetic early teaching. At the present state of knowledge there is no clear evidence that a superior IQ at preschool age, as compared to good average standing, necessarily implies a more favorable developmental status or significantly better prospects. Be that as it may, in our study cognitive test scores were consistently related to a good many other variables and by and large they provided a valuable index of developmental status.

Up to this point we have dealt with those of our major variables that could be quantified by means of established instruments to yield scores based on representative samples of the population—namely, the socioeconomic status of the family (SES index) and the cognitive development of the children (MDI and IQ). Yet the research plan also called for a determination of stable aspects of daily life experience (EP), for an assessment of the level of impulse control attained by each child (IC), and for a determination of overall—that is, cognitive and psychosocial—functioning at the age of three years. A detailed account of how we arrived at rating scores in these areas is found in the appendixes. Of the three variables mentioned above, EP is by far the most complex, so much so that a definition and discussion of experience patterns and an account of how we went about assessing them are presented in chapter 5. The remaining two variables, impulse control and adjustment status, are discussed below.

Impulse Control

In psychoanalytic ego psychology, and indeed in most other psychological theories, the capacity to control and modulate impulse is held to lie at the core of development during early childhood and to remain an indispensable component of adaptation throughout life. The literature offers a bewildering array of theoretical elaborations concerning its origins (intrinsic, acquired, or both), the processes that lead to increasingly effective and flexible ego control (structure formation, learning under the impact of reinforcement, instinctual and/or experiential vicissitudes and more), and the behavioral manifestations of impulse control (in activity-passivity, thought, affect, perceptual style, and almost every other psychological domain).

The definition of impulse control is embedded in a network of thorny theoretical issues. These need not concern us now, but they do have a bearing on the meaning of our findings and will be discussed later. For our present purposes it will suffice to say that the decision to make the degree of impulse control one of the major measures of developmental course and outcome was based on the following considerations. Much child-development research has shown that cognitive advances during the preschool years depend on the child's capacity to inhibit, delay, or modify motoric and expressive action in order that a degree of surveillance—what Werner and Kaplan (1963) called contemplation and reflection—can take place. By impulse we understand any felt compelling incitement to motoric action. The dictionary definition of "something driving with sudden force" serves as well as any other provided that the "force" arises from within, though often in response to external events. As we use the term, impulses arise in states of disequilibrium and heightened tension that—when unrestrained—lead to motoric action. Often but not always, action follows impulse so immediately as to render it involuntary or at least unintended. Such a broad view of impulse encompasses an occurrence as trivial as the impulse to scratch an itch but also an occurrence as massive as an outburst of anger that impels a toddler into an explosive temper tantrum, and all intermediate degrees.

Guided by Piaget's conception of cognitive development, the work of the Geneva school has traced the emergence of increasingly objective and increasingly abstract cognitive activity in minute detail. Piaget's term for the direction of cognitive behavior change is *decentering,* which is understood as implying an increased distance between the acting organism and the acted-upon aspect of first the concrete environment and later mental representations. The latter come to include comprehension of the necessary lawful relationships among phenomena and of the thought processes or *mental operations* whereby such understanding is applied to specific problems. Piaget (1954) demonstrated, as have Werner and Kaplan, that the transition from primarily sensorimotor operations to reliance upon symbolic systems such as language rests upon or is invariably accompanied by the capacity to interpose a delay between perception and the response to it. This all-important step of entry into the realm of symbolic thought and ideation, which also includes the emergence of imaginative play, is *the* critical developmental issue late in the second and during the third year of life. It is then that children are expected to use language in order to convey meanings beyond the expression of immediate need and to recognize and abstract from perceptual impressions such early concepts as those referring to size, form, and color. It is then, and by virtue of the same capacity, that means are clearly separated from their ends and that pictures are understood as representing real objects. In other words, the abilities and competencies measured in tests of intelligence (but not in scales of infant development) normally arise during the toddler years.

It ought to be mentioned that some degree of delay capacity emerges earlier. For instance, inhibition and modulation to some extent are necessary components of more advanced motor coordinations usually achieved late in the first and during the second year of life. Similarly, some degree of participation in adult symbolic systems of communication is found in infancy, especially in the modes of gesture and intonation. But it is only by perhaps the middle of the second year of life that the acquisition of more extensive and flexible controls, and of cognition based on the use of symbols, become the focal axis of phase-appropriate developmental transitions.

If it is true that cognitive development beyond the sensorimotor level takes place only when the requisite degree of impulse control has been achieved, one must ask how impulse control is acquired in the first place. Anyone familiar with the behavior and daily life of toddlers knows the answer. Impulsivity and its constraint are the red thread running through the life of caretaking mothers and their offspring. From early on children are asked to "wait a minute"; to moderate bodily activity and suppress screaming or joyous squealing. They are taught not to touch forbidden objects, to stay in bed in spite of resistance, to deposit excreta at the designated place, and so forth. In these and a great many other situations, toddlers are taught or required to subdue outbursts of anger and disappointment, to obey uncongenial requests, and to refrain from overt protest and defiance. Caretakers base such expectations for increasing patience and self-control upon the commonsense understanding that with growth, maturation, and increasing comprehension children are better able to tolerate constraints and to develop regulatory mechanisms that are beyond the capacity of infants.

While the establishment of impulse control is assuredly contingent upon maturation of the central nervous system and also temperamental characteristics, the arena in which the drama is played out lies in the events that serve socialization—that is, in the quality and nature of the child's interactions with caretaking adults. The ease or difficulty with which impulse control develops, the rate of its development, and the particular forms it takes all depend on the manner in which toddlers and caretaking adults live through these struggles and mutual accommodations. It is to the child's typical behavior in such situations that we turned in order to develop a measure of impulse control. We believe that impulse control is shown most readily, as is its absence, in social interactions that are often emotionally charged. It is also assumed that some degree of impulse control must be operative in everyday exchanges before it can have significant impact upon cognitive progression.

The relationship between impulsivity and cognition has been the subject of considerable study by psychologists. Most of this work was not focused on developmental changes although children as well as adults have served as experimental subjects. The most important exception is an ambitious research program conducted by Jean and Jack Block (Block and Block 1980). Over a period of some decades, these investigators studied what they term *ego control* as a significant component of personality functioning and adaptation. Their definition of ego control is identical to our definition of impulse control. They specify that in psychoanalytic writings nearly all ego functions are defined so as to involve the control and modulation of impulse. The Blocks traced the antecedents, vicissitudes, and consequences of different degrees and modes of control at various ages, from the preschool years to adolescence, and they found ample empirical support for the idea that viable adaptation and adequate cognitive development can and do take place when impulse control is *relatively* low and *relatively* high in comparison to the mode. They concluded, however, that placement at either extreme of the ego-control continuum is adaptively dysfunctional. Their results also include the finding that the degree of impulse control shown in childhood, and even in maturity, is linked to family characteristics and to the socialization procedures that had been applied to the children. Specifically, overcontrolled adults tended to come from families that emphasized structure and orderliness and in general held conservative values. Undercontrolled adults tended to come from homes that had earlier been characterized as conflict-ridden (parents held discrepant basic values) and homes in which lesser demands for conformity were placed on the young child (Block, J. 1971; Block, J. H. 1976).

In their longitudinal study of ego control, which is most relevant to our work, the Blocks made assessments of control during the mid-preschool years and thereafter—that is, at an age when some degree of impulse control has already been attained. Our effort with two- and three-year-olds was necessarily directed at very early manifestations of still quite limited control. The behavioral criteria we employed are thus quite different from those used by the Blocks.[3]

In the conviction that some degree of impulse control must have been operative in everyday life for some time if the cognitive developments that normally occur during the third year are to flourish, we developed an assessment of this capacity. Impulse control was comprehensively assessed at each age beginning with the early 2-year visit up to the last at 40 months. (The manual that guided rater judgments is reproduced in appendix B.) The procedure was for two investigators, H. H. Corman and the author, to rate each child independently for each visit. Each of us read the summary of the visit, the interview, and everything else, and prepared a written documentation of his or her judgment by citing relevant portions of the record. We agreed on 88% of the rating judgments. In cases of disagreement the material was reviewed again and discussed so as to attain a consensus rating. Nearly all disagreements arose in deciding whether or not the record contained sufficiently detailed and reliable information to justify a rating. We thought that no rating whatever was preferable to one based on invalid or minimal information. Thus it came about that for a few children impulse control could not be rated at any time. For a good many others the assessment could be made at most but not all age levels. In consequence the number of impulse-control ratings available was not the same at each age level. Data analysis was made cumbersome by this circumstance, but, on the other hand, the results are more trustworthy than if the ratings had been made on insufficient grounds.

Ratings were based on descriptions of behavior at the time of the visit and during

3. Another difference was methodological. In addition to experimental techniques, the Blocks relied on *Q* sorts. This method requires parents or teachers to select from a set of preformulated behavioral descriptions those that are more and less salient to the child.

the four to six weeks preceding it. We looked for instances in which the situational context demanded or permitted the display of behavior relevant to impulse control. These included, among many others: the appropriate reduction or suppression of motoric action; the modulation of affect expression; responding to frustration or disappointment without loss of control or behavior disintegration; tolerance for delay; persistence and patience in the pursuit of tasks or goals offering considerable difficulty to the child. Normative standards do not exist for the degree of impulse control appropriate to or typically shown at given ages. Therefore the relative maturity of impulse control (IC) had to be judged by comparison to that shown by all other children of the same age in the sample.

To a small extent the structure of the intelligence test provides normative suggestions in that many test items require the ability to delay (for instance, waiting until the formboard pieces have been aligned or until the task has been demonstrated). However, not only may test behavior be situation-bound, but IC is acquired and manifested chiefly in the course of social interactions with caretakers and other people. It is at mealtimes, bedtimes, during disciplinary encounters, and also in such social situations as family visits or shopping expeditions that the issue of control, patience, and the capacity for compromise and negotiation arises most often and most vividly. Although observation of the child in the office provided useful supplementary and illustrative material, it was never used to substantiate a rating. Rather, we compared the descriptions of one child's behavior with the descriptions of the behavior of all agemates. Behavior patterns that on this basis were judged to be age-appropriate at 28 months are likely to bespeak fairly low levels of control toward the end of the third year (34 months) and to indicate considerable immaturity in this respect at 40 months.

The IC scores are defined as follows:

1. IC is extremely low or nearly absent. This rating applied almost exclusively to deviant children.
2. IC is present to a lesser degree than in the majority of peers but within the normal range.
3. An age-appropriate flexible balance between control and impulsivity is seen. By definition, the majority of intact children received this rating.
4. The child showed greater and more consistent control than the majority. The intact children who received this rating retained a reasonable degree of spontaneity and zest though none was outstanding in this respect. Among the deviant children who received the same rating some were severely constricted and inhibited and others were not.
5. This score was appropriate to only a few among the deviant children. It was applied when a child was overly controlled some of the time and lacked control at other times. In such children a moderate degree of control was not reported or observed—they knew no middle ground.

There are obvious limitations to judgments of a central and subtle aspect of personality functioning based predominantly on family reports. The possibility that mothers' reports were less adequate than they seemed and that observation in the child's home would have led to a different rating cannot be excluded.

On the other hand, rating judgments were distilled from a wide range of behavior manifestations and were guided by rigid, predetermined criteria. Further, they were omitted when we felt unable to make a rating with reasonable confidence in its validity. We believe that the proof of the pudding is in the eating. Our IC ratings must have reflected a significant aspect of the children's functioning at the time: otherwise they could not have correlated very highly with IQ and with particular patterns of experience, as in fact they did.

An interest in the relationship between impulse control and cognition influenced the research plan from the beginning. Initially we chose to assess IC during the 28-month visit because we believed that children who were immature in this respect would also be relatively slow in early concept formation and language acquisition. At that time we thought of IC as one among many developmental variables. Our expectation was that as children inevitably move from lesser to greater degrees of control, so their cognitive abilities would grow in tandem. We also thought that a degree of control had to be operating in the social and affective realm before it could have an effect upon the rate of cognitive advance. On the basis of IC measures at 28 months we hoped to demonstrate that by the age of 34 months those who had shown age-appropriate ICs when younger would tend to have higher IQs than the rest. This expectation was borne out, but we soon learned that our view of the issue was oversimplified and hence inadequate. Nonetheless, the limited but standardized observational assessment of IC administered at 28 months is of some value (see appendix J).

Ratings were based on behavior observation during the entire developmental testing session. Two observers recorded behavior from behind a one-way-vision mirror. Eight situations likely to elicit relevant behavior and likely to arise during testing were preselected. Observers noted each occurrence of each of these situations and scored the child's behavioral response in terms of standard alternative scores. For instance, whenever an adult asked or urged the child to perform an action that he or she did not wish to execute, good control was scored if the child registered unwillingness but without a marked increase in body movement or alteration of voice quality. A relative lack of control was scored if the child showed overt distress or anger in such ways as running away, hitting, pronounced restlessness, and/or crying, screaming, using abusive language, and in general losing his or her temper. Final ratings were based on the frequency with which each type of behavioral response had been scored in relation to the number of times each situation had occurred. An overall rating based on the aggregate of scores in all situations became the final score.

Ratings of IC made in this fashion in the laboratory could be compared to the comprehensive rating of IC (based on the entire record) for seventy children at the 28-month level. (For the remainder either a comprehensive or a brief IC rating could not be made.) Of these seventy comparisons, 84% were in agreement. That is, those whose comprehensive rating was either 3 or 4, denoting appropriate or superior control, received a rating of well modulated and contained on the brief assessment. Those for whom the comprehensive rating reflected minimal (1) or less than usual (2) control also received a rating of poorly controlled and excitable for the limited-time sample observation. Of the eleven cases for which ratings disagreed, eight were well controlled during the test although their behavior at home was somewhat undercontrolled. In view of the response of most two-year-olds to strange surroundings and unfamiliar persons one can only wonder that this discrepancy was so rare. We believe that the brief assessment, though systematic, is an insufficient measure of impulse control. Yet the good agreement between the two ratings is of interest because it indicates the degree to which whatever level of control has been attained influences behavior organization even in what must be regarded as an unusual situation for the child. In addition, the disagreements that did occur testify to the fact that children whose behavior is generally somewhat deficient in control may have acquired the requisite self-regulating mechanisms but live in an atmosphere that does not encourage or enforce their application. The description of experience patterns lends substance to that assertion.

Adjustment Status

We have mentioned that some of our children proved to show deviant developmental patterns and that a distinction between neurological and behavioral deviancy was made. The diagnosis of neuropathology was of course the result of neurological examination. It is now necessary to describe how we arrived at the decision that a child showed behavioral difficulties sufficiently severe to be classified as deviant. To judge whether a two- or three-year-old is maladjusted is not an easy task under any circumstances. It cannot be overemphasized that the classification of some children as behaviorally disturbed does *not* imply a psychiatric diagnosis. It merely means that between 28 and 40 months of age these children showed emotional and behavioral disturbances severe enough to disrupt or distort ongoing adaptation and development. For the duration of such behavioral disruption the child was deviant only in the sense that his or her mode of functioning was sharply different from that of the majority of children living in similar circumstances, and that the child's behavior was functionally nonadaptive. Such a definition does *not* imply an unfavorable prognosis. (For a more extensive discussion of this issue, see appendix D.)

The assessment of what, for want of a better term, we call behavioral deviancy had to be based on reports provided by the caretaking adults and on limited direct observation. The procedure that we employed is parallel to that used in making a comprehensive IC rating. After the last research visit had taken place the author and a senior research staff member, Bruce Grellong, independently reviewed the entire record and formed a judgment as to whether or not the child should be considered deviant. Whenever one rater thought a child to be deviant, he or she prepared a document summarizing the reported and observed behaviors that led to the judgment. Subsequently we met to discuss the material and, when there was disagreement, we arrived at a consensus rating.[4]

For a clinical and developmental evaluation of this sort, a manual defining behavioral criteria and situational contexts is impractical. In lieu of a manual the appendix D furnishes an illustrative summary of the varieties of maladaptive behavior patterns that we encountered. The raters shared a conception of what constitutes adequate adaptation during the toddler and preschool years. They also shared an ego-psychoanalytic point of view concerning essential developmental trends and their behavioral manifestations. In addition, both had had extensive research experience in early child development and both had worked with families of minority ethnic backgrounds as well as with families from the entire socioeconomic range.

What was said earlier about the degree to which cognitive norms are anchored in middle-class standards is doubly true for the perception of what constitutes normalcy in the psychosocial sphere. What is normal and expected child behavior in one subculture may be rare and responded to as deviant in another. We assume that normalcy is culture-bound and that, with the exception of some severe disorders, no definition can be made applicable to all children under all conditions of existence. For our limited research purposes this knotty problem was largely circumvented by placing primary emphasis on whether or not the child's behavior differed from what was expected and appraised as normal by the child's own family and by others in the same sociocultural setting. In short, mothers, grandmothers, and others in close contact with the child had to express the belief that the child had a serious problem, that there was "something wrong" with him or her. The child's behavior during the research visits and the results of tests and assessments usually confirmed such reports. More important, it tended to exemplify the behavioral particulars of what had been described. Our observation of the child, however, was never allowed to be the sole evidence of deviancy, no matter how unusual the behavior was. We reasoned that if the atypical behavior we observed did indeed indicate malfunctioning this would inevitably manifest itself in day-to-day behavior as well.

This brings us to the second requirement for making an adjustment rating: namely, that specific and detailed accounts of the relevant behavior had to be available. It was not enough, for instance, for the family to say that the child was hyperactive (a term with which an astonishing number of our parents were familiar). Only if the description of how the child played, how he or she behaved at meal- and bedtimes, on the street, in stores, and during all phases of the day confirmed very high levels of apparently uncontrollable activity did we classify that child as deviant in this respect. The intact group therefore almost certainly

4. In a few instances the author alone is responsible for the final rating.

contained some children who were deviant as we define the term but for whom the information that we were able to obtain was too scant to permit a considered judgment. Yet even with all their shortcomings, the ratings of behavioral deviancy have face validity, for, as will be seen, they showed a clear-cut relationship to IC and also to dominant patterns of experience.

Chapter 3

Socioeconomic Characteristics of the Research Population

Many years of research have shown that the intellectual development of children reared in poverty tends to be diminished in comparison to that of children who grow up in middle- or upper-class environments. The literature is so extensive and the basic finding is so well known that a detailed review would be redundant.

A strong relationship between socioeconomic status and IQ as well as school achievement is found in low-birthweight infants as well (Drillien 1964; Drillien, Thomson, and Burgoyne 1980; Escalona 1982). Figure 3.1 may serve as a representative example. It shows the mean IQ for our sample by social class over the time span from 7 to 40 months. Sharp differences in IQ as a function of SES occurred, so that by the age of 40 months mean IQ was 74.9 for the lowest SES group and 99.5 for the highest. In figure 3.1 we present another important finding which has also been reported by other investigators (Golden and Birns 1968, 1976): namely, that social-class differences in developmental test scores are trivial until some time during the second year of life. In our data they become pronounced early in the third year, even though, to judge by other studies, they are likely to appear during the second half of the second year. SES differences become an important influence upon cognitive test scores during the same developmental phase that brings the shift from sensoriomotor to symbolic levels of functioning. There is every indication that children from materially and educationally deprived environments are as well endowed and potentially as able as all others, but growing up in poverty apparently provides less nourishment and support to the maturing mind than are ordinarily available to children in other socioeconomic strata. As yet we neither know nor understand the manner in which sociocultural impoverishment affects early development.

Some suggestions about the probable relationships between specific aspects of living in poverty and early cognitive development have been made. They include differences in speech and thought patterns, in childrearing techniques, and also in basic values.[1] For the time being, hypotheses of this kind must remain general and somewhat speculative. They are based on a statistical correspondence between overall characteristics of poor populations and overall cognitive outcome. The fact that there is a relationship between an antecedent condition (such as different

1. For a good overview see National Institutes of Health, 1968. More recently Barbara Biber (1984) has provided a helpful discussion of the relevant literature.

Figure 3.1 Mean IQ by SES Quartile for 106 Low Birthweight Infants (by Age)

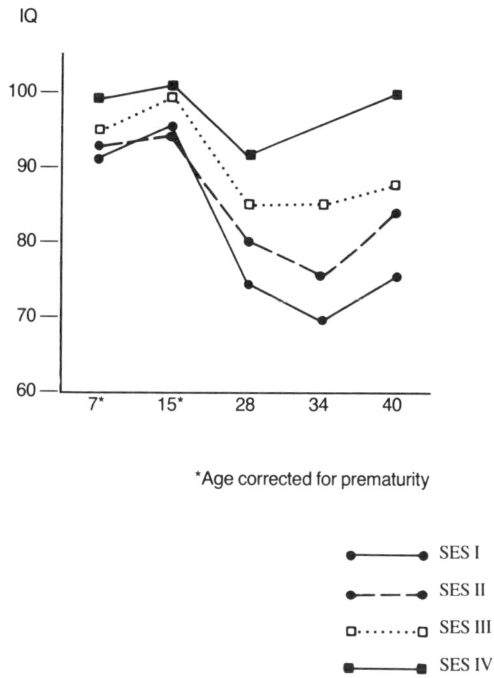

language styles) and a subsequent occurrence (such as a lower mean IQ) does not prove that a causal relationship exists between them. In this connection it is well to remember that not so many years ago the same relationship between SES (as well as ethnic background) and intelligence was recognized but was then attributed to genetic factors more than to early life experience and opportunity.

In short, what we do not know are the specific aspects of life in poverty that impinge upon cognitive development. Nor do we know the pathways through which the social environment affects development—what functions, at which stages of development, are altered in what manner by early life experience. Until the processes that link experience to developmental course have been specified, many important questions cannot be answered. For instance, even in the poorest segments of society we encounter the entire range from retardation to superior ability, and genetic differences cannot account for more than a small fraction of the wide range of intellectual attainment found among children who are reared in poverty. We ask ourselves what the differences are in life experience within the same socioeconomic group between those who do well and those whose development is impaired. Questions such as these involve basic issues in developmental theory. They address the complex problem of the interaction between the organism and its environment. This is so vast a topic that no single study can do more than explore very limited aspects of it. We shall endeavor to do just that: to inspect both the similarities and the differences in the experience of children, each as an individual within a sociocultural context, and to relate both differences and commonalities to developmental outcome. Therefore our results will be reported by comparing different SES groups as well as by delineating variations encountered within each social class.

The experience patterns that each family and each SES group generated for their young children can be understood only in light of the actual physical and social background that gave rise to them. For this reason we present the socioeconomic characteristics of the research families as an introduction to the results proper. The manner in which demographic and other socioenvironmental data were obtained by interview was described in the preceding chapter. Once all the information was at hand it turned out that our research sample was not representative of the entire population served by our medical center. By comparison to U. S. census figures for this region of the city, our research group had a significantly lower mean income and it contained a larger proportion of black and Hispanic families. Yet it also included the stable lower middle-class and upper segments of the socioeconomic scale. This composition of the sample came about at least in part because our hospital serves an area that contains some of the worst slums in the city, and the incidence of prematurity is disproportionately high among the very poor. At the same time, our neonatal care unit was the designated facility for a larger region, so that private and voluntary hospitals in nearby suburban areas transferred infants to our unit.

Our method of calculating SES was that used by the U. S. Census Bureau (Myrianthipoulos and French 1968). It is a combined index of income, vocational status, and education for the head of household on a scale from 1 to 100. Among the research families the SES index ranged from a low of 12 to a high of 94. In order to specify relationships between SES and such variables as family composition and experience patterns it was necessary to create different SES groups of equal size. All families were ranked by SES index and then divided into quartiles. Thus quartile I comprises the 25% with the lowest SES index, quartiles II and III constitute the two midgroups in this respect, and quartile IV contains the 25% of the families that had the highest SES index. In what is to follow, when we speak of the lowest or any other SES quartile (Q-), it should be understood that these designations do not necessarily indicate the same socioeconomic characteristics that are referred to in other and larger studies using the same device. In particular, our midgroups correspond to what would fall into the the low SES group in many other studies of high-risk infants. Our quartile IV is however very similar to those so designated in other publications. Nonetheless, the nature and direction of SES differences that we report are in complete harmony with all other accounts. They specify what it is that differs in the life circumstances of the very poor, the moderately poor, and those of middle-class and prosperous standing in urban populations in the United States. Somewhat to our surprise, even a measure as crude as the SES index did in fact sort out groups that differ from one another in many important ways.

As mentioned earlier, findings for the intact group of children will be reported separately from those for the deviant groups. As we intend to trace a close connection between the socioenvironmental conditions in which our children lived and the life experience these conditions brought about, the socioeconomic background data are reported here only for the families in the intact group. It so happened that the demographic characteristics of the deviant and intact groups were very similar.

In figure 3.2 we show the age, ethnicity, and educational level of the mothers in each quartile at the time of the baby's birth. The number of mothers falling within any single category is very small. The intention is to give the reader a visual

Figure 3.2 Mother's Age, Education and Ethnicity by SES Quartile (Intact Group)

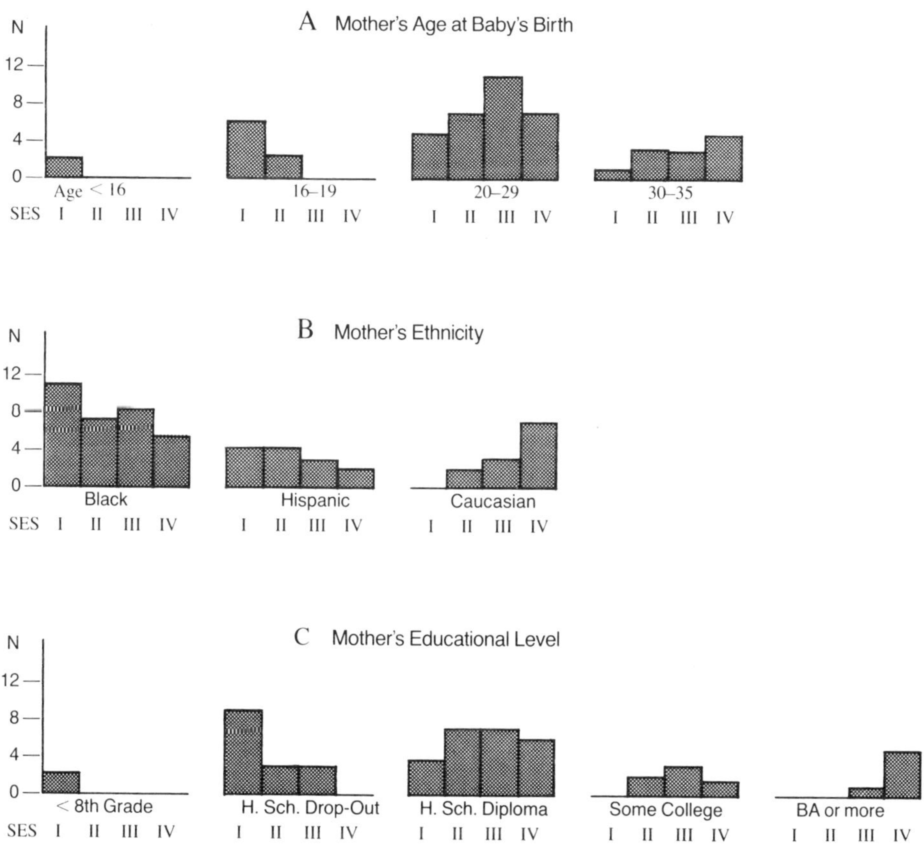

impression of major differences with little or no regard for the precise numerical distributions. From figure 3.2 it is apparent that in Q-I most mothers were teenagers, all were either black or Hispanic, and most did not graduate from high school. Quartile II mothers were predominantly in their twenties, all but three had completed high school, and all but two were black or Hispanic. All Q-III mothers were beyond their teens in age. In this group, too, blacks and Hispanics far outnumbered whites. Their educational level was about the same as that of mothers in Q-II. In the high SES group (Q-IV), half the mothers were in their thirties. As would be expected, none lacked a high school education and more than half had completed college. It is also not surprising that in Q-IV we find the largest proportion of white mothers, although exactly half were black or Hispanic. The particular composition of the research group then means that the differences in life style and childrearing practices that we found to be associated with SES cannot be ascribed to ethnic differences in our sample, or only to a very slight degree. SES differences between quartiles I, II, and III are pronounced although the ethnic composition of these groups is very similar, and even in quartile IV within-group differences are no greater than in the other quartiles.

In figure 3.3 we show who was the head of household for each quartile,

Figure 3.3 Head of Household by SES Quartile (Intact Group, by Age)

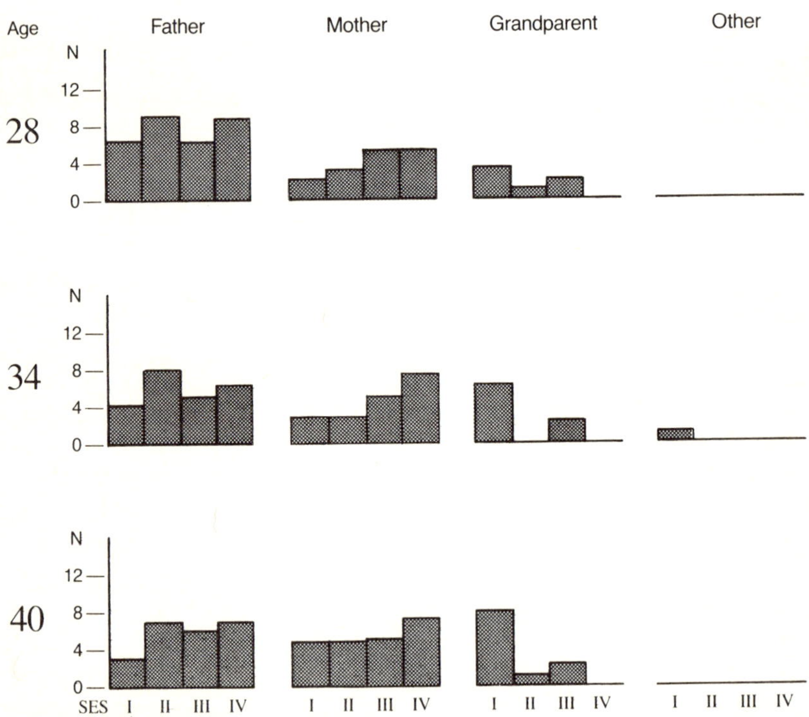

referring to the person residing in the home who was the major breadwinner and/or had primary responsibility for its maintenance. Family composition changed with time, and this item had to be updated at each visit. In quartile I the head of household changed a good deal. At 28 months it was still the baby's father in about half of the eleven cases; by 34 months two more fathers had departed; and at 40 months only three of the fathers were still in charge of the home. A glance at figure 3.4 shows that at least half of the mothers in Q-I considered themselves to be married despite the fact that by the time of the 40-month visit a grandparent had become the head of household in eight of the sixteen cases. Often these marriages were common-law arrangements. Sometimes the father also lived in the grandparents' home. More often fathers served in the army, were in jail, or, in one instance, worked in another city and came home on weekends. In any case, very few of the Q-I mothers assumed independent responsibility for their homes. As shown in Figure 3.4, the quartiles did not differ much in marital status although "never married" applied more frequently in the lower two SES groups.

As a result of these differences in family constellation, household size tended to be a good deal larger in Q-I families, chiefly because when mother and baby moved in with relatives, the home was often shared with some of the mother's sisters, who often had children of their own. In Q-I, 40% of the households

Figure 3.4 Mother's Marital Status by SES Quartile (Intact Group, by Age)

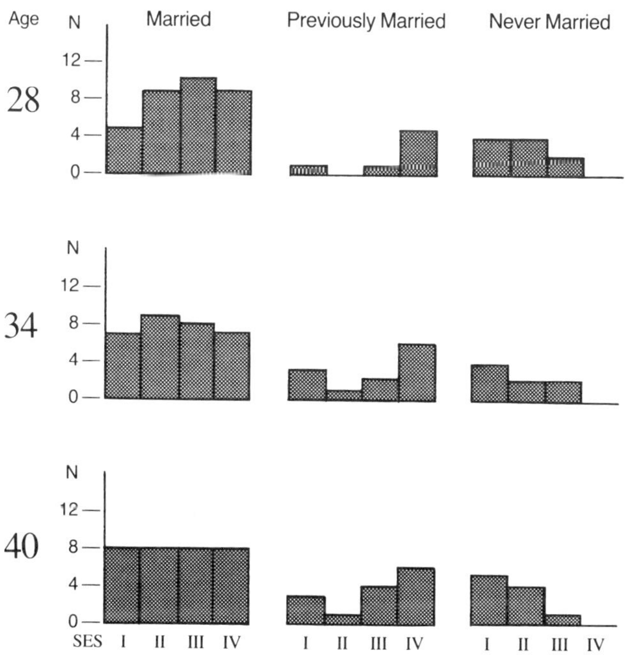

consisted of five to ten persons when the babies were 28 months old, but by the time they were 40 months old, 62% of the households were that size. The great majority of those in other quartiles lived in smaller households (two to three persons). For the same reason, more of the Q-I and Q-II babies shared a home with two or three other children below 6 years of age. In consequence, living space tended to be crowded or markedly restricted in Q-I and Q-II; only Q-IV families had ample space.

We also asked how mothers felt about their neighborhoods. As it turned out, even in quartiles I and II about 50% liked their neighborhoods well enough, as did 65% of the Q-III and Q-IV families. Scores of "bad" or "unbearable" were rare. It would have been far wiser to ask about housing. We heard innumerable complaints about failing elevator service, dirt, roaches, rats, inadequate heating, and poor security. This was almost as true among families in quartile III as among those in the lower groups. Only quartile IV families voiced no such dissatisfactions.

In figure 3.5, we show the number of families in each group receiving welfare and other forms of public assistance; it is somewhat misleading, for a variety of reasons. At times mothers were reluctant to discuss the sources of their income,

Figure 3.5 Public Assistance for Mothers by SES Quartile (Intact Group, by Age)

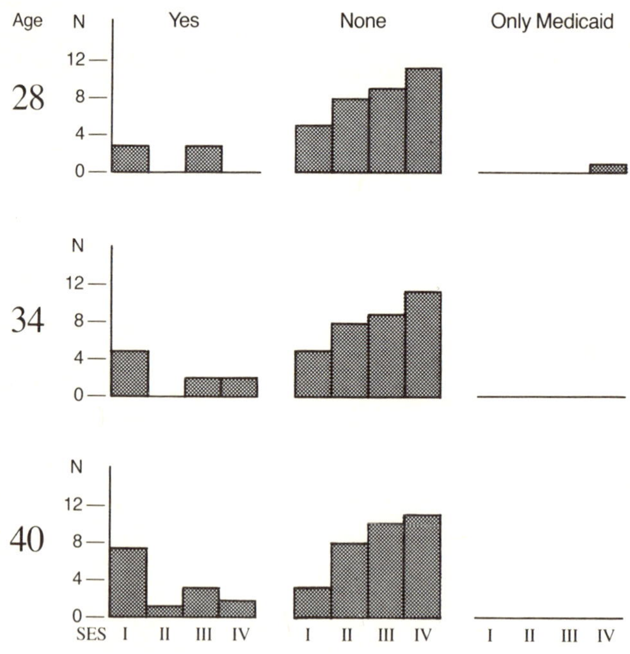

although they were quite willing to say how much money came in per week. Quite a few left financial management to others and genuinely did not know. It is certain that the number of lower SES families who lived on welfare was greater than is shown in figure 3.5, because many of the younger mothers were supported by their parents whether or not they lived with them. The families of origin did receive welfare in many cases, and not infrequently such assistance included payments in behalf of the young mother and baby.

We thought it important to find out how closely our mothers and children were interconnected with members of the extended family. In figures 3.6 and 3.7 we show how many of our mothers or parents had direct contact with not only their own parents but also with siblings, aunts, cousins, and other relatives. We found that among the intact group only one mother could be described as isolated from her family and forced to cope with life's exigencies unaided. In the first left-hand column of figure 3.6 we give a more detailed account of what was shown in figure 3.3. It tells how many of the mother-baby couples remained members of their family of origin or returned to that status after one or two attempts to establish separate households. The second left-hand column is of special interest. The category *shared life* was assigned whenever the young family functioned as members of the larger family although they had an apartment of their own. These pseudoindependent homes were located either in the same building or within two or three blocks of the grandparents' home. By sharing life we meant that these mothers (sometimes both parents) spent by far the largest part of their waking hours in the parental home and had next to no separate existence. Shopping, meal preparation and consumption, all sociability and decision making down to such trivia as what the child should wear on a given day—all were family affairs. If there was a father in the picture he might take care of the rent and some household expenses separately, but more typically family income was merged. Sharing life occurred more frequently in the lower SES groups and tended to increase over time. When the children were 28-months old, eight mother-baby pairs in Q-I remained imbedded in the larger family (note that three shared a home with the paternal grandparents, figure 3.7). When the babies were 40 months of age eleven of these mothers lived as dependent members of the larger family. A good many of the Q-II mothers were similarly situated at 28-months (seven of twelve), but in that quartile there were no changes over time. Quartile III is noteworthy because, although two mothers shared the grandparents' dwelling, the shared-life category did not occur at all. It will soon become apparent that this somewhat older and usually self-supporting group of parents tended to arrange their lives quite differently than parents in the other quartiles.

It may seem odd that quartile IV families shared life with grandparents as frequently as did some other SES groups. Here, however, the nature of the ties to the grandparents was altogether different from what has been described so far, because Q-IV families who received this score maintained genuinely separate establishments. These parents also shared meals, outings, child care, and all

Figure 3.6 Frequency of Contact with Maternal Extended Family by SES Quartile (Intact Group, by Age)

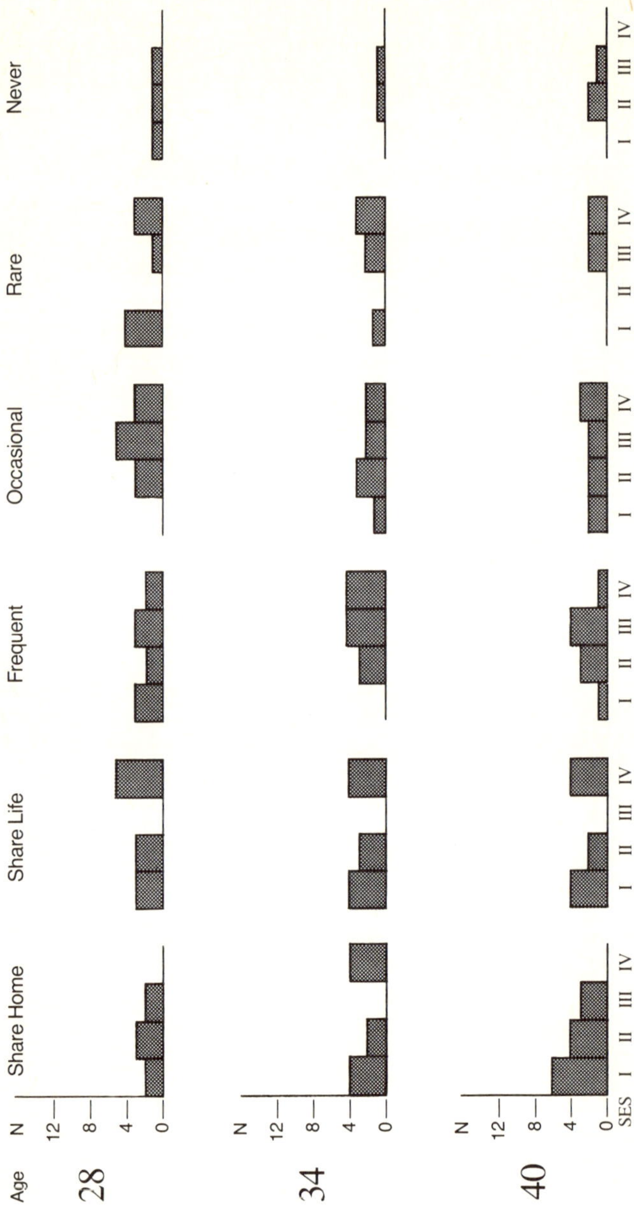

Figure 3.7 Frequency of Contact with Paternal Extended Family by SES Quartile (Intact Group, by Age)

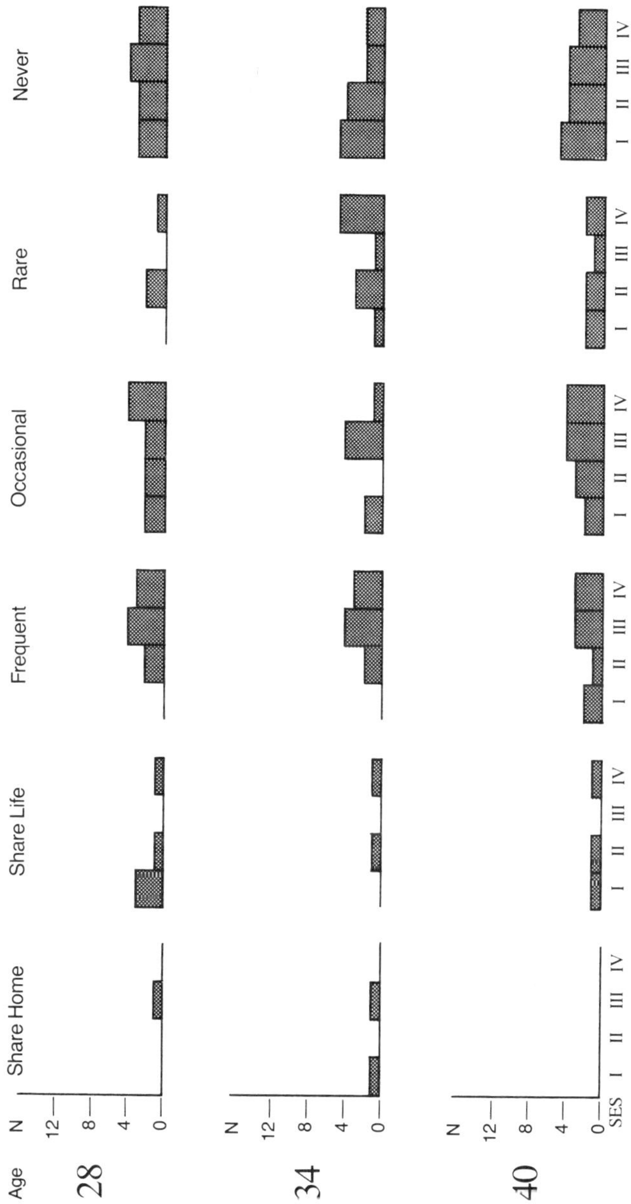

details of living, and they too spent most of the day in the company of grandparents, but they made their own decisions and tended to be dominant members of the larger family group. It was usually the younger generation that lent support, personal and practical more than financial, to their elders. At the same time, everything about the baby and family affairs was shared, discussed, and often quarrelled about to almost the same degree as in the lower SES groups.

Aside from the issue of mutual dependence, figures 3.6 and 3.7 show that most of those not as closely intertwined saw members of the maternal extended family frequently (defined as never less than twice a week and often more). Where such contact was scored as *rare* or *absent,* the reason was geographical. Contact with the extended family on the paternal side was maintained by approximately half of our mothers and was often occasional (meaning no less than once a month). Those who never saw paternal relatives were the unmarried women and some of those who were divorced. All in all, most of our children knew a great many relatives, shared all manner of situations with them, and were very familiar with the homes of relatives; their playmates were usually cousins. A sense of family beyond the nuclear constellation was cultivated for the children not only by virtue of these circumstances but also because most of our families valued and deliberately reinforced loyalty to the larger family unit.

Child care arrangements depend heavily upon whether or not mother must leave the home to go to work. In figure 3.8 we show that almost none of the Q-I mothers was employed, even after the child was 3 years old. In striking contrast, the Q-II mothers, only slightly older and not much better educated, typically held jobs, many as nursing aides in hospitals. In Q-III there was an almost even split between working and non-working mothers. The married women living with their husbands tended to stay at home. A fair number of them had several other children in addition to our index baby. Most of the working mothers in quartile III were unmarried or separated from their husbands and were in full charge of the household. A large proportion of Q-IV mothers also worked full or part time. Without exception, these women valued their professional or business careers; they worked by choice.

Given the background we have sketched, what arrangements were made for the care of the children? In figure 3.9 we show the caretaking provisions and changes in them as the children grew. By *single primary caretaker* we meant that one person was fully responsible for the child at least 80% of the time. *Shared primary caretaking* was scored if two persons between them cared for the child 80% of the time or more, provided that the time each was responsible for the child was approximately equal, and that this was a permanent arrangement. Figure 3.9 shows that at 28 months the majority of our children were reared by their mothers. With advancing age, shared primary caretaking became a bit more prevalent, at least in the upper SES quartiles. Shared caretaking was about as frequent in the highest as in the lowest SES quartile, but the form it took was different in different SES groups. Mother and grandmother jointly cared for the child in Q-I while in Q-II

Figure 3.8 Mother's Employment Status by SES Quartile and Age of Child (Intact Group)

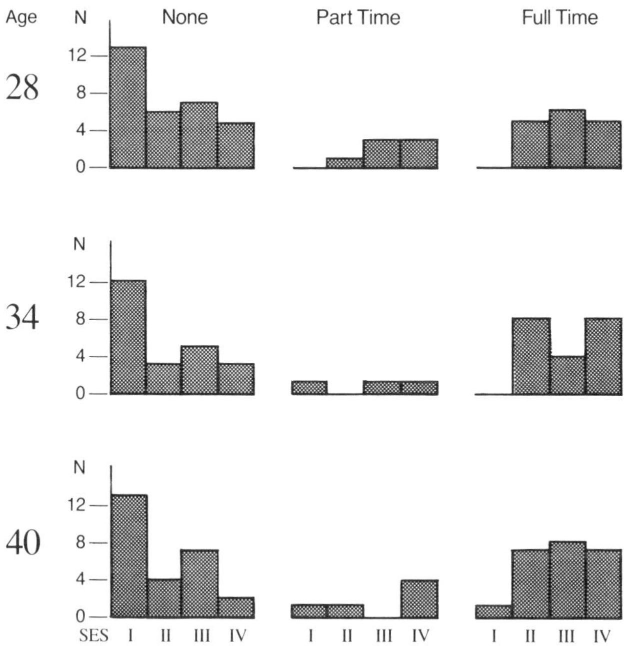

the preferred arrangement was to place the child with a sitter, usually a neighborhood woman who received payment in return for keeping the child in her home all day on weekdays. After the infants were 3 years old a few shifted to daycare centers (*Mother/Group* in figure 3.9). The working mothers in quartile III relied heavily on sitters at the beginning, but once the children were old enough to attend daycare centers these mothers much preferred to place them there, always because the child would "learn more" and always at the cost of prolonged effort to secure admission and also at increased expense. Among Q-IV families the category *Mother/Other* never referred to sitters. In this group, housekeepers or nursemaids assumed major responsibility for the child. These helpers were regarded as members of the household, and many lived with the family. Thus for Q-IV children, shared caretaking did not remove them from their home except for those who as they grew older attended preschools or daycare centers.

One consequence of the lively network provided by the extended family is that *secondary caretakers* (who regularly take over at specified times) and *ancillary caretakers* (who step in as needed) were widely used. Most of our children, more so in the lower SES groups but throughout, frequently spent afternoons, weekends,

Figure 3.9 Primary Caretakers by SES Quartile and Age of Child (Intact Group)

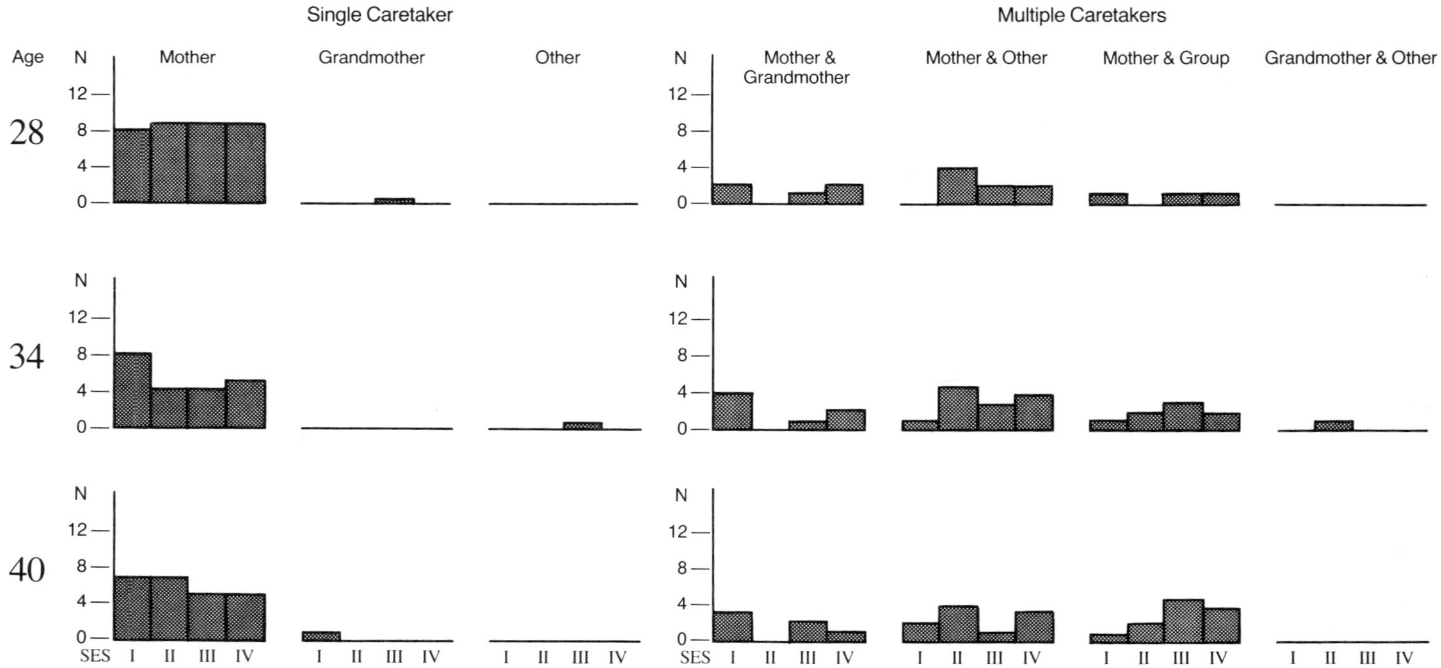

or other time periods in charge of relatives or neighbors. They were fed, dressed, put to bed, and taken on outings by many different people and in a good many different locations. The classical image of the toddler whose social world is bounded by parents and siblings was seldom realized in our research group.

In the light of these various arrangements it is of interest to look at the environmental settings provided for these children. In figures 3.10, 3.11, and 3.12 we show, respectively, the distribution of scores concerning the number and variety of playthings the child was given or allowed to handle; the frequency of excursions away from the familiar home, such as trips to stores, to the park or zoo, to visit friends, etc.; and the frequency with which the child had occasion to interact with persons other than members of the household or other extremely familiar persons. In these respects family style proved to be very consistent. It was therefore possible to add scores for the three age levels and to depict percentages which convey SES differences more accurately than do raw scores.

In all three of these dimensions, SES quartile I differed markedly from all others. At the same time differences among the other three quartiles were minimal. A great many of our children had far more toys than they could use as well as access to an astonishing variety of household objects (*abundant*). Except in Q-I, all the remaining children had what we considered to be an entirely adequate and age-appropriate number of playthings. Similarly, only in Q-I did we find that nearly half of the children (16 of 36 ratings) either did not leave the home territory at all or did so very rarely. Perhaps it should be mentioned that expeditions to the garbage

Figure 3.10 Accessible Playthings by SES Quartile (Intact Group, Ages Combined, in Percentage)

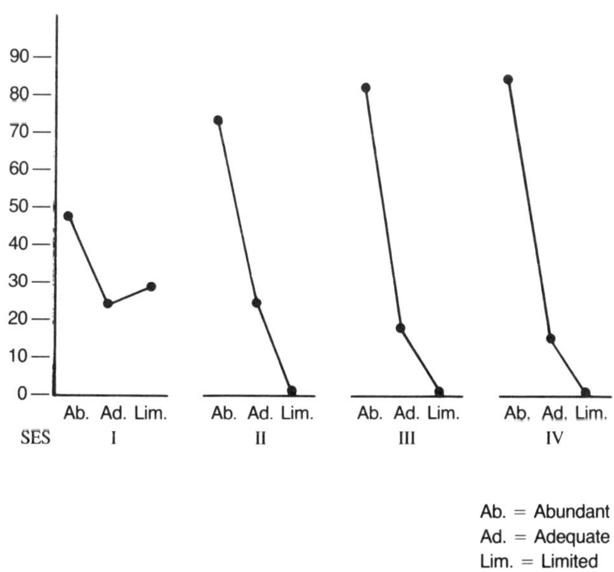

Figure 3.11 Frequency of Outings by SES Quartile (Intact Group, Ages Combined, in Percentage)

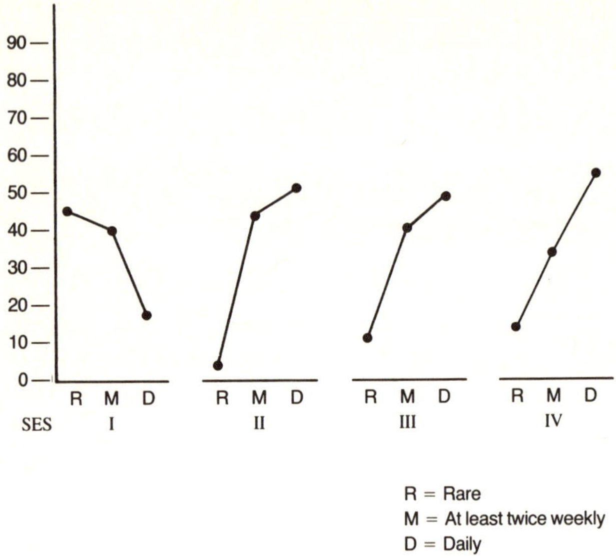

Figure 3.12 Frequency of Contact with Unfamiliar Persons (Intact Group, Ages Combined, in Percentage)

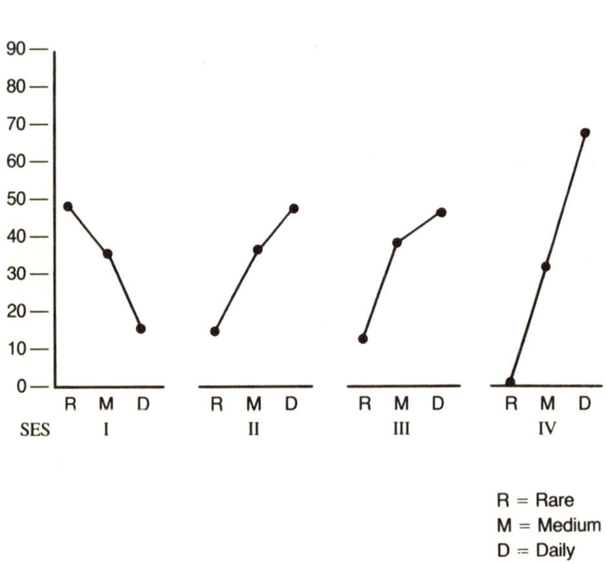

chute or brief sessions "on the stoop" in front of the house were not included here. Nor were rides in the family car if the child did not leave the vehicle at all. Further, direct encounters with fairly unfamiliar or entirely unknown persons were rare for nearly half of the Q-I children, but occurred with medium frequency or daily in the lives of all the rest. As is suggested by the almost identical percentage values on the three graphs, the same children who did not get out of their homes also had few encounters with unfamiliar persons as well as a very limited supply of objects with which to play.

Decidedly, what happened to our children from the very lowest SES group was different from the dominant patterns in all other groups. This is the more noteworthy because our Q-II families were subject for the most part to the same pressures and often hardships that beset those in Q-I. We are not the first to report that there is a radical difference in the life- and childrearing styles of what Pavenstedt (1965) has called the "very low SES" group and the rest of the population. And in Chapter 6, where experience patterns in each SES group are presented, we show that the consequences of this circumstance are critical in the development of children of the very poor.

There are a number of attitudinal and personality characteristics of mothers that influence family atmosphere as well as childrearing practices and that may vary with SES. To the extent that it was feasible to do so, and only for those mothers about whom sufficient information was available, we included such variables in the coding scheme. Scoring was based on interview data, on observation of the mother's behavior, and on all other clues that could be found in any portion of the record. As in all clinical appraisal, the investigators' judgments were based in part on the content of what the mothers said (or failed to say) and in part on the interpretation of observed behavior. What is to be reported now is less objective and factual than in earlier sections, although the manual for the socioenvironmental coding does specify criteria (see appendix A). It is with respect to some of these behavioral and attitudinal characteristics that the mothers of intact children differed sharply from those of deviant ones.

One of the scores indicates whether or not the mother felt isolated and spontaneously spoke of this. Only one of the thirty-five mothers for whom this item could be scored spoke of her isolation, and only one or two at each age level indirectly conveyed a sense of being isolated. We also recorded whether or not the mother said that she was suffering from a major emotional or psychiatric problem and, if so, whether she had sought professional help—from physicians, counselors, social workers, or clergy. In addition, we scored whether or not, in our judgment, the mother's speech and behavior indicated the presence of a psychiatric difficulty, even if it was not acknowledged. Few of the mothers of intact children reported such a problem (two of thirty-five at any one age level), and a similarly small proportion clearly manifested but did not acknowledge psychiatric difficulty.

Two other characteristics from among those included in the scoring scheme are of special interest: the degree to which the mother's recent history and current actions reflected what we called *upward striving,* and the degree to which mothers were *reflective* or thoughtful, not only about the child but in general. By upward striving we meant that mothers were resolved to improve their material and social circumstances and shaped their lives accordingly—for instance, by seeking and obtaining vocational training, by holding jobs in order to achieve goals such as better housing, or by saving toward the child's later education. To receive a score of "very much so" there had to be evidence that the mothers accepted burdens and privations as the price of a better future. By and large our mothers were anything but shiftless. The majority expended effort and made some sacrifices, whether the goal was to get off welfare or to buy a house in the suburbs. The exception was SES quartile I, where only 25% of the mothers were upward striving and 57% showed no trace of such a tendency. The remainder received a score of "more wish than deed" in that they talked of ambitious plans but did nothing to achieve their stated goals.

Reflectiveness also was present to a higher degree than might have been expected—except in quartile I. By reflectiveness we meant an inclination to think and talk about the nature and origin of things observed and things experienced. Reflective mothers wondered about how the child came to have certain characteristics (inherited, due to early illness, due to mother's way of raising them, etc.). They speculated about their relationship with their own parents and how this compared to the way they wanted things to be between themselves and their own children. They often thought about alternate ways of handling disciplinary or other issues. But they also tended to give thought to less personal issues, such as what was wrong with the welfare system and why, the reasons for inflation, the pros and cons of parochial education, and what religion meant to them. Perhaps we were unduly naive at the beginning, but we were impressed by the extent to which reflectiveness in this sense is independent of formal education. We witnessed generally inarticulate and in many ways ignorant mothers struggling to put into words trains of thought fully as complex as those expressed by some of the college-educated women. It goes without saying that interviews of the kind we held invited maximal reflectiveness. It was only in quartile I that the score of "none whatever" for reflectiveness applied to 75% of the mothers.

A very different aspect of behavior was scored under the headings of *mother expresses overt delight* and *mother expresses overt negative feeling* in relation to the child. The open display of either positive or negative feelings about the baby does not necessarily reflect the intensity or nature of what these mothers actually felt. We thought, however, that it must make a difference if in daily experience the child is subject to demonstrative signs of affection and approval or exposed to verbalized expressions of disapproval, to coldness, or to manifestations of anxious ambivalence. Once again, let it be said that scores on this behavior attribute are no more than an addition to a description of how these mothers presented themselves while we were in contact with them. Open display of negative feelings about the child was a rare occurrence among mothers of the intact group at all SES levels (the relatively highest proportion receiving this score was 12% in quartile III). Some expression of annoyance, anger, and the like, which in no way characterized their demeanor as a whole, was noted in about 25% of the mothers. The conspicuous display of enjoyment and delight in relation to the baby was more common. A score of frequent was based not only on demonstrative affectionate behavior (hugging, kissing, praising, and the like) but also on the mother's inclination to talk at length about her enjoyment of the child and to provide many anecdotes selected to illustrate how "good," "lovable," or "smart" the child was. The warmth and intensity conveyed by tone of voice and facial expression as the mother spoke also entered the final rating. By these criteria the frequent and demonstrative expression of delight was more characteristic of the upper two quartiles (61% and 71%, respectively) although it also occurred in about one third of the mothers in Q-I and Q-II. The absence of any overt expression of delight was noted in 30% of the Q-I mothers, 18% of the Q-II mothers, and extremely rarely in Q-III and Q-IV mothers. There is every reason to believe that these differences refer to cultural variations in expressive style and not to basic feelings. From what we came to know about our mothers, we consider that the less openly expressive mothers loved their children as much and were as proud of them and as committed to their care as the others.

In summary, with regard to the families of the intact children, the external life circumstances and demographic background characteristics that together define the realities of what is meant by social class varied consistently and in linear fashion from the lowest to the highest SES quartile. Aside from spelling out specific components of socioeconomic status, these data indicate that the SES index serves its purpose: it groups families appropriately in terms of sociocultural characteristics. We found that the gap between the lowest quartile and the next higher one was greater than the gap between any two of the other quartiles. Be it in family composition, employment, caretaking arrangements, or the degree to which the children were provided with cognitively and socially supportive opportunities, the lowest quartile is not only one extreme of a continuum but represents a very different way of life. Further, social-class differences were noted in some of the behavioral and attitudinal characteristics that influence the caretaking mileu, but only in the form of a marked discrepancy between the lowest SES quartile and all the rest. Some of the traits highly valued by the dominant culture, such as upward striving and reflectiveness, were amply represented in families throughout the different social strata.

PART II Results for the Intact Group

Chapter 4

Cognitive Development, Impulse Control, and Socioeconomic Status

Cognitive Development

That socioeconomic status has a strong influence upon cognitive development was discussed in chapter 2. In brief: the lower the socioeconomic status, the lower the IQ scores (for our study group we showed this relationship in figure 3.1). A closer examination of the cognitive development of the intact group is now in order. The association between SES and IQ is measured most precisely by correlating the SES index with IQ (table 4.1). At the early ages of 7 and 15 months, positive correlations were distinctly low; the amount of the total variation in MDI accounted for by SES was 10.9% at 7 months and 5.7% at 15 months. At 28 months SES accounted for 25.8%, at 34 months for 25.1%, and at 40 months for 33.8% of the total variation in IQ scores.

Somewhat comparable data have come from a very large-scale investigation known as the Collaborative Perinatal Project. Broman, Nichols, and Kennedy (1975) reported correlations between SES and IQ for a population of 26,760 infants at age 4 years. These correlations were 0.38 for whites and 0.24 for blacks. The proportion of total variance in IQ that could be attributed to SES was therefore 14.4% and 5.1% for whites and blacks, respectively. In this large population no significant correlation was found between prematurity and IQ, except that children with birthweights of less than 1500 grams had a slightly lower mean IQ. In fact, the SES index and the closely related variable of maternal education were the only single items that showed more than a trivial correlation with IQ (more than 5% of the total variance). Although the SES effect upon IQ was a good deal stronger in our sample than in theirs, it seems remarkable that our comparatively tiny group yielded results similar to those based on a major epidemiological investigation. The closer relationship between SES and IQ in our group may well be due to sample size. It may also reflect true differences between full-term and preterm infants, however, since several studies of high-risk infants have concluded that premature infants are more vulnerable to adverse environmental conditions than are healthy full-term babies (Werner, Bierman, and French 1971; Beckwith and Cohen 1980; Cohen et al. 1982; Sigman et al. 1981).

In our own data an analysis of variance indicated that at the early ages of 7 and

Table 4.1: Pearson Correlations between SES Index and IQ (Intact Group, by Age)

Age (in months)	*r*	*S*
7*	.3311	.005
15*	.2397	.038
28	.5083	.000
34	.5009	.000
40	.5812	.000

*At 7 and 15 months MDI scores were calculated on the basis of age corrected for prematurity.

15 months the association between SES and MDI scores was insignificant. Beginning at 28 months and thereafter the relationship between SES and IQ was massive and highly significant, as we show in table 4.2. It must also be noted that a decline in mean IQ occurred between 15 and 28 months in all SES quartiles.[1] In the two lower quartiles, however, the drop was massive, amounting to 19.3 and 16.0 IQ points, respectively. Consequently the mean IQ in the lower quartiles changed from average to borderline retarded (Q-I) and very low dull normal (Q-II) status. That of the children in the upper quartiles remained in the normal range even after the decline. Others who have studied early cognitive development in relatively low socioeconomic groups have encountered this phenomenon and dubbed it the "two-year slump" (Golden et al. 1971; Golden and Birns 1976; Golden et al. 1978). In the literature the main emphasis has been placed on the fact that among lower-class infant populations the deceleration in cognitive development at about two years of age ushers in a lasting disadvantage, yet relatively little attention has been paid to the apparent slowdown that tends to occur in all social groups at this age.

One interesting suggestion in regard to this phenomenon was made by Wilson (1978), who pointed out that a rapid spurt in growth occurs during the second year in the very areas of the brain that are held responsible for integration, abstraction, and all symbolic mental functions. In the association areas of the neocortex, and specifically Broca's and Wernicke's speech areas, the period from 12 to 24 months sees a change from 45% of adult surface to 70%. Wilson suggests that the transition from sensorimotor to symbolic functioning normally constitutes a labile period during which infants are especially vulnerable to a lack of appropriate environmental stimulation. We wondered whether this suggestion might be extended to apply not only to cognitive but also to overall developmental changes that occur at about this time. Certainly what mothers like to call the "terrible twos" tends to be a period of disequilibrium in the psychosocial, affective, and behavioral realms as well. The possibility that profound changes in all areas of

1. In chapter 2 we pointed out that the change from the Bayley scales to the Stanford-Binet was not responsible for the reduced cognitive scores. In fact, it was the less able children who were given the Bayley again at 28 months because the Stanford exceeded their abilities.

Table 4.2: Mean IQ by SES Quartile (Intact Group)

SES	*Age (in months)*†	*N*	*IQ*	*St.D*
I	7	16	88.7	19.2
	15	16	95.5	17.1
	28*	11	76.2	15.8
	34	14	71.5	19.7
	40	16	78.0	15.3
II	7	13	98.3	14.3
	15	12	98.5	11.6
	28*	12	82.5	14.2
	34*	11	82.6	13.1
	40*	12	88.3	13.2
III	7	15	101.4	11.3
	15	14	108.0	9.5
	28*	15	93.2	11.8
	34*	13	93.7	16.2
	40*	15	95.6	12.7
IV	7	14	104.7	14.8
	15	14	104.6	15.3
	28*	14	97.8	11.8
	34*	13	99.1	14.7
	40*	14	106.3	13.8

*F probability for SES differences was .0015 or less.
†At 7 and 15 months MDI scores were based on age corrected for prematurity.

functioning during a developmental phase that normally occurs no later than during the third year bear a meaningful relationship to changes in the nervous system in the wake of rapid brain growth should be considered. If neuroanatomical changes play a part in producing the typical two-year behavior characteristics, this might also help us to understand why an unexpectedly large number of our premature children showed behavioral disturbances at about this time. Indeed, if neurophysiological events can cause some disruption in the development and behavior of full-term infants, these same events are likely to have a more profound impact upon premature babies, largely because a degree of immaturity and hence of vulnerability of the central nervous system are characteristics of preterm infants as a group. Whether or not genetic and epigenetic speculations of this kind prove to be explanatory, the fact remains that a general tendency for some deceleration in cognitive development as measured by tests is but a transient phase for most children but has more lasting effects upon infants from low socioeconomic groups.

Mean IQs and correlations inform us about major trends but are not descriptive of the composition of each of the subgroups, as the distribution of IQ scores at each age from 15 to 40 months shows (figure 4.1). At 15 months the great majority of

Figure 4.1 IQ Distribution for SES Quartiles (Intact Group, by Age)

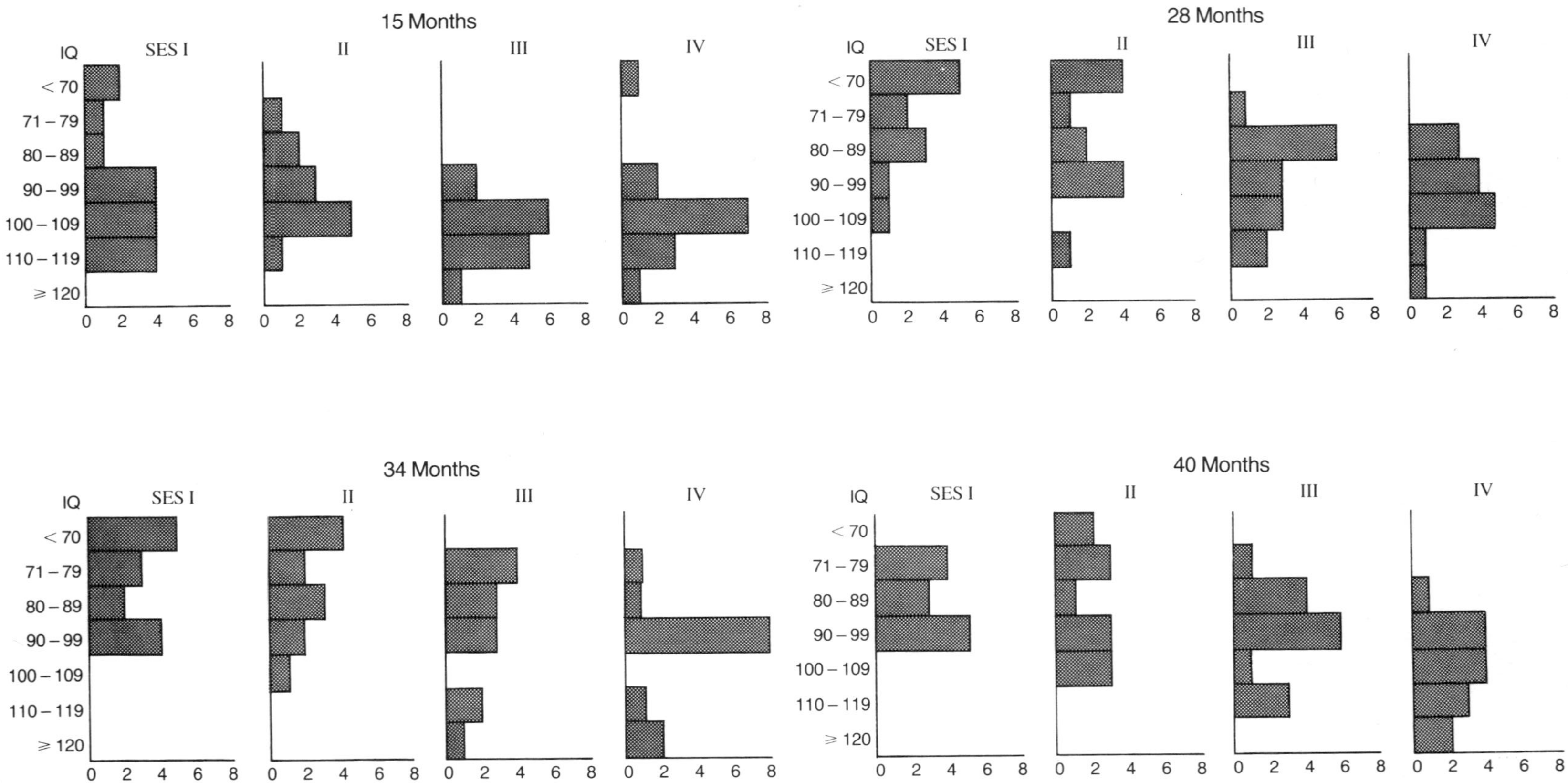

children in all SES groups had MDI scores above 90. In Q-I, for example, 75% were in that range at 15 months, but by 28 months that value had decreased to the abysmally low proportion of 18%, rising only to the still very low values of 28% and 31% thereafter. The pattern in quartile II is similar but less extreme, in sharp contrast to Q-III and Q-IV, where the majority of children had IQs above 90 at all ages. The great disparity between the upper and lower SES quartiles came about because a minority of children in each subsample departed from the normal range and, as a function of social class, they deviated in opposite directions. After 15 months of age all of the retarded children (IQ less than 70) are found in Q-I and Q-II, while not a single child in Q-III or Q-IV was retarded to the same degree. Conversely, superior cognitive development (IQ 110 or more) was found exclusively in quartiles III and IV (figure 4.1). All in all we found, as have all other studies concerned with the same issue, that socioeconomic status exerts a powerful influence upon early cognitive development but also that at least half of the children in the distinctly low SES groups functioned within the normal range by the time they were 40 months old.

The Development of Impulse Control

The rationale for selecting impulse control as a second major outcome variable was described in chapter 2, where we also described two different measures of IC: the comprehensive evaluation at each age and the laboratory assessment at the age of 28 months. The results of the two procedures were in agreement. The comprehensive score, however, was based on more inclusive and more relevant behavioral criteria. We shall therefore report results only in terms of the comprehensive score. We also mentioned earlier that the need for a more frequent and thorough rating arose as we watched our children grow over the course of the project. We then became impressed with the central importance of impulse control throughout the preschool period and for all aspects of development. In addition, we noticed how difficult it was for many children from the poorer families, compared to the others, to achieve control, and it also became apparent that maladaptive patterns typically involved over- or undercontrol of impulsivity. A rethinking of the entire issue and a reexamination of the literature dealing with delay capacity and its relationship to thought and adaptation led to the formulations contained in chapter 2.

The distribution of IC scores for the entire intact group at the three ages for which scores were assigned takes the form of a steep normal curve (figure 4.2). Fifty percent or more of the children received a score of 3, which denotes an age-appropriate degree of control. The proportions that received a 2 (undercontrol) and a 4 (overcontrol) score were nearly equal and age changes were minimal. This is the distribution that would have had to result if our definitions of what is to be expected by way of impulse control at each age level were correct and if we had succeeded in selecting those among the children who differed from the average expectable degree.

Figure 4.2 IC Score Distribution for Intact Group (By Age, in Percentage)

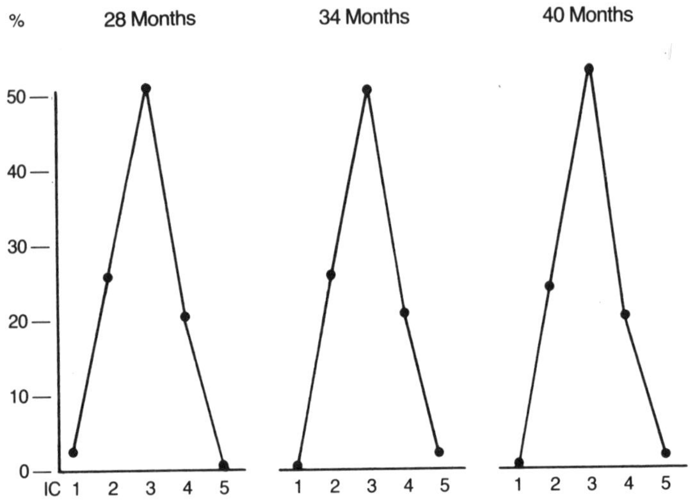

To what extent, then, does socioeconomic status exert an influence on the acquisition of impulse control? An answer to this question is given by the direct correspondence between SES and IC in that the mean SES index rises as the IC scores increase from the low (2) to the high (4) (table 4.3). The rare scores of 1 (very low) and 5 (very low and high over the same time span) occurred in the presence of low SES indices. Because there were no age changes to speak of and the number of children in each SES–IC combination was small, scores obtained at the three ages were combined (figure 4.3). The most striking fact is that the two lower quartiles contributed by far the largest proportion of low scores of 2. Conversely, scores of 4, indicating that behavior was less impulsive than that of most agemates, were contributed almost entirely by quartiles III and IV.

The initial observation that it is more difficult for children from socially and materially burdened families to acquire impulse control is amply borne out. This fact is the more striking because many of our poorer families saw the teaching of self-control as a primary goal. These parents thought about impulsivity in terms of wildness, impatience, aggressivity, and disobedience. Much of what they did for and with their young children was designed to curb what some described as an inborn tendency for "evil." Many a time we heard Q-I and Q-II families explain that the baby's initial willfulness and impatience must be "broken" very early, that failure to do so spelled parental negligence and would lead to serious trouble later on. The Q-III and Q-IV families, especially the latter, whose children tended to be well or overly controlled, were generally less concerned about their toddlers' volatile behavior. They emphasized that this was merely a stage and that matura-

Table 4.3: Mean SES Index for Each IC Rating (Intact Group, by Age)

Age (in months)	*IC**	*N*	*SES*	*St.D*	*S*
28	1	1	46.0		
	2	12	58.3	15.3	
	3	23	70.2	18.1	.01
	4	9	81.0	10.2	
		45	68.6		
34	2	10	59.3	20.9	
	3	19	71.9	16.3	.14
	4	8	76.3	9.5	
	5	1	61.0		
		38	69.2		
40	2	11	60.3	13.2	
	3	24	66.0	17.6	.04
	4	9	79.3	16.9	
	5	1	46.0		
		45	66.8		

*IC 1 = almost no control; 2 = somewhat undercontrolled; 3 = age-appropriate; 4 = somewhat or markedly overcontrolled; 5 = under- and overcontrolled at same time.

Figure 4.3 IC Score Distribution by SES Quartile (Intact Group, Ages Combined, in Percentage)

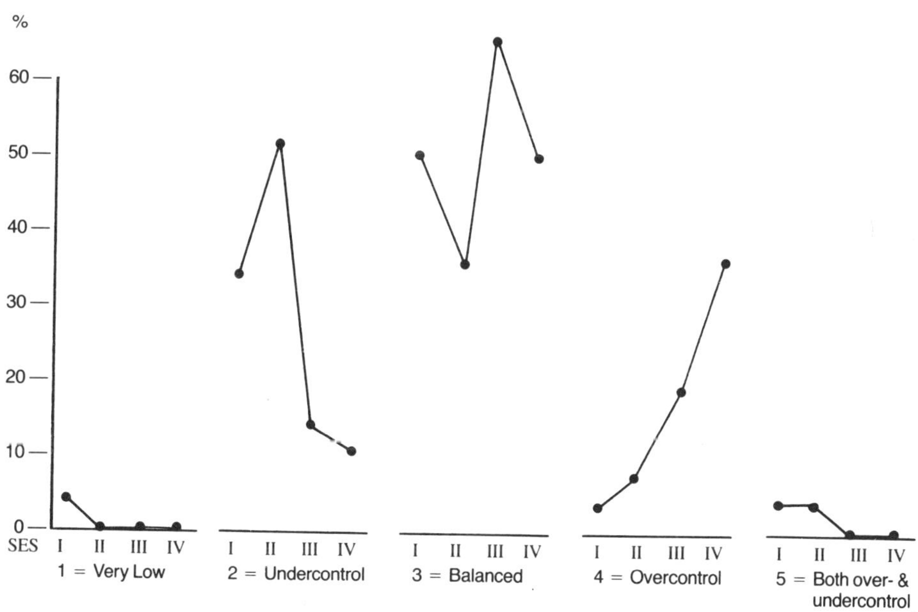

tion and growing comprehension of what was expected could be relied upon to correct the inevitable troublesome behavior.

Another striking aspect is the very great similarity between Q-I and Q-II and, with the exception of scores of 4, also between Q-III and Q-IV. There is a massive difference in IC distribution between the two lower and the two upper quartiles. This is quite different from what we saw with respect to demographic and related variables (chapter 3), where quartile I differed sharply from all others. Further, such differences in IC distribution as do exist between quartiles I and II were in the opposite direction from what would be expected. The proportion of low IC scores (2) in Q-II exceeded that in Q-I (52% *vs.* 36%). For various reasons we are not inclined to ascribe this seeming reversal to chance alone. Rather, the relatively high percentage of low IC scores in quartile II can be understood in the light of differences in the caretaking arrangements made for the children in these two groups. In both of the lower quartiles some of the mothers shared primary caretaking responsibility with another person. In Q-II the preferred pattern was to employ a sitter, whereas in Q-I a grandmother was more likely to be the second primary caretaker. From all descriptions it appears that the sitters used by our mothers usually dealt with their little charges in a friendly and perhaps somewhat indulgent manner. At the same time they provided little more than physical care and a comfortable existence. They were not expected to participate in teaching and training the child, nor did they provide varied experiences or cognitive stimulation. The relative barrenness of this variety of family day care stands in marked contrast to the intense involvement with the child and his or her upbringing that mothers and grandmothers typically showed. It seems likely that impulse control emerges partly in response to life situations that are often arousing, challenging, and demanding, as is usually the case when mother and close relatives are in charge. The more placid, less intense atmosphere we have described for sitters' homes is probably not as conducive to the early development of impulse control.

For the children in SES II, we looked at the distribution of IC scores separately for those solely in their mother's care and those whose weekdays were spent with a sitter. Unfortunately the number of children for whom no IC rating could be made is exceptionally large among the children looked after by sitters. Working mothers often did not know enough about how the child behaved in their absence, and sitters could not accept invitations to the laboratory. Nonetheless, when ages are combined, sixteen IC scores are available for children entirely in mother's care; of these nine, or 56%, received the age-appropriate score of 3. Among the seven ratings available for children cared for by sitters only one, or 14%, received the same rating (3). It does appear that family day care of the type we described does not encourage the development of ego control.

This is as good a place as any to digress in order to explain why we chose occasionally to splinter our sample and report on very small groups or even individuals. In order to discern what can be learned from a large mass of heterogeneous information, we found it necessary to support hypotheses and interpretative ideas by relying on what some philosophers of science have called *multiplicative corroboration*—that is, the assembly of similar or identical items of evidence in many different instances (Pepper 1942).[2] In so doing it is necessary to demonstrate the consistency of relationships between the same variables in many different contexts. Exceptions to the overall data trend are then of special interest. The greater frequency of relatively low ICs in quartile II than in quartile I is such an exception, as it runs counter to the otherwise consistent relationship between SES and IC.

Exceptions do not prove the rule, but they can be compatible with the explanatory assumption that lends meaning to the rule. The thus-far unspoken assumption here is that when caretakers feel a strong personal investment in the child's development *and* are able to provide supportive care, impulse control will emerge normally. By and large the evidence suggests that more members of low SES groups cannot or do not provide supportive care to the same extent as do most mothers in the middle and higher SES groups. Knowing that the exception—that is, lower IC scores in Q-II than Q-I—applies only to children cared for by sitters is entirely compatible with our understanding of SES differences in relation to IC. In this example, even conditions that prevail for a single child can be relevant. It so happens that the one child who spent his days in a sitter's home and yet obtained an IC score of 3 at 28 months was soon thereafter transferred to a group day care facility. His mother had a strong investment in early education, as demonstrated by, among other things, the fact that she removed him from the sitter's home as soon as it was feasible to do so from a practical point of view.

Socioeconomic status does not by itself determine the degree of impulse control a child is likely to attain, no more than it predicts IQ for individuals. Most of the children in our study group showed the age-appropriate level of control by the age of three years. We recognize that the relationship between SES and various measures of developmental progress has no explanatory or other theoretical significance, although it is of great practical importance. We chose to trace the association between SES and IC or other developmental indices because such an analysis provides a convenient framework within which to explore what it is about the life experience of young children that has an impact upon specific aspects of development.

Impulse Control and Cognitive Development

Are impulse control and cognitive advance linked directly to each other? If low IC tends to impair cognitive development, much of the SES difference in IQ can be accounted for by the greater frequency of low IC among the children from the poorer families. Two somewhat separate things will have to be established: first, that there is a strong association between IC and IQ when social class is disregarded; and second, that within social class, variations in IQ correspond to variations in IC.

2. In an unpublished paper, Peter H. Wolff (1964) discussed the application of multiplicative versus structural models to psychoanalytic developmental research.

We give the mean IQ for each IC rating for the entire group of intact children for whom IC ratings were available (table 4.4). At each age the mean IQ is seen to rise as IC ratings rise from less to more than the usual. By far the largest shift in IQ occurs with the transition from undercontrol (ratings of 1, 2, or 5) to age-appropriate or higher levels of IC (ratings of 3 or 4). In view of the significance of these results, it is safe to conclude that a relationship between IC and IQ does exist.

As a first step toward learning whether or not variations in IQ within any one social group correspond to IC variations in the same quartile, we present the basic data in the form of a scattergram (figure 4.4). It plots separately for the four quartiles the IQ scores that occurred within each IC category. The higher IQ scores are seen predominantly where IC ratings were either 3 or 4. Similarly, most of the IQs that fell below the mean are found in association with IC ratings reflecting less than the usual degree of control. Figure 4.4 shows with equal clarity that there is not a one-to-one correspondence between ego control and IQ. Among the well-controlled children several had relatively low IQs, and some of the undercontrolled children had IQs above the mean value for the sample.

Unfortunately, a stringent test of the magnitude or significance of the association between impulse control and cognitive status is impossible to perform with data of this nature. We can make an approximate estimate of the magnitude of this effect by comparing the distribution of IQs for well-controlled children with that for children with low or very low ICs (figure 4.5). For the age levels combined, superior IQ scores (100 or more) were obtained almost only by children who were

Table 4.4: Mean IQ Index for Each IC Rating (Intact Group, by Age)

Age (in months)	*IC*	*N*	*IQ*	*St.D*	*F*
28	1	1	66.0		
	2	12	77.1	7.85	
	3	23	94.1	10.13	0.000
	4	9	100.2	13.94	
		45	90.4	13.89	
34	1	0			
	2	10	74.9	19.32	
	3	19	93.8	14.79	0.007
	4	8	97.8	12.11	
	5	1	73.0		
		38	89.1	18.85	
40	1	0			
	2	10	86.0	12.85	
	3	24	94.6	12.45	0.005
	4	9	105.7	14.08	
	5	1	73.0		
		44	94.3	14.42	

Figure 4.4 Scattergram of IQ Scores for Each IC Rating by SES Quartiles (Intact Group, by Age)

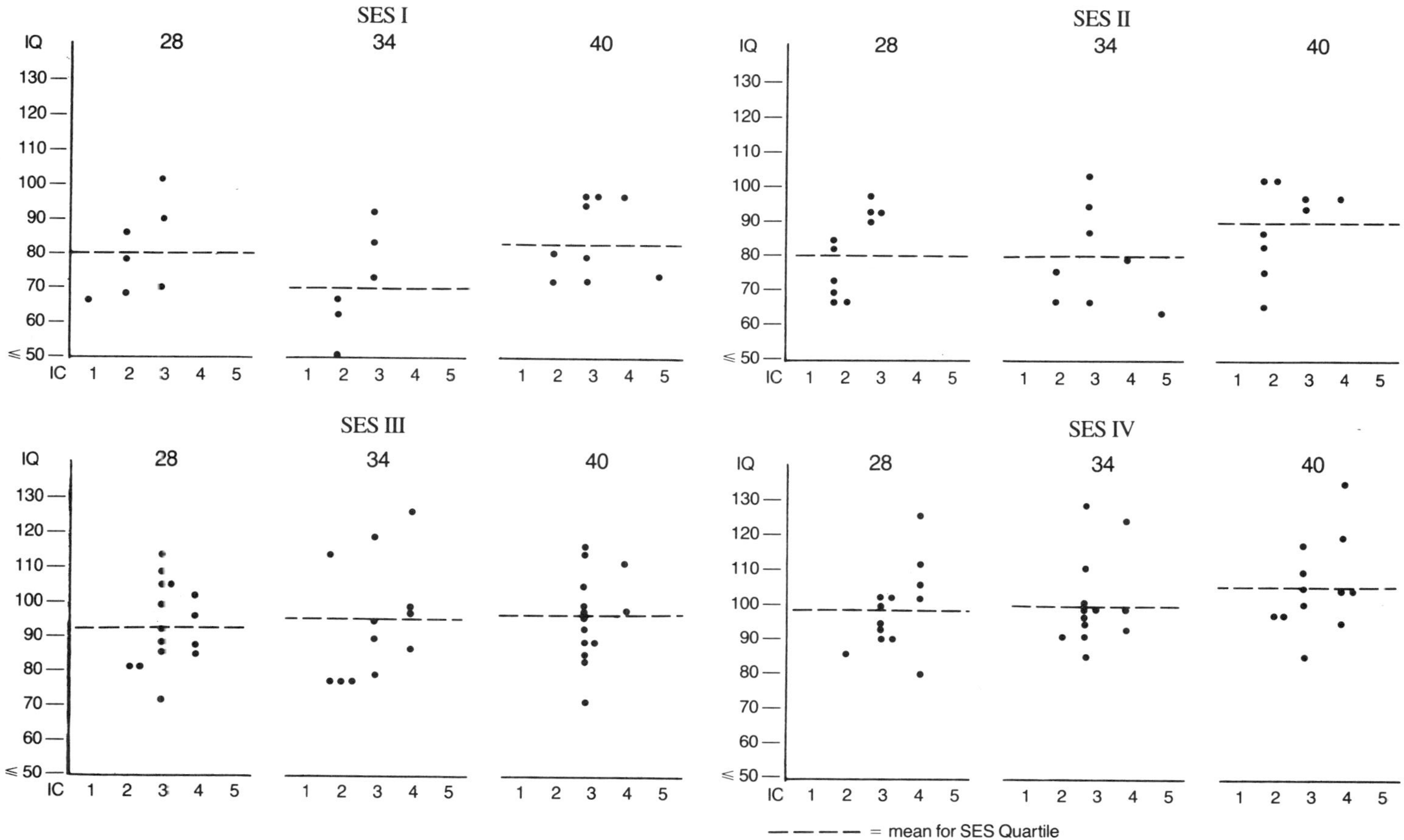

Figure 4.5 **IQ Distribution for Well-Controlled and Ill-Controlled Children (Intact Group, Ages Combined, in Percentage)**

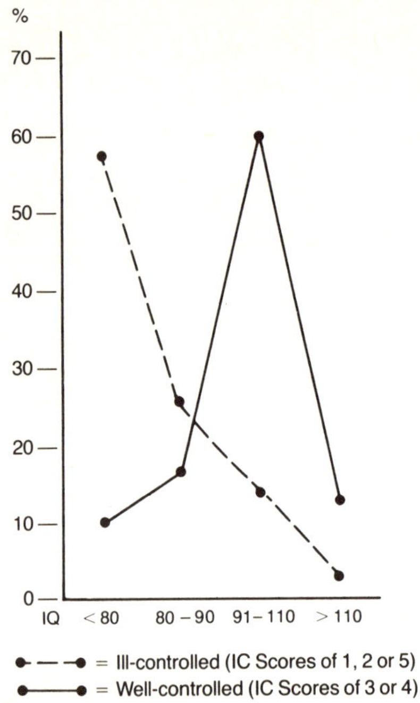

well controlled, and the proportion of IQ scores below 80 was higher among the children with low ICs (figure 4.5). At the very least we can conclude that a lack of age-adequate control can and often does impede the expected cognitive advances.

Figure 4.6 and table 4.5 are intended to reflect the interrelationships of cognition, impulse control, and socioeconomic status. In table 4.5 we show the mean IQ for each IC rating separately for each SES quartile. In figure 4.6 we show for each quartile the mean IQ for those who, to one degree or another, showed less impulse control than is usual and contrast it to the mean IQ of those who showed at least age-appropriate control. Within each quartile the undercontrolled children had markedly lower mean IQs than did those with good control. Yet SES effects upon cognitive development were pronounced even when IC was held constant. For the well-controlled children, mean IQs ranged from 87 (Q-I) to 102 (Q-IV). For poorly controlled children the range was from 79 (Q-I) to 93 (Q-IV). In figure 4.6 we also show, in yet another way, the association between low SES and low IC. In the two lower quartiles the mean IQ for the entire sample fell about midway between that for the under- and the well-controlled groups. In the two upper quartiles, on the other hand, the SES sample mean and that for the well-controlled group were nearly the same. As we already know, and as is shown again in table 4.5, well-controlled children constituted barely half of the SES quartile in Q-I and Q-II whereas they

Figure 4.6 Mean IQ by SES Quartile for Well-Controlled and Ill-Controlled Children, and Mean IC for Each SES Quartile (Intact Group, Ages Combined)

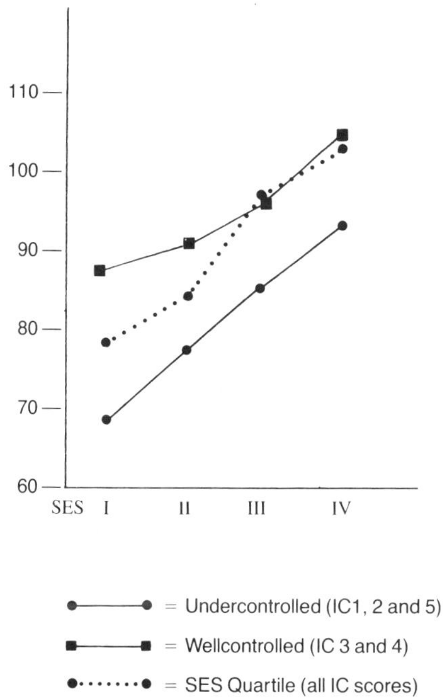

accounted for more than 80% of quartiles III and IV. Thus the mean IQs in the two upper quartiles chiefly reflect the performance of the well-controlled children. In the two lower quartiles the mean IQ reflects the performance of under- and well-controlled children to an equal degree.

In summary, we have reported that, for the intact children, cognitive development as well as impulse control are strongly linked to SES. Developmental progress in both these areas tends to be slower and more frequently impaired when SES is low. For our research sample there is a direct relationship between impulse control and cognitive development in all social groups. Test scores throughout are relatively low for children who had less than age-appropriate impulse control, and this discrepancy was somewhat greater in the lower SES groups. Last, we found that the relationship between socioeconomic background and cognitive progress remains marked even when age-appropriate levels of impulse control have been attained.

We conclude from this that for two- and three-year-old children impulse control is a mediating variable between social class and cognitive development. It accounts for a considerable portion of the differences in IQ between the upper and lower ends of the socioeconomic range. It appears that, at least during the early

Table 4.5: Mean IQ for Each IC Rating by SES Quartile (Intact Group, Ages Combined)

	IC	*N*	*IQ*	*St.D*
SES I				
	1, 5	2	69.5	4.95
	2	8	69.2	14.23
	3	11	85.9	11.04
	4	1	96.0	
		22	78.8	14.50
SES II				
	1, 5	1	62.0	
	2	14	78.2	13.26
	3	10	90.8	9.93
	4	2	87.0	12.72
		27	82.9	13.50
SES III				
	1, 5	0		
	2	6	85.0	14.28
	3	25	95.0	13.26
	4	7	102.5	12.20
		38	94.8	13.88
SES IV				
	1, 5	0		
	2	4	93.2	5.85
	3	20	99.5	10.62
	4	13	107.6	12.97
		37	101.7	12.97

preschool years, less than age-adequate impulse control is an impediment to age-appropriate cognitive development. When impulse control is adequate or superior the distribution of IQ scores takes the form of a normal curve, similar to what is seen in any unselected population. When impulse control falls below the expected level, the IQ distribution curve is severely skewed, with a disproportionate number of scores at the low end of the range. We think that the close connection between impulse control and cognitive development may be limited to the early preschool years. It is the transition from primarily sensorimotor to primarily symbolic functioning that requires delay capacity. Without it, the necessary degree of separation between the acting organism and the acted-upon environmental field cannot be achieved.

The view that impulse control has a unique function in relation to early forms of abstraction and to symbolic functioning in general is in keeping with the theory sketched out in the introductory chapters. It is also in keeping with empirical results, also mentioned earlier. In their extensive studies of ego control in somewhat older children, Jean and Jack Block (1980) found little difference in intelligence between somewhat less controlled and somewhat more controlled individuals. Yet their results on markedly under- or overcontrolled older children are parallel to what we found for toddlers.

Although the immediate and strong influence of weak or delayed impulse control upon cognition is time-limited, impulse control at the early ages can have important consequences. IQ at 3 years is correlated to school-age IQ and also to school achievement, whereas this is not the case with developmental test scores obtained at younger ages. It is therefore likely that impaired or delayed cognitive development early on can be a lasting disadvantage at later ages.

Some additional support for this assumption comes from follow-up studies of our children. At the age of 6 years the children whose IC at 40 months had been adequate (IC 3 or 4) had a mean IQ of 105; those whose IC scores at 40 months had been low (IC 1, 2, or 5) had a mean IQ of 91. This difference was not due to social class either at preschool or at school age. In the six-year-sample the SES difference between the two groups was very modest, largely because more of the children from the poorest families did not participate in the follow-up. It is also of interest that at school age only three of the seventeen children in the low IC group had IQs below 80, and of these only one was severely retarded. That is, there was a distinct improvement in mean IQ between the ages of 3 and 6 years for those with low preschool ICs as well as for the others. Such a change might be accounted for by an improvement in the socioeconomic situation of the family (not the case here), by school attendance, or by an increase in impulse control, which almost certainly occurred during the intervening years. We think that during the interim years impulse control, initially delayed, reached and surpassed the threshold required for more abstract and more objective mental functioning. If so, formal learning in the classroom should have become effective. Yet, a difference of 14 points in mean IQ at age 6 between those with initially low ICs and the others is not altogether trivial. We interpret these tentative results to mean that the relatively low preschool IQs of children with low impulse control did constitute a handicap in their further cognitive development. On the assumption that the earliest phases of cognitive development in the symbolic realm are important, we shall proceed to identify some aspects of children's daily life experience that have a bearing on the development of impulse control as well as upon cognitive functioning when requisite levels of control are present. These patterns or aspects of experience vary greatly among social classes and thus enter the chain of reasoning that leads from SES to developmental outcome.

Chapter 5

The Experience Patterns

Definition and Rationale

In our previous research concerned with the interaction between environmental and intrinsic factors in development (Escalona 1968), it was useful to draw a sharp distinction between that which determines a child's experience and the experience itself. In young infants it was possible to show that individual differences in response to the same environmental situation are related to organismic characteristics such as activity level and perceptual sensitivity. Among inactive placid infants, for instance, the most intense and complex social responsiveness of which the infants are capable occurs in response to intense social stimulation involving vigorous touch and sound as well as vivid visual presentation of the mother's face and other interesting spectacles. The same variety of intense approach made to markedly active infants leads to less than optimal social response on the infants' part. Their optimal response typically occurs when the playful approach is low-key. In short, an infant's response to a given set of environmental stimuli, as well as his or her more stable behavior characteristics, were found to be determined by the objective environmental circumstances, but also by the intrinsic and acquired characteristics of the infant organism.

Observations of this nature could be systematized in such a way as to yield typical constellations of infant experience over time, which in turn could be related to developmental patterns and outcome characteristics (see Escalona and Corman 1974). The end result of these and other research efforts—one might say our experience while engaged in such research—led to the formulation of a model that differs somewhat from the customary one.

We concluded that the most effective strategy in linking antecedents to developmental outcome is to assume that what shapes development is the nature and sequence of the child's actual experience, regardless of how it came about. By experience we mean that which the child perceives, does, and feels in so far as these have a degree of stability and consistency over time.[1] In application our

1. Patterns of experience as here defined are but a part of the totality of significant life experience. One time events can have major traumatic or enabling consequences and, if so, will affect subsequent experience patterns. Beyond that it is axiomatic that subjective experience cannot be communicated or inferred in full.

model dictates that such objective variables as social class, childrearing practices, and biological attributes of the child *not* be seen as the direct cause or antecedent of development and adaptation. Instead a systematic relationship is sought between prominent aspects of the child's past and present experience and subsequent child characteristics. In consequence, what constitutes a single step in most child development research is transformed into two separate lines of inquiry. Thus, in studying the relationship between social class and cognitive development, the first step must be to determine how and to what degree membership in different SES groups yields different patterns of experience. The second step is to determine the relationship between all known patterns of experience, which are the product of much more than social class, and cognitive development. Insofar as experience patterns found to be more (or less) conducive to intellectual development are found more frequently in some social classes than in others, a more differentiated and concrete picture of the relationship between SES and cognition can be formulated than would otherwise be possible. The same approach applies to all other determining factors. With our premature infants, for instance, we tried to trace the impact of neurological impairment upon experience patterns where this was possible.

Selection and Assessment of Experience Patterns

From what has gone before the reader knows that our ability to document prominent and salient features of the experience of our children was severely limited. For a determination of how the children lived and functioned we depended upon what mothers and others communicated during interviews, supplemented by what could be observed during family visits to research quarters. Most of the participating families were willing and able to provide detailed information about everyday life events. Yet, under the best of circumstances, what emerged on this basis was a far cry from knowledge of the actuality as lived by the child. Our assessment of patterns in each child's experience was a compromise between what was desirable and what was obtainable. We gambled that accounts of frequent and typical behaviors under known circumstances would reflect underlying patterns of experience sufficiently to provide meaningful clues—which is all that could be hoped for. With all their imperfections, most of the experience patterns we were able to identify did prove to be associated with external variables (SES) and with developmental outcomes.

The selection of aspects of experience to be assessed was based on what we regarded as developmentally relevant but also on the type of information most mothers could provide on most occasions. In many ways the procedure for the assessment of experience patterns (henceforth EP) was like that described for the rating of impulse control and adjustment status. Seven aspects of experience were selected and defined, rating criteria were specified in a manual, and H. Corman and the author independently rated each child at each age. Again, both raters produced written documentation for their judgments, disagreements were discussed, and a consensus rating was made. As with the other ratings, a score of "unknown" was given whenever the information available to us was insufficient or unreliable. It will surprise no one to learn that on this complex issue rater agreement was not as good as it was for impulse control and behavioral deviancy. In 28% of the ratings it was necessary to review and discuss the material a second time before achieving consensus. Disagreements arose most frequently as to whether or not sufficient information was available. Usually the "unknown" score was assigned if either of us continued to doubt the adequacy of the data.

Ratings of experience patterns were based on a comparison between each child and all agemates in the sample, much as had been done for impulse control. For ICs, however, a normal distribution was built in by definition, whereas for several of the EPs there was no way of knowing in advance how the high, low, and medium ratings would be distributed within the sample.[2] The rating manual specified the behavioral criteria and the situational context in which they were to be applied (see Appendix C). These criteria were developed from our general knowledge of child behavior as well as from a preliminary survey of the material in the research files.

Another distinguishing characteristic of the EP ratings was that the rating of 2 (present but not prominent) covered a wide range, whereas ratings of 1 and 3 each comprised a fairly homogeneous group with respect to the variable in question. It was necessary to give wide latitude to the in-between region in part because the data did not allow for a more finely differentiated scale. In addition, the midposition rating had to encompass a variety of patterns because so many of our children spent their time in different settings and with different people. For instance, a child cared for by grandmother as well as by mother may be exposed to sharply different situations and caretaking styles in the two settings. Even if the youngster's way of responding to given circumstances remained constant, his experience would vary as a function of living in two different environments. Similarly, children who attend daycare centers may lead very different lives at home and away from home. Such combinations had to be included or somehow condensed into a single rating. In practice this meant that a child whose life while in mother's charge would have justified a 1 or a 3 rating was rated 2 if what happened at other times differed markedly from the event structure at home. Probably for this reason it proved that with some of the EPs meaningful results were obtained only for the extreme ratings.

As we move into a description of each experience pattern it will be noted that some EP ratings are completely tied to concrete facts and thus approximate the goal of basing judgments on overt behavior in specific contexts. Others require a degree of interpretation of behavioral manifestations and hence inferences based on what mothers said and on qualitative aspects of observed behavior. It will be seen that the less firmly anchored judgments were contributory, but it was the experience patterns defined exclusively by overt criteria that yielded the most useful data.

2. For the two youngest ages we had included freedom and movement as one EP. It turned out that movement restraint beyond that required during caretaking procedures did not occur at all. Freedom of movement was high for 100% of the children!

The Experience Patterns

Eight different aspects of everyday experience were assessed. (One of these, the amount of body contact between mother and child, was relevant only up to 15 months and will be omitted from this account.) The manual (Appendix C) provides a detailed description of each experience variable. Below we combine a brief summary with a discussion of the relevance of each EP to development and adaptation.

Intensity of Mother's[3] Emotional Involvement with the Child

This EP refers to the degree to which mother's feelings, interests, and actions were focused on the child, with the implication that other concerns and commitments were thereby diminished or excluded. The intensity of such involvement was judged in disregard of the quality and nature of the bond: a mother who was totally absorbed in the child but in an anxious and troubled manner was rated "very prominent" on this variable, but so was a mother whose loving and delighted feelings for the baby dominated her existence. What we hoped to gauge was the degree to which the mother conveyed to the child a sense of his or her overriding importance to her.

Of all the dimensions of experience that were rated, this one was the most inferential. The manual does specify behavioral and other criteria, but much depended on the rater's evaluation of the material, which in turn depended on clinical acumen and also on common sense. The manner in which a very strong involvement with the child finds behavioral expression varies greatly even among mothers whose life revolves around the child to an unusual degree. The behavior correlates of a relative lack of such involvement are easier to discern.

The decision to stress the degree to which the child appears to be at the center of mother's inner and outer life rather than the quality of her attachment was made because, on the basis of clinical and research experience, we became convinced that the sense of being a vitally important object to the mother is itself supportive of ego development in very young children. Or better, a sense of maternal indifference and a lack of close connectedness with the mother are destructive to ego development. This is not to say that an unduly strong concentration of a mother's life energy on her child cannot be harmful to personality development. Nonetheless, psychopathology that has its roots in an ambivalent, conflictual, and painful early mother-child relationship is ordinarily not so devastating in its consequences as is the absence of any close bond to the mother. The former can lead to neurotic disturbances of great severity but—in the absence of other vitally disruptive experiences—does not prevent the progressive development of ego functions and defenses, however distorted these may be. The lack of a maternal presence, in the absence of potent compensatory experience, can lead to a failure to develop some

3. Here as elsewhere the term *mother* refers to the person or persons who function as primary caretakers.

of the complex and integrative ego functions altogether. It can lead to primitive and largely ineffective modes of adaptation and/or to a sort of inner emptiness such as is seen in some psychoses and in massive inadequacies of the sort familiar to us from contact with certain delinquent and criminal populations and from the study of hard-core unemployable and often unschoolable groups. For this experience variable it is assumed that a position at either extreme, and especially in the low group, constitutes an obstacle to normal development.

Frequency of Overt Conflict between the Child and Significant Adults

Conflicts between toddlers and the adults with whom they live are an inevitable byproduct of normal development in the setting of the family. The frequency of such open and usually angry confrontations varies greatly from occasional to many, many times each day over a period of months or even years. The criteria for what constitutes high and low frequency of conflict, specified in the manual, take into account the fact that oppositional behavior typically increases during the third year and usually subsides somewhat during the fourth. The phase-specific waxing and waning of mother-child conflicts was thus built in.

Overt conflict was defined as episodes during which child and adult expressed open antagonism and hostility toward each other. Therefore episodes during which a child responded to scolding or punishment by plaintive crying, withdrawal, or efforts to beguile the adult were disregarded. Similarly, some mothers are able to meet their child's outbursts with composure and unaltered friendliness, and such episodes also were not counted as conflicts. We made no attempt to judge whether nonhostile behavior on the part of child or adult might nonetheless mask underlying hostile feeling.

This experience variable afforded an especially clear example of behavioral events that vary in intensity and frequency as a function of the child's state and disposition quite as much as they vary as a function of family atmosphere and childrearing practices. There were children who displayed anger, defiance, and a combatant attitude at the slightest interference with their wishes, and some who went beyond this by clearly provoking unoffending mothers as though they sought an opportunity to give battle. When this was the case, even the calmest and most skillful mothers, who accepted difficult behavior without rancor, became embroiled in conflict as we defined the term. What we assessed was the end result regardless of how it came about.

The developmental relevance of how much conflict typically occurs is a topic to be explored; there are no foregone conclusions. Certainly among well and normal children one encounters the entire gamut, from those for whom the preschool years were tumultuous to those who lived through this period in a fairly tranquil manner. Cultures and families differ in the degree to which they tolerate and perhaps even cultivate the energetic expression of assertion and aggression. There can be little doubt that a child's image of the world and of his place in the scheme of things is shaped in part by the role of hostility in everyday life and by how conflicts are actually resolved or terminated. Clinically speaking, we know that a young child who fails to show protest, defiance, and anger during the early preschool years is either very immature or lacks the degree of assertiveness and spontaneity expected of children in our culture. Further, the frequency of oppositional encounters during the formative years is also an important feature of the relationship between the child and significant adults.

The Degree of Structure in the Child's Life

Any aspect of the child's life that serves to provide a stable and predictable environment and goal-oriented, organized activity for the child contributes to structure as we use the term. On the simplest level, daily life is structured by the regularity with which recurrent events take place. Mealtimes, bedtimes, and the like shape the day's events. Thus the presence of a schedule and the rigidity with which it was adhered to were always considered in evaluating structure. A great many other things also contribute to the degree of structure prevailing over time. These include relative consistency in the adults' response to the child's behavior. Caretakers who maintain certain standards of behavior in such a way that some actions are consistently approved while others remain unacceptable lend structure to daily life. Homes where the same behavior on the child's part is sometimes ignored, at other times reprimanded, and at yet other times applauded for its entertainment value fail to structure this dimension of the child's life. Under the latter condition it is difficult for the child to form any expectations about the consequence of his actions before praise or disapproval actually occurs. Another important way in which toddler experience is structured is by the establishment of customs, habits, and little rituals in relation to routine procedures. For instance, bedtime rituals, the custom of not serving food until everyone sits at his or her appointed place, particular ways of accomplishing such tasks as getting dressed or bathed, and innumerable others lend form and consistency to how things are done. A play hour after dinner, a distinction between party clothes and garments suitable for play—all such stabilities in time and place are ways of structuring a child's experience.

Structuring also takes place on another level. A child who lives in a well regulated household where childrearing practices are consistent may yet lack structure in other dimensions, namely, in the degree to which caretaking adults play a regulating, channelling, and guiding role during what might be called free hours, when there is nothing special that has to be done. Ordinarily the youngster is expected to spend such time in play. An extreme and yet frequently observed example of lack of structure in this respect is a state of affairs in which the child is left entirely to his or her own devices and attracts attention only if and when the child causes mischief or danger. In the absence of suitable playthings, and especially in the absence of some help in getting started and in the transition from one activity to the next, most two- and three-year-olds cannot cope for long and become subject to restless boredom. They are apt to turn on faucets, climb furniture, empty drawers, create havoc among adult possessions, and the like; in short, their actions become more random, short-lived, and inappropriate and sooner or later lead to trouble. Alternatively, their behavior becomes primitive and stereotyped—for instance, endlessly rolling a toy car back and forth, tearing paper to shreds, or sitting before the TV screen but not attending to it. Or the child may clamor for adult attention hardly knowing what it is that he or she wants.

We have used the term *mini-structure* to denote adult behavior that lends content and meaning to the child's activity. Among the ways of supplementing the child's resources and thereby providing mini-structure are: providing or suggesting interesting things to do; intermittently joining the child as participant or interested observer of his or her play; and encouraging the child to "help" with household tasks. In short, we refer to any of the thousand and one ways in which adults can interest a child in a meaningful, goal-directed activity. Be it play, conversation, an outing, or shared activity, all serve to fill the vacuum that is likely to occur if two- or three-year-olds remain without attention for more than brief periods of time.

We have gone into such detail about the nature of this variable not only to avoid possible misunderstanding (for instance, a confusion between monotony and structure) but also because we believe that for young children structure as here defined is a crucial condition for well being. The developmental changes that occur during the third and fourth years of life revolve around the emergence of cognitive and other structures that support increasing cohesiveness, self-regulation, and increasingly complex reality-attuned adaptation. The here-and-now existence of the sensorimotor phase is gradually replaced by a mode of functioning that includes awareness of past and future as well as the capacity for goal setting and goal striving. The child begins to evaluate his own behavior and that of others, as well as the environment at large, in a more highly differentiated manner. Appraisal is no longer limited to the distinction between that which is pleasurable and that which is unpleasurable. Two- and three-year-olds begin to realize that something pleasurable in itself may entail disapproval and hence displeasure. Simultaneously they begin to feel responsible for their own actions and to hold mother or anybody else responsible for what that person did (quite often on the basis of an erroneous belief). Part and parcel of these changes is the realization that an environment exists which is independent of the child's participation, so that events occur that he or she cannot control or influence. Children also begin to know that there are reasons or causes for whatever happens, and they come to know that their own wishes and those of their mother may not coincide.

These developmental changes could not occur without major transformations in the cognitive domain. They rest on the child's growing ability to classify things and people in terms of categories that are in fact simple concepts. With this capacity for abstraction comes the recognition that objects within a single category and designated by the same word may nonetheless have different attributes: for instance, balls may be of any size or color. In other words, the toddler moves into a world that affords a bewildering manifold of events, causes, intentions, agents, attributes, and affective qualities. Much of what he perceives and recognizes is as yet incomprehensible to him. Expectations are often disproven by events, and uncertainties arise. Thus, while new interests and abilities emerge, so do new sources of stress and anxiety.

Adaptation to an enlarged and more complex environment, and to a more complex inner life, is facilitated by the existence of signposts, signals, and concepts that lend order and stability to an otherwise fluid field. Maturing cognitive capacities, combined with intrinsic tendencies toward mastery, assertion, and an emerging clear sense of self, support both the need and the ability to organize and comprehend events, objects, relationships, and feelings. It is as participants and as observers of everything in their surroundings that children establish meanings and contextual groupings that lend coherence to day-by-day existence. A life pattern that is in fact irregular and unpredictable, and that often leaves the child without assistance in organizing his own behavior, fails to provide many of the props and pathways that aid in the development of appropriate internal structures and behavior strategies.

The Degree of Accommodation to the Child

Here we refer to alterations in the behavior of adults that are guided by and attuned to behavior signals emanating from the child. We use the term *accommodation* to denote flexibility in many aspects of childrearing, in distinction to *indulgence*, to be discussed later, when immediate caretaking goals are relinquished in the face of the child's resistance. The hallmark of accommodation is that the means are flexible while the purposes and end results remain intact. Accommodative behavior serves to reduce avoidable stress and/or displeasure for the child or to help him achieve satisfaction in whatever activity he is engaged.

Accommodation can take place in any situation and through an infinite variety of ways. An adult who is more comforting and less demanding than is his wont at moments when the child is very tired is accommodating. Providing a night light to a toddler who fears the dark is accommodating, and so is masking unpleasant medicine with applesauce. A mother who plays with a child in such a way as to compel him to use a toy (or any other thing) only in what she holds to be the proper way or who herself performs the toy manipulation instead of allowing him to do so is, for the time being, not accommodating. Play in which a mother enables a child to carry out his or her own intention, helping just enough so that the child can complete the action unaided, is playing in an accommodating style. If a child fears the toilet seat it is accommodating to try a pottie.

Experimenting with different methods of motivating a child is a primary arena for accommodation. For instance, finding that loud scolding does not work, the mother may try to speak softly but emphatically; if that does not work, she may send the child to the bedroom for a little while. Accommodation can consist of altering certain expectations, as in continuing partially to dress a child when it becomes apparent that he cannot cope with sleeves and trouser legs. In all instances it requires the adult to observe and interpret the child's behavior signals. It also requires a reasonably good understanding of what may be expected of children at a given age or developmental level. Among our parents who provided next to no accommodation were a good many whose beliefs concerning the skills and comprehension to be expected of a two- or three-year-old were grossly erroneous on developmental grounds alone. In order for adult behavior to be considered accommodating for rating purposes, we required evidence that by and large such efforts were successful—in other words, that discomfort was in fact reduced or that the child's behavior integration was facilitated.

Accommodation so defined encompasses much of what is generally held to be effective mothering. It reflects an important way in which the mother and others create a social environment adapted to the child's immediate and long-range needs. It is more than likely that mothers' feelings about themselves in the maternal role play a major part in enabling them to "read" their children well and act accordingly. As always, however, our ratings disregarded underlying attitudes and focused on what caretakers did and the impact this had upon the child.

The Degree to Which Didactic Experience Was Provided

This rating specifies how often and how intensively the children were taught cognitive skills by someone in their customary environment. In many homes didactic endeavors begin with the teaching of words and picture recognition. A bit later such things as numbers, the alphabet, and the use of pencils or crayons are added. The use of puzzles, shape boards, and other educational toys is relevant insofar as adults spend time with children teaching the requisite skills. We included story telling and the joint inspection of picture books as well as the teaching of nursery songs with words. If viewing of educational television programs was strongly encouraged for the older children, this also contributed to didactic input. We excluded varieties of teaching that were not directly related to cognitive functions, such as teaching gross motor skills, or social conventions like the correct use of cutlery, and also teaching children what *not* to do—for instance, to refrain from touching the stove. In didactically oriented homes the appreciation of cognitive advances typically finds expression indirectly also. New-found abilities and skills are noticed and praised, books and similar materials are treated as valuable objects, and conversation with children tends to be extensive and explanatory.

It was not difficult to ascertain factual information about the extent to which adults tried to teach but also the extent to which the child actually engaged in the cognitive activity, whether or not what was taught was developmentally relevant. One extreme of didactic intent that was not scored was an instance where a mother patiently taught her little daughter how to write her name, persisting over many weeks, although the child (who was retarded) was barely able to produce a random scribble.

Didactic teaching is of course one mode of structuring a child's experience and influenced the assessment of that variable as well. It was scored separately because of its obvious importance in relation to test scores. If cognitive level as judged by test scores were almost entirely a function of how much the child was taught, a detailed consideration of the relationship between other variables and IQ would become meaningless.

The Amount of Focused Social Attention the Child Received

The definition of this experience variable specifies just one variety of social situation: occasions when an adult (arbitrarily defined as anyone over 16 years of age) devotes all of his or her attention to the child and therefore behavior is directed exclusively toward the child. Almost invariably such a situation leads to reciprocal interaction between the two. A child's experience when an adult is wholly focused upon him or her differs from that in many other social situations, not least because the potency or vividness of one-to-one encounters is much greater. At first glance it may seem as though in any family such exclusive child-adult interactions must be frequent, even when they are largely limited to caretaking routines. Such events as being dressed, toiletted, or bathed often involve mutual focused attention as do some varieties of play and also episodes of conflict. Such social transactions can be more casual, however; for instance, the adult may simultaneously keep an eye on other children, watch television, or carry on an unrelated conversation. We learned that there are children who live animated social lives, who are frequently responded to and addressed, and who yet have few opportunities for concentrated involvement with just one person at a time. All of our children did experience focused social attention, but the difference between those for whom this situation was very frequent and those for whom it was much the lesser part of the social transactions that occurred proved important. We included this aspect of daily life because we think that highly focused one-to-one encounters with adults play a unique role in the development of interpersonal relationships and, at the same time, can provide prime learning opportunities.

Selected Styles of Discipline

No attempt was made to assess the great variety of ways in which children were taught to conform to caretakers' demands. Instead, three styles of discipline were selected, each representing an extreme. These were overall patterns of dealing with the child which we think have an effect on the totality of the child's experience that is massive and perhaps specific in its developmental consequences. The majority of children in the research group were not subject to any of these three selected patterns of discipline and received a rating of *inapplicable*. As might be expected, of those to whom one of these ratings did apply, the greater number fell into the deviant group.

MARKED SEVERITY AND HARSHNESS THROUGHOUT. This rating was assigned to children whose families maintained unusually demanding standards of behavior and punished what they interpreted as misdemeanors more harshly than is common in our sample and in general.

MARKED INDULGENCE THROUGHOUT. This rating was assigned to children who could justly be described as spoiled. It applied when in dealing with the child the family made next to no effort to provide guidance or control. The child's wishes were gratified if at all possible, impulse expression was not checked, and no incentives were provided for more mature or desirable modes of behavior. Such lack of direction or control could occur when caretakers were indifferent or apathetic and found it easier to let things go. It could occur on the basis of profound ignorance and inexperience on the part of caretakers who knew neither what to expect nor what to do with children of toddler age. It could also be an unfortunate manifestation of unbounded acceptance and affection coupled with ignorance.

Appendix C includes examples of what is meant by this pattern, and more discussion will be required when we turn to the deviant group. At the moment it is enough to specify that children who received this rating were those who met no opposition when they insisted on eating only when and what they wanted (caretakers might find themselves cooking midnight meals on demand) and were allowed to stay up until all hours because they did not want to go to bed (sometimes keeping a parent from his much needed rest). In the supermarket caretakers bought these children nearly everything they asked for, even if the child threw it away at once. Any demand or prohibition addressed to the child was abandoned as soon as it was resisted, often for fear of the temper tantrum that would otherwise occur. Since disappointments are inevitable, families such as these went all out in efforts to pacify their offspring, offering food, petting, gifts, and the like as consolation. Whenever we have seen this pattern in existence consistently over an appreciable period of time it has led to infantilization of the child accompanied by developmental arrest in at least some areas of functioning.

A COMBINATION OF MARKED SEVERITY AND MARKED INDULGENCE. In the extreme form which defines this variable the pattern is rare even among deviant children, but milder versions of combining severity with indulgence are fairly common in some subcultures.[4] In order for this rating to apply it was required that children be severely punished and subject to high standards of behavior in some areas while they were grossly indulged in other important behavioral domains. Typically it was obedience, good manners, and outward tokens of respect for elders that were highly valued and harshly enforced. At the same time, an indulgent stance was maintained in such areas as eating, sleeping, destructiveness, and the expression of movement impulses and affect. The same child who could with impunity run through the supermarket sweeping objects off the shelves might find himself beaten with a belt should he say no to his father or fail to kiss a relative on demand.

Such a combination of severity and indulgence constitutes an obstacle to normal development during the toddler years and beyond. Most of the conditions that

4. In retrospect we wish that our definition of this experience variable had been less stringent. The developmental consequences of this pattern when it occurs in milder forms were discernible in a good many instances.

make for a secure relationship with the mother, for impulse control, and for cognitive learning are not present. Paradoxically, the demands made on children in a setting such as we have described could be met only if the child had achieved fairly high levels of impulse control. Yet the indulgent style of responding to much of the child's behavior provides minimal opportunities for the youngster to acquire the self-regulating mechanisms needed to achieve control and to conform to parental expectation. We learned that within this pattern children may or may not become fearful or intimidated, but invariably they are immature for their age and, if the pattern persists, come to function in maladaptive ways.

A word is in order about the degree to which these patterns of experience may be independent of one another. There are overlaps between structure, didacticism, and focused social attention. For example, a high rating on any one of these patterns may preclude a low rating on one or two of the others. In addition to the probable overlap among these aspects of experience we assume that a central unitary combination of external, familial, and intrinsic factors is at the core of the totality of each child's experience at any given time. Regarded in this light, our separate assessment of several aspects of experience may be likened to an inspection of the interior of a house by peeking through different windows, thus gaining several perspectives on the very same thing. Assuredly, life does not come in separate compartments. Cohesiveness among all EPs existing at a given time, both those that could be assessed and those beyond our reach must be assumed. By looking at different behaviors in different situational contexts and by employing different criteria for each, however, it is possible to obtain a more differentiated and more concrete description of each experience syndrome than would otherwise be possible. We shall later have occasion to report on a quantitative analysis of the degree of interdependence among different EP ratings. It will be possible to ascertain which of these patterns are relatively autonomous, which tend to go in tandem, and also which of the EP constellations have similar, or unlike, developmental consequences. The separate assessment of various facets of a child's daily life experience is an abstraction. It is little more than a device intended to shed light upon major developmental trends as they are influenced by diverse experience.

Chapter 6

Experience Patterns and Developmental Outcome

The EP Ratings

An overview of the distribution of EP ratings for the intact group is provided in figure 6.1. The distribution remained virtually the same from 28 through 40 months. It is therefore possible to report some of the results for the three age levels combined.

We mentioned earlier that the criteria were constructed so that ratings of 1 (rare or absent) and 3 (frequent and prominent) identified the children who, for the pattern under consideration, were like one another in that they either lacked or abundantly experienced the life situation that was being rated. A rating of 2 (present, not prominent), however, encompassed a wide range of circumstances. Children who received that rating were a somewhat heterogeneous group even with respect to the pattern in question. Therefore the fact that a rating of 2 was by far the most frequent for all EPs does not necessarily imply a normal distribution for these aspects of experience. Our EP ratings represent a continuum but not a scale. What is of interest in scrutinizing figure 6.1 are the differences among the EPs with respect to the frequency with which extreme ratings occurred. For instance, ratings of either 1 or 3 were fairly frequent in the areas of structure and accommodation (40% of all ratings). By contrast, for didacticism and focused attention, a scant 20% of all ratings occupied an extreme position. The distribution of ratings for frequency of conflict differed from all others in that minimal conflict with adults was not uncommon (30%) yet a high frequency (for age) was almost never found. Last, very few of the intact children experienced any of the preselected patterns of discipline, and these are therefore reported by the number of such ratings that occurred. Pervasive severity was not found at all, although overall indulgence as well as a combination of indulgence and severity were applicable in a very few instances.

The EP ratings were undertaken in order to describe, in systematic terms, some aspects of the everyday experience of young children as it varies from family to family and from one socioeconomic level to another. This information was put to use to trace the interconnections between SES, experience-pattern ratings, impulse control scores, and IQ. We already know that IC and IQ are associated with each other and that both of these vary as a function of SES. Do the EP ratings fall into the same pattern?

Figure 6.1 Distribution of EP Ratings for Intact Group by Age

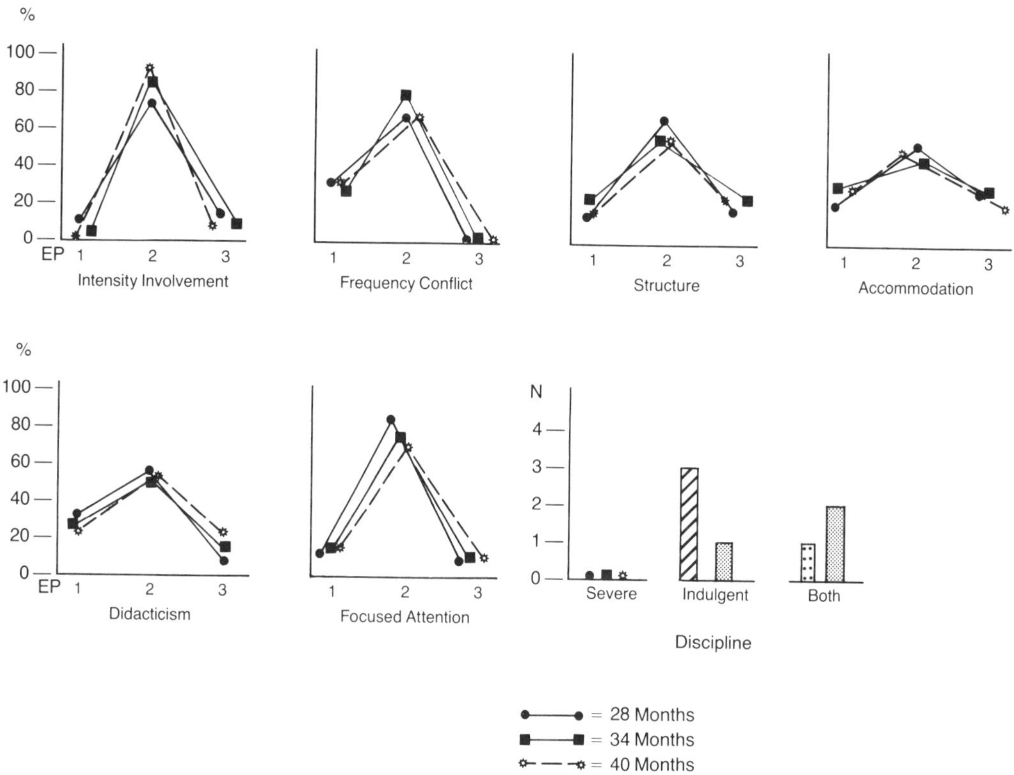

EP Ratings and SES

The most precise appraisal of socioeconomic status available to us is the SES index. In table 6.1 we show the mean SES index for each rating within the six aspects of experience that were rated. There is no reason to suppose that social privilege or disadvantage affects the extent of a mother's emotional involvement with her baby, and table 6.1 shows no such difference on this EP, within the limits of what can be ascertained when extreme ratings are very scarce.[1]

Concerning the frequency of conflict between child and adults, there is a trend for less than the usual amount of conflict to be associated with higher social status. We can think of many instances to the contrary and were not at all surprised that the SES difference failed to achieve statistical significance. Ratings on structure, ac-

1. Some of the literature describing teenage mothers suggests that their emotional immaturity makes it difficult for them to develop maternal feelings. As it happened, the teenage mothers we came to know typically showed strong affection accompanied by something like fierce possessiveness toward their babies.

Table 6.1: Mean SES Index for Each EP Rating (Intact Group, by Age)

		28 Months			*34 Months*			*40 Months*		
EP	*Rating**	*N*	*SES*	*St.D*	*N*	*SES*	*St.D*	*N*	*SES*	*St.D*
Intensity of Involvement	1	4	57.2	13.7	1	59.0		0		
	2	37	69.1	18.4	34	68.2	23.6	42	66.6	19.2
	3	8	63.0	17.7	5	62.0	23.6	5	61.0	22.1
		49	67.1	18.0	40	67.2	19.0	47	66.0	19.4
Conflict	1	16	70.5	14.1	12	71.6	14.1	16	70.0	20.1
	2	31	63.8	19.3	32	63.8	19.9	32	63.2	18.4
	3	1	91.0		0			2	45.5	0.7
		48	66.6	18.0	44	66.0	18.7	50	64.7	19.1
Structure†	1	9	41.8	18.4	11	42.6	14.7	11	41.2	15.8
	2	33	70.0	15.7	28	66.3	17.3	29	68.7	17.8
	3	10	73.2	15.9	12	76.1	15.6	13	74.6	11.9
		52	65.7	19.4	51	63.5	19.9	53	64.4	20.0
Accommodation†	1	10	43.5	21.9	13	47.2	21.9	13	47.8	21.1
	2	24	70.2	11.3	21	67.9	14.6	23	65.2	15.7
	3	13	74.3	17.0	11	74.2	16.5	10	77.2	14.6
		47	65.6	19.3	45	63.5	19.5	46	62.9	19.9
Didacticism†	1	18	54.9	19.6	16	46.2	15.7	12	38.8	12.7
	2	29	68.4	16.2	26	69.5	14.4	30	67.5	16.8
	3	5	87.2	9.6	8	83.0	10.4	12	79.8	9.6
		52	65.5	19.2	50	64.2	19.4	54	63.9	20.4
Focused Attention†	1	4	48.7	7.2	5	41.2	17.6	7	36.0	14.9
	2	34	63.1	19.8	31	66.7	16.9	30	66.4	16.9
	3	4	89.0	10.1	5	84.4	9.2	6	76.5	21.0
		42	64.2	20.2	41	65.8	19.3	43	62.9	20.9

*1 = absent or minimally present; 2 = present, but not prominent; 3 = very prominent.
†F probability = .001 or less for all ages.

commodation, didacticism, and focused attention on the other hand, are significantly related to SES at all ages. In particular, a minimal presence of these experiences is associated with distinctly low socioeconomic status. The differences in the SES index when these experiences are of medium as compared to high prominence are in the same direction though of lesser magnitude.

A clearer picture of the manner in which experience patterns are related to social class is given by the distribution of EP ratings for each quartile (figure 6.2). This graphic representation departs from the customary format, but it has the virtue of combining all relevant information. For each experience pattern the columns represent the distribution of ratings within a given quartile, and the quartiles are aligned in rows. For instance, under the heading of accommodation a comparison between the extreme left-hand and right-hand columns shows that in quartile I fully half of all ratings were 1 and all but two of the remaining ratings were 2. The reverse distribution is seen in quartile IV, where we find only two ratings of 1, fourteen of 2, and seventeen of 3. To find the relative frequency of a given rating in

Figure 6.2 Distribution of EP Ratings by SES Quartile (Intact Group, Ages Combined)

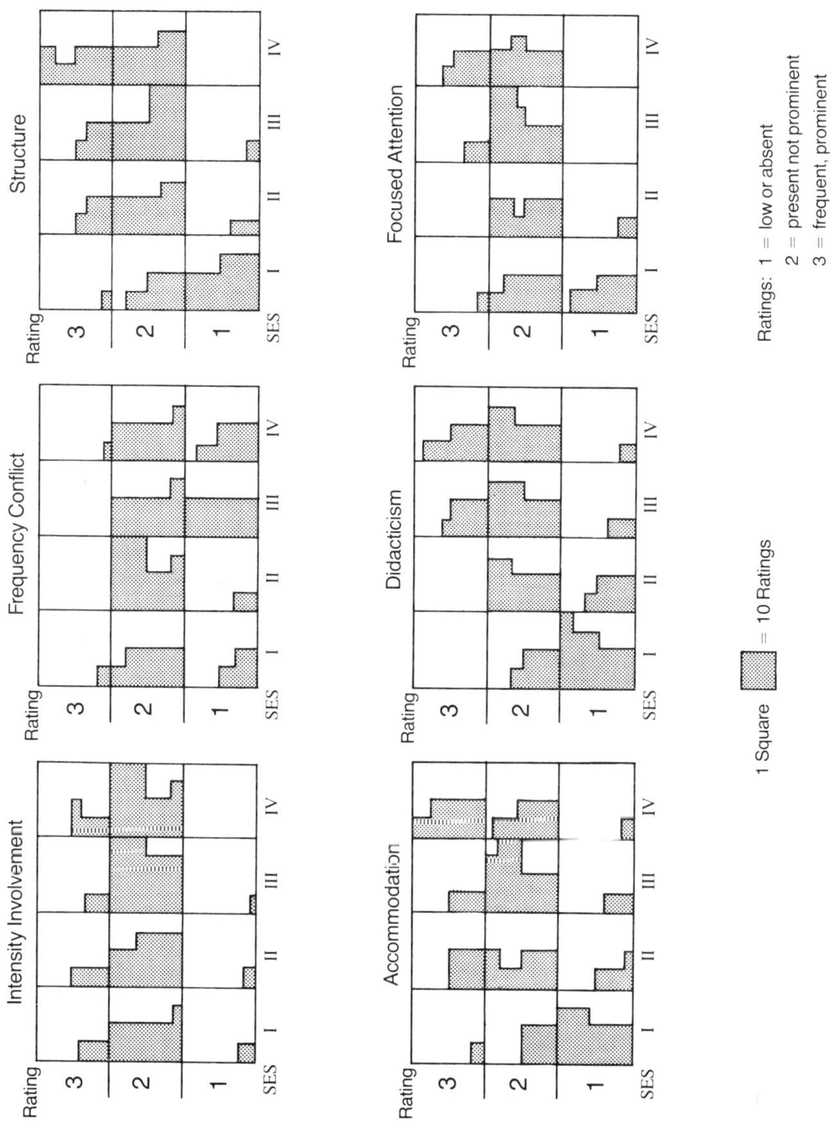

different quartiles one looks from left to right in the same row. The high rating of 3 for structure, for example, increases in ladder-like fashion from quartiles I to IV. What is learned from figure 6.2 can be summarized as follows: The extreme ratings of rare or absent and frequent and prominent are strongly associated with social class. In all areas, ratings of 1 (denoting a marked lack of the experience) were scored mostly for quartile I children and a few in quartile II. With one exception (accommodation), this had its counterpart in the distribution of the ratings of 3, which denote abundant experience in the area. Such ratings came chiefly from Q-IV and secondarily from Q-III. Quite as important as the uneven distribution of ratings 1 and 3 as a function of social class is that the rating of 2 (present, not prominent) was assigned about equally often in all social groups, from the lowest to the highest.

We were struck by the fact that although the absence of accommodation was concentrated in the low SES groups, a highly accommodating style of caretaking was as frequent in Q-II as in Q-IV. Our predilection for the scrutiny of out-of-pattern findings then led us to consider maternal characteristics that may relate to accommodation. As we define the term, accommodation always involves reflection concerning the meaning of the child's behavior and the best way of dealing with a situation, but reflectiveness is only one of several requirements for the creation of an accommodating childrearing atmosphere. The fact that maternal reflectiveness was present to equal degrees in all quartiles except Q-I accords well with the finding that accommodation is the only one of the SES-linked experience patterns for which ratings of frequent and prominent were well represented in one of the low SES groups.

The primary result of an examination of the influence of social class on EP ratings is that all but one of the six experience variables are lacking or minimally represented in the lives of children from the lower SES groups and tend to be more highly represented the higher the socioeconomic status of the family. The next step was to see whether all or some of the experience patterns had a bearing on impulse control and on IQ.

EP Ratings and Impulse Control

The essential information on this issue is presented in figure 6.3, in which we show the relationship between each EP rating and IC scores. Because EP ratings were distributed in virtually the same way at each age level (figure 6.1), we used percentages based on the sum of scores for the three age levels.

A rough index of the relationship of EP ratings to IC is found at the left-hand side of figure 6.3, where mean IC scores are plotted for each EP rating. Of the six experience patterns, only one, intensity of maternal involvement, showed no discernible relationship to impulse control. We mentioned earlier that the frequency of overt conflict with adults is, among other things, a behavioral expression of the child's level of impulse control. Thus those children who had developed better than average ego control were by and large also the children who had relatively few conflicts with adults. Among the great majority of children who showed considerable but not excessive frequency of conflict the distribution of IC scores followed a normal curve.

For structure, accommodation, didacticism, and focused attention, the mean IC showed a sharp increase from the very low level (1) to a medium rating (2) and a slight increase with the shift from 2 to 3. In short, minimal experience in these four dimensions was accompanied by a delay in the development of impulse control. When these experiences were very amply present there was a trend toward precocious levels of impulse control.

On the right-hand side of figure 6.3 we show the distribution of IC scores for each EP rating. Because at times percentage values were based on very small numbers, the number of ratings is shown beneath each EP category. The different experience patterns do not relate to impulse control in quite the same manner. When life was minimally structured, more than half of the children were undercontrolled. With medium levels of structure the proportion of undercontrolled children dropped to 25%. When structure was of a high order, only 9% received that score. The close connection between structure and impulse control is further indicated by the fact that low structure was never associated with unusually high control (4), a score of which was present in 20% of those with medium structure and rose to 34% of the children who led highly structured lives.

The relationship between didacticism and control was somewhat different. Here too low impulse control was most frequent among the children who received almost no teaching. But whether didactive experience was massive or moderately prominent made no difference: The distribution of IC scores was about the same under these two conditions. Children who were accommodated minimally or not at all also were much more likely to have low IC scores than the others. And, as was the case with the amount of didactic input, whether accommodation was present to a medium or high degree did not affect the frequency of unusually mature ego control. The relationship between accommodation and impulse control did have one unique feature however: an IC of 3 (age-appropriate balance between control and impulsivity) outnumbered all other scores only among those children who experienced very high levels of accommodation. In the other patterns the score of 3 was equally frequent whether the experience in question was present to a medium or to a high degree. This special feature of accommodation makes good sense when one considers that it is defined as an overall style of caretaking that minimizes stress, avoids coercion, and is therefore likely to foster impulse control while supporting spontaneity and hence a degree of impulsiveness.

Last, the amount of focused attention the child received showed a clear-cut relationship to impulse control. The proportion of undercontrolled children decreased and the proportion of somewhat overcontrolled children increased as the amount of one-to-one social attention shifted from minimal to moderate to very prominent.

From this material we concluded that by and large fairly stable aspects of experience differ markedly for children whose control of impulsivity was low for

Figure 6.3 Mean IC Score and Distribution of IC Scores for Each EP Rating (Intact Group, Ages Combined, in Percentage)

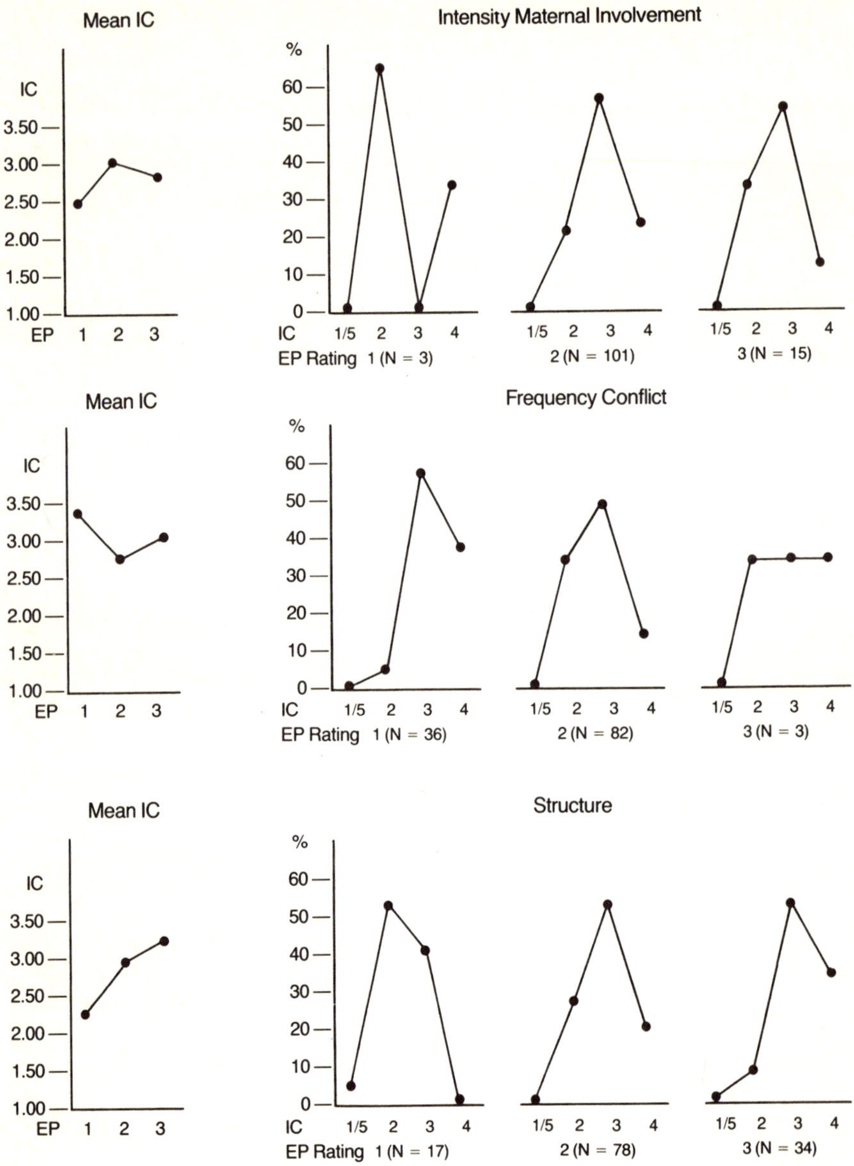

Figure 6.3 *(cont.)*

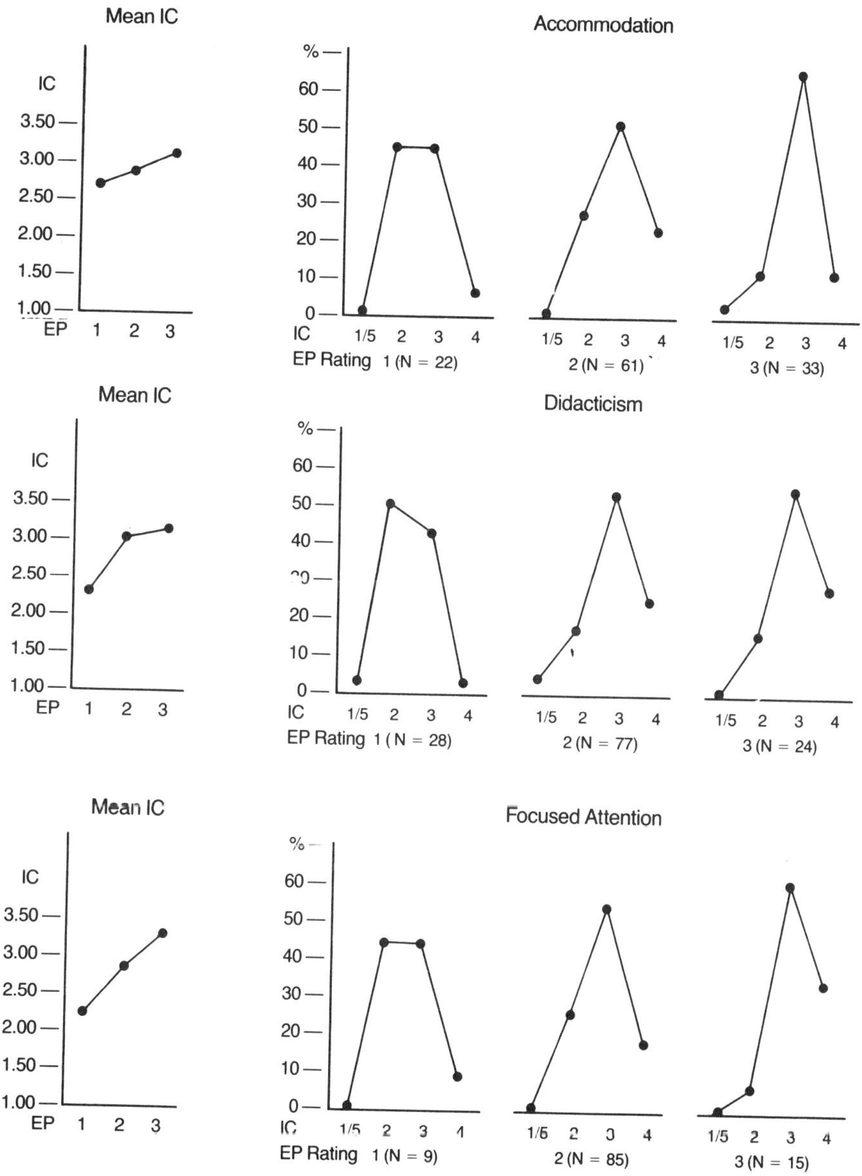

their age and those whose control was age-appropriate or unusually mature. The undercontrolled children were predominantly those who led less structured lives, were not taught as often or as much (or were unwilling to engage in cognition-related activities), were seldom if ever subtly accommodated, and had less opportunity to experience focused social attention. Nothing in our data suggests a stringent and direct relationship between any one of the stable patterns of experience and a normal and adequate development of impulse control. In fact, about 40% of the children who received a low rating on any one of the experience patterns also received an age-appropriate IC score of 3. At these early ages then, a relative lack of experience in these areas carries with it a greater likelihood that impulse control will be delayed or comparatively poor and good impulse control will be nearly impossible to attain when experiential support is lacking in all the EP areas.

EP Ratings and IQ

There proved to be a strong association between cognitive development and the degree to which the variety of experience being rated was present in the life of

Table 6.2: Mean IQ for Each EP Rating (Intact Group)

		28 Months			*34 Months*			*40 Months*		
EP	*Rating*	*N**	*IQ*	*St.D*	*N**	*IQ*	*St.D*	*N**	*IQ*	*St.D*
Intensity of Involvement	1	4	65.0	16.7	1	66.0		0		
	2	38	93.0	12.5	35	91.8	15.7	43	94.3	15.5
	3	8	82.0	14.7	5	96.6	11.2	5	94.2	12.3
Frequency of Conflict	1	16	93.1	17.7	12	92.4	27.5	16	96.1	19.7
	2	32	86.5	14.8	32	84.1	17.7	33	91.7	16.1
	3	1	93.0		0			2	76.5	4.9
Structure†	1	9	68.2	11.9	11	67.7	15.9	11	73.8	14.4
	2	34	90.8	12.1	29	89.1	14.1	30	95.0	16.8
	3	10	96.4	16.4	12	96.9	23.0	13	98.7	11.0
Accommodation†	1	10	77.4	8.6	13	70.6	18.8	13	76.8	17.1
	2	25	90.0	12.2	21	87.0	12.8	23	92.7	13.9
	3	13	98.5	14.6	11	79.8	23.6	10	105.1	7.0
Didacticism†	1	18	77.1	15.0	16	72.3	15.9	12	76.5	10.3
	2	30	91.4	11.5	27	90.5	16.9	31	93.2	14.4
	3	5	108.4	13.8	8	99.5	20.4	12	102.4	15.8
Focused Attention†	1	4	63.0	13.3	5	56.2	15.3	7	73.5	18.2
	2	35	88.3	12.0	32	90.0	16.9	31	94.7	14.2
	3	4	113.0	10.7	5	105.6	15.7	6	103.8	20.3

*The N for each rating is larger than on figures 6.2 and 6.3 because this table includes all ratings, whether or not IC scores and SES were available.

†Significance (F) is .001 or less.

these children. In table 6.2 we show the mean IQ for each EP rating. Differences in mean IQ corresponding to differences in EP ratings were substantial and significant in the dimensions of structure, accommodation, didacticism, and focused attention. These are of course the same experience patterns found to be associated with IC and with social class. In all four areas the difference between the ratings of rare (1) and present but not prominent (2) were accompanied by a massive difference in mean IQ. The shift from the midway rating (2) to frequent and prominent (3) brought a modest increase in IQ in the areas of structure and accommodation but substantial increases in the areas of didacticism and focused attention. (The one reversal in accommodation at 34 months is an artifact that arose because one subject who received maximal accommodation had a very low IQ.)

The children who had relatively few conflicts with adults also had higher mean IQs in comparison to the rest. It would be absurd to believe that frequent episodes of conflict were somehow responsible for a slower pace of learning. More likely, the children whose impulse control was good for whatever reasons, and who could therefore avail themselves normally of learning opportunities, were less inclined to engage in oppositional behavior. That the intensity of maternal involvement

Figure 6.4 IQ Distribution for Each EP Rating at 40 Months (Intact Group, Scattergram)

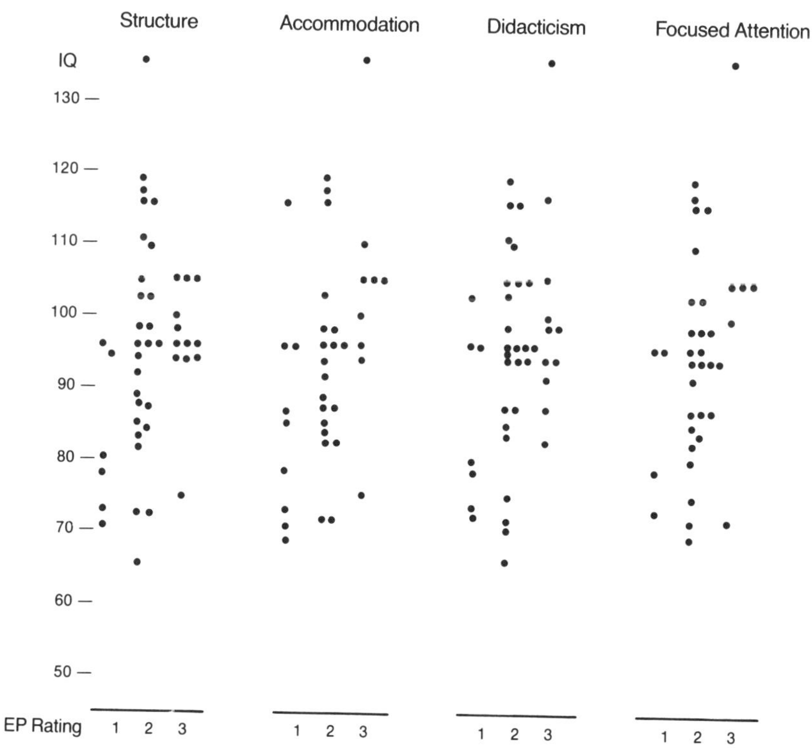

with the child made next to no difference in mean IQ would be expected if for no other reason than that this experience pattern bore no relationship to any other variable.

In figure 6.4 we supplement what was learned from table 6.2 by plotting the IQ distribution for each rating on the four EPs that are strongly related to IQ. We chose to present this material for the 40-month age level because IQs are relatively stable after the age of three years. The correspondence between EP ratings and IQ is far from perfect. Some of the children whose experience in one of these areas was minimal nonetheless attained IQs in the normal range and, at the opposite end, maximal exposure to these experience patterns did not preclude impaired cognitive development, though both of these departures from the general trend were rare. By far the largest group, those receiving a rating of present but not prominent, showed the entire gamut of IQ scores from retarded to superior. One way of looking at these distributions is to say that, with respect to cognitive test scores, a lack of these experiences is a handicap, abundant experience is favorable, and moderate experience has no bearing on the issue.

Interconnections between SES, IC, and IQ

In piecemeal fashion we have presented evidence to show that: (a) social-class differences exist in relation to IQ, to the level of impulse control, and to EP ratings; (b) IC scores and IQ scores are associated with each other both across and within SES groups; and (c) EP ratings are directly related to IC scores as well as to IQ. In short, the global variable of social class, the experience patterns prominent or lacking in each child's life, and the developmental variables of impulse control and cognitive development are highly intercorrelated. Our interpretation of these findings is that social class is a major determinant of the experiences provided for the child, that typical and prominent aspects of experience play a role in the development of impulse control, and that, during the toddler years, normal and optimal cognitive development depends heavily upon the presence of an age-appropriate degree of impulse control.

Two assumptions cannot be bolstered by further manipulation of the data: that the nonpsychological variable of social class largely determines the experience patterns, which are codetermined by psychological and organismic characteristics, and that the developmental changes reflected by IC and IQ scores are the resultants of experience. What can be offered in support of our understanding of the matter is a demonstration that all the facts and observations contained in the research data are *compatible* with the assumptions we have made. Figure 6.5 is our final effort to present a cohesive picture of all major findings. It brings together the mean SES index, the mean IC score, and the mean IQ as these values differ, or fail to do so, for the different ratings on each experience pattern. That all three of these scores are altered in the same direction as a function of different EP ratings needs no further comment. Figure 6.5 is designed, however, to highlight differences between experience patterns in their relationship to the other variables.

Figure 6.5 Mean IQ, IC, and SES Index for Each EP Rating (Intact Group at 40 Months)

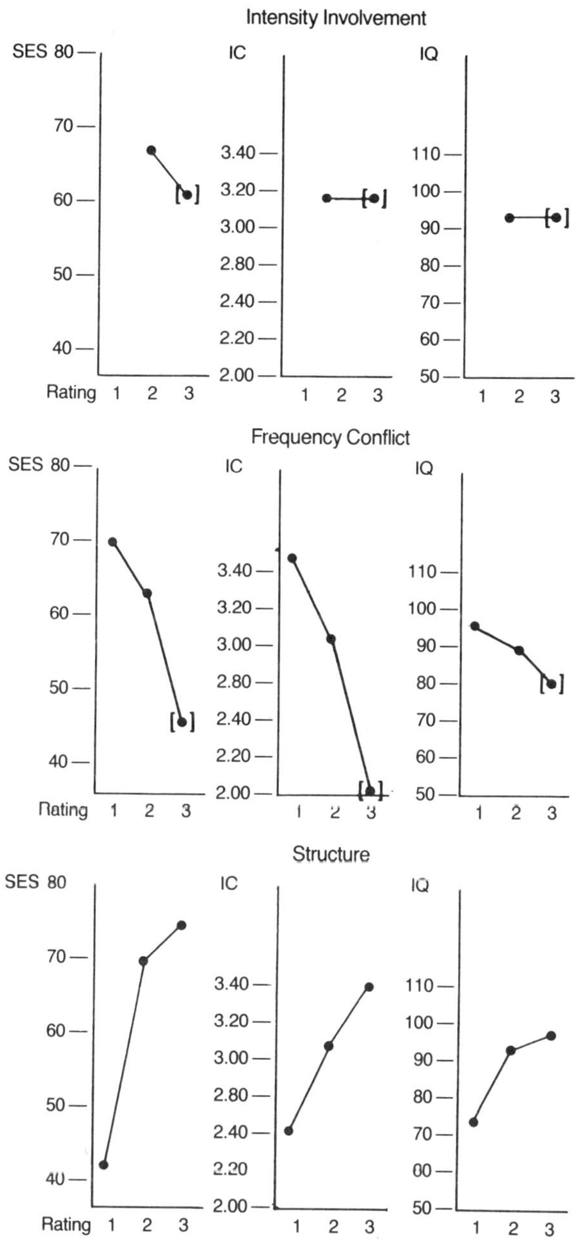

Figure 6.5 (*cont.*)

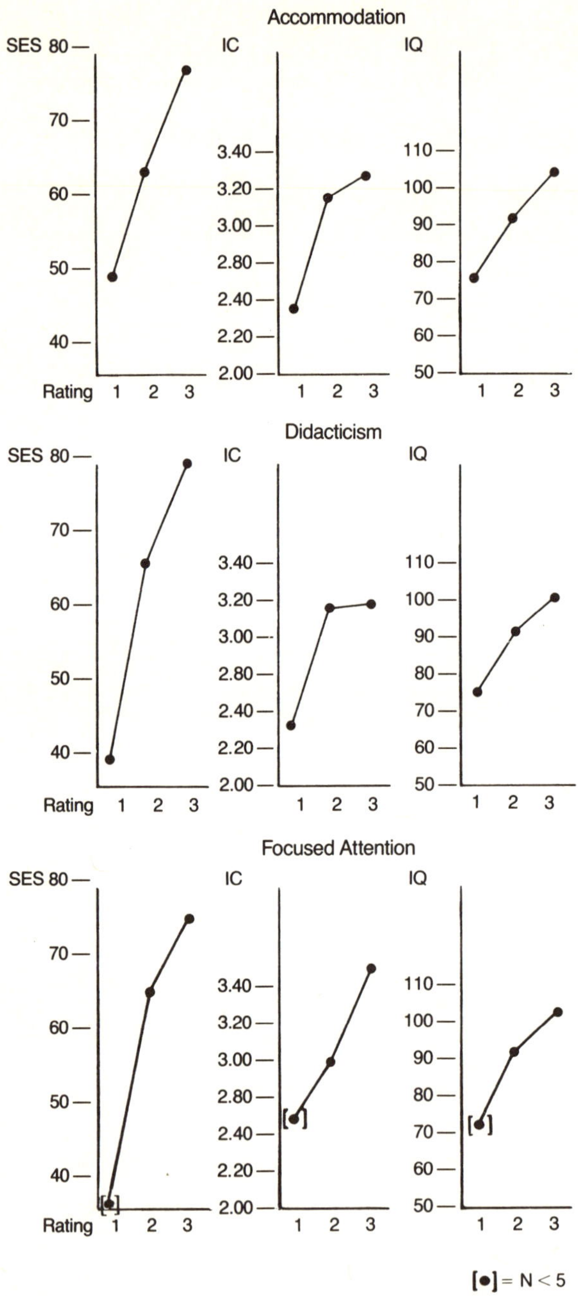

Frequency of conflict was associated with an appreciable difference in ego control in that those with few such conflicts had a mean IC above the age-appropriate level and those who experienced such conflicts about as often as most of their peers had a mean IC indicating slight immaturity. Cognitive development was not affected by this difference and the SES index differed but little.

Whether or not the child's life was *structured* to at least a medium degree was almost entirely a function of SES, though this was not at all the case for the difference between medium and high levels of structure. IC scores rose sharply as structure ratings shifted from the minimal to a moderate degree. And last, a relative lack of structure was associated with impaired cognitive development, but whether structure was medium or high made no difference in the mean IQ.

The degree of *accommodation* experienced by the child was strongly influenced by social class and had a clear influence upon IQ, which ranged from a mean of 77 for rare to 92 and 105 for moderate and very frequent, respectively. Yet impulse control was much the same for medium and very high levels of accommodation, with only the children who largely lacked this variety of experience rated as markedly undercontrolled.

Didactic input was also massively influenced by social class. When didacticism was minimal, impulse control was distinctly poor and cognitive development well below age expectation. Although the difference between medium and high amounts of teaching corresponded to a marked difference in SES, didacticism had no effect on impulse control and very little on mean IQ.

For *focused attention* comparison can be made only between those who had this experience with medium frequency and those who had it with high frequency. It was the families of higher social status who tended to provide focused attention very frequently. IC scores tended toward the overcontrolled side for the children who received the very frequent rating, whereas those with a medium rating showed a slight trend toward undercontrol. The difference in mean IQ for these two groups was small.

Interdependence of Experience Patterns

Up to this point we have dealt with each experience pattern separately, as though it had the same meaning regardless of the constellation of EP ratings within which it occurred. In actuality the aspects of experience that were rated are but part of the totality of events that form the matrix for the child's development. Even within the confines of those domains of experience that we rated, we had to assume that the impact of any one component would be affected by the total profile of ratings. For instance, a high rating for didactic input is not as likely to have the same effect if focused attention and accommodation are minimally present as when these other facets of experience are also prominent. Further, it is difficult to know to what extent a rating on any one EP captures an aspect of the child's life that is reasonably distinct from the texture of his experience in other EP areas that were rated. If it is not distinct, the particular rating makes no independent contribution to the sum total of experience pattern ratings. In other words, we had to ask if our ratings merely specified different behavioral and situational manifestations of a single characteristic or did the aggregate of ratings describe meaningful variations in the combination of relevant aspects of life experience? Whatever the case, information about six different aspects of experience provides a richer picture of what each child's life was like than could possibly be conveyed by any single, more global expression. What we wish to explore is whether clusters of EP ratings do more than specify different consequences of the same attribute.

Many questions arise in this connection. In a hypothetical extreme case where at least five of the six ratings referred to essentially the same pattern, each child would receive the same rating on all patterns. If the ratings dealt with different aspects of experience that implied one another to some degree, a given rating on one pattern would always appear in combination with the same rating on one or more other patterns. For instance, if very prominent didacticism were possible only when structure was also very prominent, a rating of 3 for didacticism would always be paired with a rating of 3 for structure. In the equally extreme case that none of the EP variables is associated with any other we would expect the distribution of ratings to be dictated by chance. It is impossible to calculate precisely the degree to which these ratings are independent of one another, largely because the number of ratings in the two extreme positions (1 and 3) is so small that a matching of two ratings across several patterns would occur by chance whether or not an intrinsic and meaningful relationship exists between the experience variables that received this same rating.

It is, however, possible and worthwhile to consider the degree to which ratings for a single child are concordant with each other. When ratings on all five experience patterns are combined at 40 months, 62% are concordant. Discordant ratings are more frequent for the extreme positions on the scale than for the midposition. Specifically, the concordance rating for the present but not prominent rating (2) was 74%; that for the rare rating (1) was 48%; and for the rating of very prominent (3) it was 35%. For about half of the intact children at 40 months, if any one of the experience patterns was minimally represented, several others were also under-represented. If any one of the experience patterns was assessed as being very amply present, others received equally high ratings in about one third of the instances.

The association among all of the ratings is less interesting than the description of which of the EPs tend to go together and which are more often disparate. For instance, does the degree to which a child's life is structured ordinarily accord with the degree to which he or she is accommodated? A rough measure of the degree of concordance between all possible combinations of two EPs is shown in table 6.3. (Ratings for the intensity of maternal involvement are omitted from this and some other tables because only five of the forty-nine children received a rating other than 2 at 40 months, which constrains concordance values to the point of absurdity.)

Table 6.3: Concordance between Ratings for All Combinations of EPs (Intact Group, 40 Months)

EP *Combination*	*N Ratings*		*Percent*
	Total	*Same**	*Same**
Accom. + Foc.Att.	39	30	76.9
Struct. + Accom.	44	33	70.2
Didac. + Foc.Att.	44	30	68.2
Struct. + Foc.Att.	43	29	67.4
Struct. + Didac.	53	35	66.0
Confl. + Foc.Att.	41	24	58.5
Didac. + Accom.	47	25	53.2
Struct. + Confl.	48	24	50.0
Confl. + Accom.	43	21	48.8
Didac. + Confl.	48	21	43.7

**Same* refers to the number of cases in which the same rating was given to both EPS.

Table 6.3 shows that the proportion of identical ratings on two EPS ranged from 77 to 44 percent. Accommodation and focused attention were most closely tied to each other, with structure and accommodation next. Conflicts between children and caretaking adults can arise under very different circumstances and for very different reasons and so it comes as no surprise that ratings for frequency of conflict were not associated with ratings on any of the other experience variables.

In order to look more closely at the issue of congruence between EP ratings, we compare the ratings on each experience pattern to the ratings the child received on all other patterns (table 6.4). Thus, in the first row under the didacticism heading we see that of ten children who received a rating of 1 for accommodation and for whom ratings on didacticism were available, nine, or 90%, of the cases received the same low rating for both EPS. Of the twenty-four children who received a medium rating for accommodation, fourteen, or 58%, also had a medium rating for didacticism. When the rating for accommodation was very prominent, the rating for didacticism was also 3 in 40% of the cases. Table 6.4 highlights what was suggested earlier: When two EPS receive the same rating in an extreme position, such concordance is far more likely to occur at the lower than at the upper end of the scale. That is, a child who received a rating of 1 on one EP also received a rating of 1 on another dimension of experience relatively often. One who received a rating of 3 on one EP was not as likely to be rated as 3 on another. The reason for this circumstance is not difficult to find: For each of the experience patterns, the rating of rare or absent applied primarily to children reared in poor and minimally educated families. It is more than plausible that a childrearing milieu that provides impoverished experience for a child in one respect will also entail impoverished experience in other areas. That unlike ratings were more often found in the medium and high ranges is consistent with the greater range of sociocultural circumstances that yielded these ratings. The high ratings were

Table 6.4: Concordance between each EP Rating and All Other EP Ratings (Intact Group, 40 Months)

					Accommodation				
	1			2			3		
	N	N=*	%=†	N	N=	%=	N	N=	%=
Foc. Attention	9	6	67	20	19	95	10	5	50
Structure	12	10	83	22	17	77	10	8	80
Didacticism	13	9	69	21	14	67	10	4	40
Conflict	11	0	—	22	18	82	10	3	30
					Focused Attention				
	1			2			3		
	N	N=	%=	N	N=	%=	N	N=	%=
Accommodation	6	6	100	27	19	70	6	5	83
Structure	7	6	86	30	19	63	6	4	67
Didacticism	7	7	100	31	20	64	6	3	50
Conflict	7	0	—	28	21	75	6	3	50
					Structure				
	1			2			3		
	N	N=	%=	N	N=	%=	N	N=	%=
Accommodation	11	10	91	21	17	81	12	8	67
Foc. Attention	9	6	67	22	19	86	12	4	33
Didacticism	11	9	82	29	20	69	13	6	46
Conflict	10	0	—	25	21	84	13	3	23
					Didacticism				
	1			2			3		
	N	N=	%=	N	N=	%=	N	N=	%=
Accommodation	10	9	90	24	14	58	10	4	40
Foc. Attention	11	7	63	22	20	91	11	3	27
Structure	12	9	75	29	20	69	12	6	50
Conflict	10	3	30	26	18	69	12	0	—
					Frequency of Conflict				
	1			2			3		
	N	N=	%=	N	N=	%=	N	N=	%=
Accommodation	2	0	—	28	18	64	13	6	46
Foc. Attention	2	2	100	26	21	81	13	0	—
Structure	0	0		31	21	68	15	8	53
Didacticism	2	0	—	31	18	58	15	3	20

*Number of same ratings.
†Percent of same rating.

contributed as frequently by families in quartile III as by those in quartile IV and, on some EPs, occurred among quartile II families as well.

When only the proportion of like ratings between two experience patterns is considered, as was done in table 6.3, the result can be misleading. The interdependence of accommodation and focused attention is a good example. When ratings for focused attention are aligned with those for accommodation (second section from top in table 6.4) there is indeed a close correspondence between the two, but when accommodation ratings are aligned to those the child received for focused attention (first section at the top of table 6.4), there is little correspondence for either the high or the low ratings. In other words, accommodation ratings depend heavily on those for focused attention, but the reverse is not true.

That the minimum or maximum presence of focused attention had greater impact on ratings for accommodation than the other way around would be expected from the definition of these experience patterns. Accommodation refers to only one style of interaction between child and adult. Focused attention, on the other hand, refers to any manner in which the child receives undivided and sustained adult attention. In order to accommodate a child to a high degree it is necessary to observe closely and interact with him or her, and this usually also involves focused attention. Yet a child can be the focus of adult attention in a manner that is not in the least accommodating.

A similar inspection of which EP in any given combination exerts the greater influence upon the ratings of the other EP can be summarized as follows. Ratings for structure and accommodation were very similar. In this case the tie seems to be more fully mutual; the degree of conformity is about the same whether one or the other pattern is regarded as the baseline. The exception is that children whose lives were very highly structured were not necessarily accommodated to a high degree. Accommodation and the amount of didactic experience the child had were more disparate. Quite a number of the children received different ratings for these two EPs. We noted especially that of the children who were accommodated to a high degree less than half received more than the usual amount of teaching. There was also a considerable discordance between the ratings for structure and focused attention. Of those who received high structure ratings, 66% experienced medium amounts of focused attention. In addition, a marked lack of structure in the child's life (rating of 1) could be accompanied by the rating of focused attention typically received by the majority (2). As for the relationship between structure and didacticism, we found that low ratings usually coincided, but ratings of 3 on either of these variables were not strongly associated with equally high ratings on the other. Frequency of conflict ratings appeared to be largely independent of the other four EPs.

Overall the experience-pattern ratings that refer to accommodation, focused attention, and structure tend to be coordinated with one another, though there are enough discrepancies to assure us that different aspects of experience were assessed under these headings. Didactic experience, on the other hand, was relatively independent of other facets of experience, and frequency of conflict even more so. There is reason to suppose that of those EPs that are related to our outcome variables each contributes something different to the end result, although a degree of overlap as well as an inherent affinity exists between some of them.

In light of the fact that ratings on the five relevant EPs did not imply one another and that each of the EPs was shown to be related to the outcome variables, we explored the relationship between the sum total of EP ratings and the level of impulse control as well as cognitive development. For each child we constructed a composite EP score consisting of the sum of all EP ratings that he or she received at a given age divided by the number of ratings. Those children for whom fewer than four of the five relevant EPs were rated, as well as those for whom no IC score was available, were excluded from this calculation. The correlation between composite EP scores and IQ proved to be .70 at 28 months, .59 at 34 months, and 0.60 at 40 months. These are strong and significant relationships, but they can hardly be accepted at face value as an index of a direct relationship between composite EP scores and IQ. Low EP ratings were dominant among the lower SES quartiles while high ratings were contributed primarily by the two upper quartiles. It is conceivable that these correlations are a reflection of the relationship between SES and IQ. In other words, SES characteristics not necessarily identical with those that entered the EP ratings could indirectly lead to a high correlation between composite EP and IQ, since both are closely related to SES.

In order to interpret these and similar findings, it is necessary once more to return to our basic model insofar as it concerns the relationship between SES and IQ. We stated that to a large extent SES differences in IQ are the result of SES differences in prominent experience patterns and also that IQ differences within a given SES group are largely a function of differences in experience within that group. If this formulation is correct the correlation between composite EP scores and IQ should be greater than that between SES and IQ. As reported in chapter 4, the correlation between SES and IQ was .51 at 28 months, .50 at 34 months, and .58 at 40 months. Our expectation was amply fulfilled at 28 months (.70 *vs.* .51), it was met at 34 months (.59 *vs.* .50), but it broke down at 40 months (.60 *vs.* .58).

When a single result is out of keeping with the rest one wonders whether the incongruous result is due to some extraneous factor, so that it has no bearing on the main issue. Inspection shows that at the age of 40 months, for example, all but one of the very low composite EP scores—those between 1.00 and 1.75—were contributed by children in quartile I. It is no wonder that the correlation between the lowest composite EP scores and IQ is the same as that between IQ and SES; of the fifteen quartile I children, however, six, or 40%, had composite EP scores in the intermediate range (1.80 to 2.40). The mean IQ of these six children was 89.6, in contrast to a mean IQ of 75 for the nine children in quartile I who had low combined EP scores.[2] Thus we have an indication that the stronger association between

2. Statistically minded readers will recall that the correlations of SES and IQ were based on the SES index, which is more differentiating than are SES quartiles.

composite EP scores and IQ than between SES and IQ obtains at 40 months as well. It is of incidental interest that medium scores were generated in all social groups. Of the twenty-six children with intermediate composite EP scores, quartiles I and IV each contributed 23%; quartile II, 19%; and quartile III, 35%. Of the seven children with very high combined EP scores (from 2.60 to 3.00) one came from a Q-II family and the others were evenly divided between Q-III and Q-IV.

In table 6.5 we provide the mean values for IQ, SES, and IC for each of the three groups of composite EP scores. What was amply demonstrated for each individual experience pattern also holds for total EP scores, which are consistently related to SES as well as to the outcome variables. At each age level, IQ and IC are distinctly low when composite EP scores are low and rise as the EP scores shift from low to intermediate and high. As has been true of all the other material we reported, the gap between the low and intermediate groups is much wider than that between the intermediate and high groups. This applies to SES as well as to the outcome variables. In table 6.5 we also see something not previously reported, although it was hinted at as probable: mean IC values are the same whether combined EP scores are intermediate or high. This is in contrast to mean IQs, which rise as EP scores move from intermediate to high.

It may also seem that IQ and IC should rise and fall together, so another glance at the relationship between impulse control and cognitive development is in order. We have postulated that during the early preschool years normal and optimal cognitive development depends upon the presence of an approximately age-appropriate degree of impulse control. This is not to say that adequate control in itself facilitates cognitive advance. Rather, we think that a certain degree of impulse control is necessary to enable toddlers to utilize fully whatever learning opportunities are provided experientially. It is when impulse control has reached this minimal necessary level that differences in the richness of appropriate experience,

Table 6.5: Composite EP Ratings and Mean IQ, SES, and IC (Intact Group)

Composite EP	*Age (in months)*	*Mean*		
		IQ	*SES*	*IC*
Low	*28*	*77.5**	*52.0**	*2.57*
1.00–1.75	*34*	*72.4**	*47.1*	*2.22*
	40	*80.3**	*46.9*	*2.50*
Intermediate	*28*	*92.3**	*71.2**	*3.00*
1.80–2.40	*34*	*93.9**	*73.0*	*3.16*
	40	*93.4**	*67.0*	*3.00*
High	*28*	*100.0**	*75.3**	*3.11*
2.60–3.00	*34*	*95.4**	*76.7*	*3.00*
	40	*103.0**	*76.6*	*3.10*

*Difference between EP groups S = .003 or less

and probably also differences in endowment, come into full play and most clearly affect the rate and pattern of cognitive development.

To evaluate the material in table 6.5, another complication must be recognized. Impulse control has been treated by and large as an outcome variable, but, although it is a developmental acquisition, it is also a codeterminant of experience patterns. A child's experience is jointly shaped by what exists in the relevant environment and by the child's characteristics, of which impulse control is one. Once a degree of impulse control has been acquired in the course of ego development, it also affects cognitive development in an indirect manner through its contribution to the shaping of experience patterns.[3] These patterns will affect the further development of impulse control and thereby also the subsequent patterning of experience.

3. These considerations also apply to the changing level of cognitive functioning with development. The same environmental circumstances will be perceived and responded to differently by an older and a younger child, and differently by a dull and a bright one. It is the essence of the developmental process as we understand it that very nearly all resultants of development are antecedents of subsequent developmental changes. This is never a straight sequence; rather, each component interacts not only with all others but also with innumerable external and intrinsic conditions and events. We acknowledge with regret that the interpretation of empirical results in this arena of research cannot help but be an oversimplification and distortion.

First Interlude: *Vignettes of Six Children from the Intact Group*

It is now time to turn away from numbers and generalities and to acquaint the reader with some of the individual children and their life circumstances. What follows are vignettes of some of the intact children and their families selected from among those with low, medium, and high composite experience-pattern values. In the interest of confidentiality some details and external circumstances have been altered or omitted. The vignettes are nevertheless faithful accounts of what was reported and observed, as integrated by clinically-informed perception. Although they are based entirely on fact, these essays convey the author's sense of the quality, and to some extent the meaning, of the things we came to know about each child and family.

I begin with two children whom we named Rosie and Tony. They were chosen as examples of what we also saw in a good many others: good adaptation and reasonably good intellectual and personality development within a setting of chronic poverty.

Rosie: A Well-Endowed Child in An Impoverished Setting

Background

Rosie's mother was 17 years old and still in high school when her little girl was born. Members of her large family occupied several adjacent apartments in the same building. The mother, father, and baby lived in one of these but spent most of each day and every evening in the apartment of the maternal grandmother. From the beginning, her grandmother's place was a second home to Rosie; later it became her primary abode. The extended family, consisting of at least eight adults and from four to six children (relatives with children moved in and out at intervals), functioned as a single household. Only one dinner was cooked and shared by all; financial affairs (welfare plus intermittent contributions from family members who were working at the time) were in the grandmother's hands. All members of the family group were deeply involved in each other's affairs and none seemed to strive for a more independent existence. Family style was lively, noisy, quarrelsome, and affectionate. The paternal grandparents, whom we did not come to know, lived just across the street.

Rosie's parents were not married. Within a year of the baby's birth the father had become an occasional visitor, and within another year he disappeared from the scene altogether. Thereafter the household consisted of women and children, which seemed entirely acceptable to all concerned. All these people had much contact with little Rosie. They spent time with her, spoiled her, and helped to take care of her. The grandmother became so possessively attached to the baby that she tended to take over, at first much to the mother's distress. By the time Rosie was three years old her grandmother was clearly the primary caretaker and was recognized as such by her mother, who had accepted this arrangement, though not without resentment.

Ratings at 40 Months

Impulse control. Rosie was described as a most impatient child possessed of a terrible temper. When anything displeased her she screamed and cried, and tantrums occurred every day. When confronted with something difficult she either abandoned the task or insisted that someone do it for her. The reports of her uncontrolled behavior in the home environment were detailed and internally consistent. They were entirely credible to us, especially as they were confirmed by observation during research visits, but we also saw another side of her. In direct interaction with staff members who were highly supportive she became engrossed in some activities and then coped with delays and (very slight) disappointments reasonably well. Although we knew that she had the capacity for somewhat better modulation and control, she received an IC score of 2 (fairly low).

Structure. Household routines in this home were neither regular nor chaotic but, because her whims were catered to, the pattern of Rosie's life was erratic. For instance, she snacked at will during the morning, often refused lunch in consequence, but then asked for and received a meal some time during the afternoon. Not surprisingly, she had no appetite at dinner time, and an evening meal was served to her much later than to the others in the home. Sleep patterns also varied from day to day as there was no fixed bedtime and as she often chose to sleep in her grandmother's bed. The most organized periods in her life were the occasions when her grandmother took the child on shopping trips, to the park, or to the front of the house where Rosie could ride her tricycle. Otherwise Rosie entertained herself as best she could at home. Much time was spent in conflict with her little brother (who was two-years younger) and with her mother, who tried to put a stop to such activities as climbing on the windowsills or messing up adult belongings. Toys or games of the kind that lend content to a young child's activity (puzzles, blocks, picture books) were not in evidence, though many other toys were bought for her and soon broken. We did learn that on occasion, usually when separated from her brother and mother, she could and did play by herself. For instance, she might dress, pet, feed, and scold her dolls in the same way that she had observed her little brother being treated. The adults either could not (mother) or did not wish to (grandmother) discipline the little girl or guide her in any way. One example of this state of affairs is that although she was perfectly capable of using the toilet, Rosie often urinated wherever she happened to be. Grandmother cleaned up without remonstrance; mother did no more than voice disapproval. The EP rating for structure was 1 (minimal).

Accommodation. A good deal of what has already been described also defines a lack of accommodation. Rosie was not expected or encouraged to overcome such difficulties as she had. That nothing was done to stop the day- and nighttime wetting is but one example. An especially striking manifestation of an unaccommodating stance on the part of the caretaking adults was that Rosie was not allowed to dress herself unaided.

Although she had been clamoring to do so for some weeks and typically cried and protested while it was being done for her, her mother refused to let her try because she felt it was too time consuming and her grandmother thought the child was too young. Thus both adults dressed the child even though both acknowledged that she was eager to do it for herself. A similar attitude on the part of the adults found expression in relation to self-feeding. Except for snacks consumed on the run, Rosie sat and waited to be fed. To the grandmother this was as it should be, whereas for the mother it was not, but she could think of no way to cause her child to eat except to feed her. In other ways as well, Rosie's gradual progression toward greater self-sufficiency was not appreciated as part of normal development.

From what we were told and could observe, it seemed to us that the caretaking adults often failed to notice what went on before their eyes, or they failed to understand the meaning of the child's behavior. For instance, when Rosie began fighting with her brother in our presence, her mother sat watching passively. She volunteered that this went on all day long and that there was no use in spanking the children because it did not help. She failed to notice how the younger child slyly provoked his older sister. She also did not realize that there was nothing for either child to play with or to do (they settled down somewhat better when we provided toys). At no time were we told of occasions when either mother or grandmother acted in such a way as to forestall boredom, unruliness, or any other undesirable condition. Both caretakers responded to the child's actions only *after* the event. If what Rosie did was undesirable, the grandmother responded by comforting or offering a treat and the mother by very pointedly ignoring her or by threats and scolding. The EP rating for accommodation was 1 (minimal).

Didacticism. The idea of teaching cognitive skills to a young child had no houseroom in this family. Certainly Rosie's many toys did not include any of the educational variety. Television was not regarded as an educational resource, and play of the sort that teaches vocabulary, picture recognition, and the like did not take place. The EP rating for didacticism was 1 (minimal).

Focused attention. Rosie undoubtedly received a great deal of attention from her grandmother. How much of it was reciprocal and sustained in conformity with our definition of this variable was difficult to judge. From descriptions one could feel fairly certain that in situations when Rosie was being dressed, bathed, or fed, she often absorbed all of her grandmother's attention. The EP rating for focused attention was 2 (present, not prominent).

Frequency of conflict. The mother claimed that conflict between Rosie and her grandmother did not occur at all "because she gives her everything she wants." On the other hand, the mother felt that she and Rosie clashed incessantly. She added that she never approached Rosie except when she felt very angry; otherwise she tried to ignore Rosie's presence. We were not inclined to take either of these assertions at face value. From anecdotal data we knew that Rosie did get angry at her grandmother, and not infrequently. Though this was often met by gentle remonstrance rather than antagonism, it can safely be assumed that some of these episodes were perceived as conflictual by both participants. There can be no doubt that Rosie did fight with her mother often and that conflicts with other adults in the home occurred every day. The EP rating for frequency of conflict was 3 (very prominent).

Intensity of maternal involvement. This aspect of the child's experience proved impossible to rate. The grandmother's jealous possessiveness probably reflected a more than ordinary degree of emotional involvement with the child. So much of the relevant information came from the mother rather than directly from the grandmother that the evidence is weak. As far as the mother's feelings about Rosie are concerned, she spoke as though the child were nothing but a burden. Yet the fact that she intervened so often and that she found so much to complain about indicates that she was by no means indifferent to the child. All this is so speculative that it could not be used for rating purposes. For what it is worth, the clinical impression was that Rosie must have felt herself to be an important person to those who cared for her, as much from witnessing impassioned quarrels about herself between the two adults as from affection and attentiveness on the part of at least one of them. The EP rating for intensity of maternal involvement was ? (unscorable).

Developmental Course

As an infant Rosie was exceptionally alert and well organized. Her MDI was 101. She was hypersensitive to sound and highly reactive to stimulation in all modalities. As her environment was overstimulating by any standard, it is no wonder that she spent a good deal of time crying (largely from exhaustion, we thought). Yet joyous excitement was an equally prominent feature of her waking hours during infancy.

At 15 months Rosie again presented herself as a thriving, well-endowed infant. Her MDI was 111, and her behavior closely corresponded to what Mahler and others have described as typical of toddlers during the early (hatching) phase in the individuation-separation process. Thus, her response to the *open space* situation[1] was to leave mother happily, without a backward glance, at sight of the invitingly large corridor. She wandered far enough to have to be retrieved, as she gave no sign of returning of her own accord. During the *play session,* while mother, seated on a couch close by, conversed with the examiner, Rosie readily manipulated most of the large supply of toys that had been placed on the floor. Often she looked briefly at her mother, and occasionally she directed her gaze to the examiner. In typical toddler fashion she sometimes left the toy area to approach and touch her mother, only to move away from her toward the toys again (four times in ten minutes). Her sensorimotor play was rather complex. As yet she seemed to have little need for intentional communication with her mother across a distance. Of the seven simple gestures or words that are included in the scale of *conventional communication* signals, she employed only one, holding up a toy for mother to see and acknowledge. It should be remembered that at this early age her mother was still the chief caretaker and the mother-child relationship was not unduly troubled.

Unfortunately Rosie was not brought in for the 28-month visit and when we saw her again at 34 months great changes had taken place. Her IQ was now 76, largely because she was unfamiliar with many words and situations that are known to most children at

1. See the appendixes for a description of the Open Space procedure, as well as other assessments mentioned in the text.

this age. In addition, it was difficult to arouse her interest except for some activities that happened to involve dolls. On the *concept formation* scale, which requires that objects of the same kind (keys, toy shoes, small animals) be matched, she was unable to understand the task despite many demonstrations. This was not a matter of unwillingness—she was highly pleased with the activity of dumping (the wrong) objects into boxes. Her scores on the *Achievement Motivation* procedure were consistent with this behavior in that there were next to no indications that she took pleasure in achieving a difficult goal. That is, she was as pleased by the accomplishment of very easy tasks as she was by success in something difficult. She tended to avoid or refuse tasks that required effort and perseverance. All this was done in a perfectly friendly manner, quite unlike her unruly behavior at most other times.

Her response to the *Level of Aspiration* experiment, designed to assess the response to success and failure, told the same story. In choosing a distance from which to throw a ball into a basket she returned to the same spot after each trial whether or not she happened to hit the target. It was as though she ascribed the result to chance rather than to her own skill or lack of it. Last, when asked whether she wanted to climb up on a sofa (with her mother's permission) to get a much desired cookie or to have it given to her, she chose the latter. Most two-year-olds in our group were delighted at the chance to get at the cookie without adult help.

In the play session she fared better, though much of her play was immature; the most developmentally advanced behavior occurred during a brief spurt of imaginative play that consisted of serving make-believe tea. As on previous occasions, she maintained close contact with her mother, mostly by addressing questions and requests to her. Yet, from a structural point of view, her play was less mature than that of most of her peers in that she did not create a play area within which the play action took place (*microplay*, in Erikson's terminology) but moved through the room with or without toys (*macroplay*). Neither could she tolerate separation from the mother. As her mother moved toward the door, explaining that she would be "right back," Rosie cried so loudly and ran after her mother so energetically that we abandoned the attempt.

At this time Rosie's relationship with her mother had deteriorated, and the grandmother had assumed the lion's share of the caretaking responsibility. During the interim a baby brother had arrived. We thought that Rosie's current difficulties might have been intensified by her jealous feelings, although her mother did not believe this. Her explanation was that grandmother's overly indulgent and possessive manner encouraged Rosie to defy her own mother with impunity. For whatever reason, the descriptions left no doubt that Rosie had become a household tyrant and—at the same time—received such compliance with her wishes that she behaved "like a little princess," as one investigator put it. Certainly at the age of 34 months she was distinctly immature in the psychosocial as well as in the cognitive sphere.

When Rosie returned at 40 months of age the pattern of cognitive functioning was much as it had been on the previous visit (IQ 80), as was her tendency to avoid tasks that seemed difficult to her. But there were some important changes. One or two tasks among those used in the Achievement Motivation assessment interested her greatly. For instance, buttoning a doll's dress was exceedingly difficult for her, yet she pursued it with determination and hugely enjoyed her final success. Her mother commented that Rosie had never had occasion to button anything. Here it is important to remember that the issue of being allowed to dress herself unaided was a major source of conflict in the home. That the child had reached the point in her development where she appreciated the result of her own efforts was also shown by her response during the Level of Aspiration experiment. After failure she reduced the distance from which to throw the ball, and after success she increased it, trying to better her performance. This time she also chose to climb for the cookie.

Our version of the *World Test* uses a very large array of miniature toys and the invitation to build something with them on a large square board placed on the floor. On this task Rosie performed at a more mature level than did many other children in the sample. Interestingly, she began by placing human figures all around the periphery of the board (a ''world'' bounded by people) and then placed clusters of similar objects, such as trees, fences, and animals, on the inside.

In spite of these gains, Rosie remained woefully inept when it came to the comprehension of verbally mediated concepts. In her vocabulary ''knife'' and ''fork'' were used interchangeably, she could not point to the larger of two balls, and once again she was unable to sort objects by category but instead combined the toys in ways that were meaningful to her.

Discussion

In Rosie at 40 months we saw a child who demonstrated considerable competence in relation to practical problems and to nonverbal tasks provided that these concerned materials and ideas that are part and parcel of everyday family life. She had next to no information about the larger world. Animals, other places, and stories such as are contained in picture books or shown on children's television programs were not within her ken. Nor had she been introduced to ways of perceiving and using objects in terms of their invariant attributes, such as size and shape. She had not been involved in naming things or in identifying pictures as activities in their own right, and she had never been engrossed in working at a puzzle. To the best of our knowledge no game with rules had been played with her. Life at home took place in a somewhat turbulent atmosphere, and she experienced a good deal of conflict, but also many pleasurable and gratifying situations. She had not been expected or taught to subdue momentary inclinations in the interest of later satisfaction or in order to obtain the approval and affection of important people in her life. Much of her everyday behavior could be understood as an effort to find interesting things to do and also to impose her will on all about, and this led to a good deal of interpersonal strife. Yet, in the company of an attentive and supportive adult (research staff) and with interesting things to do, Rosie was a delightful child. At such times her behavior was appropriately modulated and quite planful. That this was a function of the immediate situation and not of being away from home is indicated by the fact that during the same research visit we also witnessed the immaturity, impulsivity, and irritability that had been described to us. Invariably this occurred when staff members became inactive observers while the mother was in charge.

We thought that in her home the style of social interactions between Rosie and caretaking adults tended to counteract the inherent tendency to develop impulse control. The slowdown in her intellectual development as reflected by test scores seemed inevitable in view of poor ego control coupled with very restricted learning opportunities.

When she was seen again at the age of 6 years, after she had been through kindergarten and a half year of grade school, Rosie had an IQ of 92, well within the normal range. This lends support to our earlier suggestion that this intrinsically able child made good use of such opportunities as came her way. At the same time her behavior style was and remained well adapted to the somewhat unusual pattern of relationships within the home.

Tony: A Boy Splendidly Adapted to His Life Circumstances

Background

Tony's mother was 19 years of age when she gave birth to her first child. The fact that she lived with baby's father on and off without planning to make the union permanent was easily accepted by the large extended family. The marital and financial arrangements in this black family tended to be loose, informal, and variable. The mother was a high school dropout and before her pregnancy had been employed sporadically. Her relationship with her own mother had always been troubled and tempestuous. Nor did she express fondness for the baby's father; on the contrary, she hoped the father would "split" sooner rather than later. Yet the mother maintained warm and cordial relationships with several other relatives. Throughout the time we knew this mother-baby pair they lived in a small apartment that lacked basic amenities. Plaster peeled off the walls, heat and elevator service frequently broke down, and neither cleanliness nor security was maintained in the building.

From the first day this young mother greatly enjoyed her infant. As time went on she appeared untroubled by the demands he came to make on her or by the high activity level and unruliness that were typical of him during the toddler years. The father as well was "crazy about the baby." In spite of his inability to get along with the mother and the fact that he lived at home only intermittently, he spent much time with his son and, while living at home, played with him every afternoon. Later he took the child on many outings. Tony was also an important personage to both sets of grandparents and to other relatives. These people loved him and helped to take care of him. Tony's social life was contained within "the (housing) project" where all maternal relatives had their homes. He was cared for in an affectionate and tolerant manner.

Ratings at 40 Months

Impulse control. At 40 months Tony had overcome rather serious problems with impulse control that had been conspicuously present when he was younger. At the supermarket he now helped rather than racing about and causing havoc, as had been his wont. He could watch television attentively for as much as an hour at a time. Although he remained fidgety and distractable, he was no longer overactive. Tantrums had become rare. He still became angry very easily but expressed it in a more modulated manner. During developmental testing he could be helped to curb impatience although it remained most difficult for him to persevere on difficult tasks. The family was proud of how well he had controlled his fear during a visit to the dentist. The IC score was 3 (age-appropriate).

Structure. Tony was one of the few children who was never at loose ends although his environment lacked structure. His mother customarily slept very late in the morning, often well into the afternoon. Tony might rise as early as 9:00 A.M. but on other days might sleep until noon. If, as was usually the case, he awakened before his mother, he helped himself to cereal and milk, though at times she got up to fix him a bite to eat and then returned to bed. Tony was content to amuse himself provided that the television was on. Although there were some programs that he knew and watched attentively, for the most part television was a necessary background noise (as it was for his mother also). Except for dinner, which was a cooked meal served some time between midafternoon and evening, Tony chose when and what to eat throughout the day.

His afternoons and evenings were spent with his mother, who often took him to a nearby park and kept an eye on him as she chatted with neighbors. There were other children there, but he seldom played with them, he was said to be too bossy to get along with peers. A stop at McDonalds on the way home was also likely. Instead of the park excursion or sometimes in addition to it, one of his parents (never both together) might indulge his passion for bus riding. He requested this treat urgently and often. When his mother or father took him on a bus, they had no destination in mind—the idea was to give him pleasure. Evenings at home were long. Again the television was on, and there were frequent animated interchanges with the mother. Many were playful and of the mutually teasing kind, but many others consisted of unpleasant encounters when things did not go his way and he was scolded and threatened with the belt.

Relatives were constantly in and out of the home. Tony might also spend part of the day or an occasional night in one of their homes, but most of the time mother kept him by her side. The bath and other routines took place at whatever time happened to be convenient. Tony went to bed when he chose, usually after midnight. He no longer shared mother's bed but, depending upon his mood, he might sleep in his own bed or join his father on the living room couch if he happened to be staying over. There was a sort of rhythm to this child's life as he easily swung along with the mother's activities and moods. But neither major divisions of the day nor moment-by-moment activities were organized sequentially, stable, or filled with purpose.

Some of the things that lend structure to the existence of most three-year-olds rarely if ever happened to this little boy. For example, he had few toys, although some picture books or magazines (mother used the terms interchangeably) as well as paper and pencil were made available to him, and he had access to most household objects. But it seems that no one ever played *with* him or shared practical tasks. He was joked with, his comments were responded to, he was hugged, scolded, praised, given things, and seldom ignored when his mother was awake. Yet prolonged enquiry yielded no instances of someone playing ball or games of any kind with him or showing him how to do things. This extended to such areas as learning how to dress himself. Mother laughed tolerantly at his failures and neither interfered with his attempts nor helped him. In short, overall structure was minimal by comparison to most others in this age group, and ministructure in terms of behavior organization throughout the day was very nearly absent. The EP rating for structure was 1 (minimally present).

Accommodation. The style of child care practiced in this family is best described as laissez-faire; it seldom provided accommodation as we defined the term. Two possible exceptions are that mother did get a night light when Tony showed reluctance to remain in his darkened bedroom, and she restricted fluid intake in the evening to reduce the incidence of bedwetting. She referred to these changes as a convenience to herself rather than as things done for him. We never heard the mother say that Tony responded better when things were done one way rather than another. Mother conveyed the impression that, in her perception, children grow and learn like Topsy. She was entirely unaware that his speech development, play, and social behavior were delayed, although at 28 and 34 months he was manifestly retarded. She either disbelieved or managed to screen out our explanations about the areas in which he did not meet normal expectations.

In the absence of a particularized notion of developmental progression against which to gauge his progress, and without thought that children learn as they are taught, she had little reason to deliberate about his needs or requirements beyond his physical health. This family expected children to be noisy, willful, and demanding, and Tony did not disappoint them in this respect or in any other. For this mother-child couple, under these circumstances, there was little need for accommodation on her part. Tony was a lively, sociable child, friendly as long as he was not thwarted and as long as few demands were made that might have taxed his powers. The EP rating for accommodation was 1 (minimal).

Didacticism. It is apparent that none of the adults with whom Tony lived tried to teach him anything, certainly nothing directly relevant to cognition. His mother thought he had learned his numbers from a television show, but actually he would recite numbers in arbitrary sequences, such as 1–2–5. The family believed him to be at least as bright as his little cousins were. There was talk of enrolling him in a daycare center, but solely to enable mother to take a job (we later learned that this never happened). The EP rating for didacticism was 1 (minimal).

Focused attention. Tony lived in a highly sociable milieu, and it is certain that he was not ignored. Yet, as we examined the accounts of what happened during the day and anecdotes descriptive of his behavior and of how adults behaved with him, we could find few instances when anyone gave him undivided attention more than transiently. Many items that led to a low structure rating were also relevant to this experience variable. In particular that there were verbal exchanges but no connected conversations, no joint looking at picture books or television, nor was there reciprocal play. Interactions consisted of a single comment or action responded to in the same brief manner. Focused attention of the type we had in mind requires longer sequences during which what each partner does remains responsive to the other. This mother was usually casual and intermittent in her responses and approaches to the child, as, it appears, from descriptions, were other members of the family as well. The EP rating for focused attention was 1 (minimal).

Frequency of conflict. By the time Tony had reached the age of 40 months head-on antagonistic encounters with his mother, father, or other relatives occurred several times each day, but they tended to be brief and seldom developed into full-blown tantrums. When frustrated or disappointed he might hit the offending adult, speak angrily in a loud voice, or throw himself on the floor and remain motionless and mute in a manner suggesting stubborn resistance rather than distress (we witnessed this performance repeatedly). Mother reciprocated by scolding and threatening him with the one disciplinary device she did use, the belt. These episodes were soon forgotten, however, especially as the mother seldom persisted in her demands. The frequency of conflict with adults fell near the upper end of the medium range. The EP rating for frequency of conflict was 2 (present, not prominent).

Intensity of maternal involvement. Tony was valued by his mother and was clearly a very important person to her, in much the same way as was seen in the majority of mother-child pairs. All interviewers felt that her relationship with Tony was as close as any she could muster. It certainly was more important to her than her relationship to Tony's father and quite possibly even more important than that with her own mother. Tony had every reason to sense his mother's continuous interest and emotional investment in him. The EP rating for the intensity of maternal involvement was 2 (medium).

Developmental Course

At birth Tony weighed less than 1600 grams, and, as he was only moderately premature, a diagnosis of small for gestational age (SGA) was made. His course on the intensive care unit (ICU) was uneventful. When his mother was allowed to take him home she found that her apprehension about caring for a tiny baby was unwarranted. Indeed, Tony was then and remained a vigorous and healthy baby. Developmental tests placed him in the average range at 7 and also at 15 months (MDI 99 and 101). At the time of the visit at 28 months, the Stanford-Binet test was too difficult for him; when the Bayley Scales were administered again his MDI proved to have dropped to 69. Thereafter intelligence quotients slowly increased to 73 at 34 months and 78 at 40 months. Except for gross motor coordination, which was always excellent, the developmental lag was fairly uniform. It affected language, perceptual organization, memory, and attention to about the same degree.

Social and personality development, on the other hand, progressed in a very normal manner and at the expected pace. At 15 months he gleefully left his mother without a backward glance when confronted with the open space situation. In roaming the corridor, he happened to encounter a passerby to whose advances he responded in a friendly manner while mother was out of sight. During the play session he at once made for the toys and played with them throughout at a considerable distance from his mother. He did look at her frequently, although the person whom he approached directly many times was the staff member seated on the sofa next to his mother. It was as though, having just gone through the developmental testing, he perceived the examiner as a play-person. He used a variety of conventional communication gestures across a distance, and these were directed exclusively at his mother. For instance, he knew how to point at a toy saying "dat" while looking at mother for affirmation and he also held out toys for her to look at (11 times in 10 minutes). Further, he once called her from across the room and once attempted to pull her toward a certain spot. Like many 15-month-olds he loved to climb and refreshed himself with such activity between bouts of play with toys.

During the 28-month visit both mother and child were very tired, neither of them being accustomed to early rising (our reminder call found both asleep). Nonetheless, Tony participated in all procedures with enjoyment. On the assessment of *body awareness* he demonstrated better understanding than a good many of the children in our sample. As would be expected at this age, he easily pointed to different parts of his own body on request and could do the same when asked to point to them on a doll. When the procedure was repeated in front of a large mirror and he was asked to identify body parts on the reflection (which he recognized but could not name as himself), he unerringly pointed to the appropriate portion of his own anatomy but—and this is where he excelled—while doing this his gaze was fixed on the area of the reflection where he could see his pointing finger. In view of his cognitive immaturity, and also because during developmental testing he showed no perseverance whatsoever, the assessment of Achievement Motivation was omitted. The matching task (Concept Formation) also was much too difficult for him.

The procedures designed to tap patterns of interaction with the mother showed him to have developed very normally in that component of the psychosocial sphere. All the more formal assessments as well as observation placed him in the phase of the individuation-separation process that Mahler has called rapprochement. Thus, in the open space situation he took a few steps away from his mother, immediately turned around to look at her, and did not budge until, after quite a while, she came to join him. The attempt to separate him from the mother failed. As soon as she announced her intention to return almost at once while moving toward the door, he protested energetically and ran toward her. In other words, as we expect of normal two-year-olds, he now showed much greater dependence on mother's proximity than when he was a toddler.

For the 34-month visit he was in fine fettle. Yet neither his cognitive level nor his behavior style showed much change. He evaded tasks that seemed difficult to him and very seldom persevered even with much encouragement. Much as he enjoyed playing with the ball, he altogether failed to understand the Level of Aspiration situation. What mattered to him was the act of throwing the ball, at any target, not how well it was done. He also preferred to have the cookie given to him rather than to get it for himself. During the play session some of his activity was more complex than previously observed in that he assembled toys by category (matching cars and doll house furniture) and also showed a brief bout of imaginative play, serving make-believe tea. In contrast to the preceding session, he now tolerated separation from the mother. In response to her explanation he said "OK" and continued to play as before. At this time he was reported and observed to be an exceedingly active child who needed close supervision because his heedlessness endangered himself as well as household objects. He was easily angered, impatient, and by and large unresponsive to the brief spankings administered by mother. The medical and psychological research staff agreed that his behavior was best accounted for by immaturity of the central nervous system (CNS). Fortunately, he was basically a friendly child, and the mother attributed his difficulties to exuberance and lack of judgment. Thus she made few demands upon her son, seldom punished him, supervised and protected him carefully, and enjoyed his company.

At the time of the 40-month visit Tony's cognitive status still remained much the same, which means of course that he had continued to learn at his own pace. Both functional and expressive language were now age-appropriate, but he had barely begun to comprehend or use verbal concepts. He still could not point to the longer of two lines, his vocabulary was limited to items in daily use, and what were called his drawings consisted of scribbles and dots that did not represent anything and at which he did not look after they were finished.

In other ways he had made a lot of progress. He now evaluated his own performance by objective standards (Achievement Motivation). Although he still preferred to avoid difficult tasks, he now could persevere if given a good deal of encouragement. In areas where he apparently felt inadequate the value he placed on success was shown as much by occasional cheating (claiming success on tasks he knew full well he had not accomplished) as by real pleasure when he did succeed on a difficult item. The Level of Aspiration experiment uses a skill with which he felt more at home. He not only understood the situation but made sure of success by proceeding gradually but persistently. After each success he remained at the same level of difficulty for a while but then moved to the next more difficult position. After failure he again remained at the same distance but kept on trying until he succeeded, and then he terminated the activity while he was ahead. He also understood the matching task (concept formation), since he matched correctly immediately after the demonstration, but when he was left to his own devices, he made a good start only to become confused so that soon objects were assembled in random fashion. The World Test was abortive. He played with the toys but could see no reason to place them on the board; therefore the play session was given once again. He was now able to generate longer sequences of imaginative play (still limited to food serving). He also created a delimited area to use as an arena for play with miniature toys (microplay). He easily separated from the mother without disruption of his play activity.

Discussion

All in all we saw in Tony a three-and-a-half-year-old whose cognitive development was slower than that of the majority although his social and personality development progressed at a normal rate. He was well adapted to his life circumstances, gave and received a good deal of pleasure and satisfaction, and learned what there was for him to learn well enough. In his case, poor impulse control during the third year and the corresponding cognitive slowdown were probably due to a lag in the development of the CNS. The fact that he was not exposed to formal teaching or to demands for more control may well have been to his advantage. At any rate, he was spared the stress of encountering demands he could not meet, and the close and harmonious relationship with mother remained undisturbed.

After he had attended kindergarten we saw Tony again when he was in first grade, at which time his IQ was 92. He was a somewhat tense and restless child who loved to play with peers above all else and was still close to his mother. His perceptual functioning and graphic products now showed deficits of the kind frequently seen in low-birth weight children. When seen again at nine years of age Tony was doing moderately well at school but showed many behavior characteristics typically associated with minor CNS deficit. His mother and also his teachers described him as very restless, impetuous, impatient, and experiencing attention difficulties. He was as friendly and likable as ever, but some of his intrinsic weaknesses had caught up with him; he was no longer the happy-go-lucky young boy we had known earlier.

Next we tell the stories of Freddie and Gene, two little boys who have in common perinatal complications that left their mark upon the organism; both differed from healthy full-term babies in several respects and were especially vulnerable in infancy and early childhood. Freddie's family was under so much stress that they never even recognized his special needs and would have been unable to meet them if they had. Gene's family, on the other hand, was able to provide their little boy with what we thought to be the best possible experience for him. The two vignettes also provide a vivid demonstration of what everyone knows as a generality, yet few professionals have occasion to witness directly: that poverty always takes its toll but nonetheless allows for infinitely varied patterns of living.

Freddie: A Vulnerable Child in a Constricted and Stressful Environment

Background

Freddie was born into a setting that might serve as a classical example of an urban welfare family. His father was unemployed and had had minor brushes with the law. The family moved from one deplorable apartment to another (nine times within three-and-one-half years) and between moves shared cramped quarters with one or another set of relatives. Such as it was, their social life took place exclusively within the family. Mother had her first child at the age of 16 and was only 18 at the time of Freddie's birth. But unlike most of our teenage parents, Freddie's remained together and the father fully accepted responsibility for the everyday maintenance of family life.

The mother consistently described herself as unsociable and lethargic. On many occasions she explained to one or another interviewer that she was unable to enjoy her children, had no desire to get out of the house for either work or entertainment, and often felt tired, drowsy, and dizzy to such a degree that most of her day was spent resting. This young woman, who lacked education and experience, was remarkably articulate as she spoke of being an unfit mother, of not knowing what she wanted, and of her regret that she could not feel affection for her children. Yet she expressed warm appreciation for relatives on both sides of the family who were always ready to help out, in small ways as well as large. She appeared to trust her husband and to rely upon him though she never spoke of her relationship to him.

Her self-description was largely accurate and confirmed by other members of the family. Throughout the time we knew her she seldom rose from bed before noon and spent much of the afternoon on the sofa, rousing herself only to do what was absolutely necessary when the children got into trouble or to prepare the evening meal. It was the father who did the shopping and who often saw to dressing and bathing the children. No matter where they lived, it was always close to relatives who also helped to take care of the children.

Ratings at 40 Months

Impulse control. Freddie was one of the very few children who was poorly controlled most of the time but showed a very high level of self-restraint in one recurring situation. His high level of activity and general unruliness often led to friction with adults. If he became very angry, as happened nearly every day, he typically displayed implacable resistance of the passive variety. He might refuse to eat or speak and remain sullenly withdrawn for hours or even a whole day. Another of his repeated responses to annoyance was quietly to carry his plate of food to the garbage can and dispose of it there. (An interesting sidelight on the inner life of small children is afforded by the fact that, during the *symbolization* procedure at 22 months, Freddie's imaginative play consisted of calling the upended cup a garbage can and throwing imaginary food into that receptacle.) The impulse control score was 5 (both over- and undercontrolled).

Structure. Freddie and his brother usually slept until about noon, rising when mother was still asleep. As the boys foraged for food (the brother was 5 years old) they made enough noise to awaken their mother, who usually did not get up, although she would speak to them. During this period the father was not home during the day so that the boys were left to do what they wished much of the time. The one regularly recurring event was supper after father's return. On most evenings Freddie watched a favorite television program. Mother said he spent most of his time "tearing about," which led to plants and furniture being upturned and also involved throwing toys and objects, often destructively. In his father's presence there was less of this because he exercised some control by using the belt. The mother felt herself to be so ineffective that she had to "let him be" except when real danger was involved, as in his various attempts to light the gas stove with a piece of burning paper. Thus there were virtually no rules or other requirements that were enforced.

Freddie was not a participant in organized or structured activity of any kind and therefore lacked what we have called ministructure to an unusual degree. The father did play with the boys of an evening, but this was described as excited roughhousing. Several times a week Freddie spent some time in a grandmother's apartment. She had recently declared that because of his "roughness" she would not keep him for more than a few hours at a time. From this one guesses that the grandmother's home probably also failed to provide more organized or purposeful activity. In short, it is difficult to imagine how a three-year-old could lead a less structured life than Freddie did. The EP rating for structure was 1 (minimally present).

Accommodation. It is possible that during the limited time that he spent with his grandmother Freddie was accommodated in minor ways, though by and large this experience variable seems irrelevant in his case. This active child was given next to no opportunity for outdoor play; he was not helped to learn or play (mother said she tried picture books but he would have none of it); nor was anything done about his destructiveness and ready anger. It is doubtful that either parent was aware of his immaturity and cognitive retardation. The mother did recognize his disobedience and irritability, but her behavior attested to the truth of her repeated statement that, being unable to alter her son's behavior, she had "given up on him." It was our impression that normal development and learning were not recognized as a process or a goal. Hence the idea of furthering developmental progress could not occur to these parents. The EP rating for accommodation was 1 (minimally present).

Focused attention. Concerning the time Freddie spent with his grandmother all evidence is indirect, and therefore a question mark was attached to our rating. She apparently did not take him out of doors, and there was no mention of toys or games in her home. All we heard was that the grandmother's efforts to relieve the mother had to be time-limited because Freddie was so difficult. In his own home altercations with his mother provided attention, but not of the focused variety. The description of these mother-child interchanges made it clear that they were neither prolonged nor reciprocal. Typically both participants were too aroused to permit this. The EP rating for focused social attention was 1 (minimally present).

Didacticism. A low rating is implied in what has gone before. Not only was this child not taught, but neither parent ever spontaneously reported that he had learned something since we last saw him (other changes were reported in detail). When staff members commented on his new skills this was courteously acknowledged but received with little interest. Opportunities for incidental learning were also scarce. To the best of our knowledge Freddie had never been inside a playground and had not been taken to a restaurant or store. The EP rating for didacticism was 1 (minimally present).

Frequency of conflict. By all accounts Freddie at this age was so irritable and so resistant that openly angry encounters with adults were frequent. We were told that previously his behavior with persons other than his mother had been relatively more compliant whereas more recently he resisted and fought back almost as much with everybody else as he had always done with mother. His behavior during the research visit bore this out. The EP rating for frequency of conflict was 3 (very prominent).

Intensity of maternal involvement. Mother's feelings about her boy were so complex and puzzling that any rating could only be misleading. In spite of her apparent apathy and withdrawal this mother knew her child quite well. She was able to describe his behavior in detail, and whenever another person could be asked he or she confirmed her report. She was plagued by the difference between what she thought she ought to feel about him and what she actually felt. She spoke about this issue with considerable affect during most of our interviews with her. Freddie was important to her, yet neither her thoughts nor her actions were dictated by concern for him to any marked extent. Even when, at a younger age, Freddie had clung to her and resisted separation from her, his mother thought of this as but another example of his willfulness. The EP rating for intensity of maternal involvement was ? (unknown).

Developmental Course

Freddie's development was stormy and uneven. On coming home after five weeks in the ICU, and for most of the first year, he was exceedingly inactive, "no trouble at all except for his crying." During the early months he slept most of the day and night, awakening or being awakened for a bottle about four times during the twenty-four-hour day. His one waking period was between midnight and 2:00 or 3:00 A.M., and even then he did not move about much. Crib rocking began in early infancy. He invariably rocked himself to sleep then and for as long as we knew him. At 7 months the developmental test score placed him in the moderately retarded range, and he was quite as placid as we had been told.

By the age of 15 months things had changed. Although he still slept somewhat more than is usual, his waking hours were exceedingly active. Having learned to walk between 12 and 13 months he spent his time running around the house, often throwing himself to the floor as if angry or distressed. The parents were troubled by his frequent and inexplicable crying spells. They found no way of consoling him—he had to rock until he calmed himself. He was said to disregard his toys. Yet during the office visit he presented himself as a lively and socially responsive youngster, only slightly more restless than most peers. Both gross and fine motor coordination were good for his age, and his MDI score was 98, which was something of an overestimate as, had he been two days older, the same performance would have yielded an MDI of 88. He thoroughly enjoyed himself and neither cried nor fussed.

Because of the persistent rocking, and also because some nonspecific neurological signs had been noted, he was among the children who were seen again at 22 months. By this time he was reported to "cry over every little thing" and to have rather frequent and severe temper tantrums. His parents thought that he really hurt himself as he forcefully threw himself to the floor. Also, he now would not allow his mother to leave him, even to leave him with father, without becoming severely upset. Crib rocking was as severe as ever. Developmental evaluation revealed a pronounced unevenness in his functioning. Motor coordination and functional speech were good. Referential speech, however, was virtually absent. He was unable to point to a single part of his own body, and the only object he named on request was "shoe." Yet in other ways he had made good progress. During the symbolization procedure as well as the play session he engaged in reasonably well-organized play with enjoyment. He was capable of simple imaginative play, in the form of serving pretend coffee using toy dishes. He did need help in maintaining his composure when things did not go as he seemed to expect, but we saw none of the irritability and negativism that had been described so vividly.

His response to the situations designed to tap the level of the mother-child relationship was very much as would be expected at this age. When his mother left during the play session, explaining that she would return soon (separation), he looked dismayed but turned to the examiner for comfort. Standing with his mother in a doorway that faced a very large hallway (open space) he immediately walked off but, having traversed a considerable distance, did a "double take"; that is, suddenly realizing that mother had been left behind, he turned back and ran to rejoin her without any sign of distress.

We next saw Freddie at the age of 34 months. Since the previous visit family life had been seriously disrupted by many moves and other upheavals and finally by a serious injury to the father, who was in the hospital. Very recently mother and the boys had moved in with a cousin's family, and this involved extraordinary crowding. The mother's distress about her inability to deal with Freddie was at its peak. Against her will she found herself extremely angry and reduced to yelling and hitting him, to no avail. The rocking habit had not diminished. Yet mother reported that toilet training (by the expedient of refusing to give him a diaper) and that no longer offering him a bottle had not been unduly difficult. Possibly it made a difference that at this time Freddie was cared for almost entirely by one of his mother's cousins, as his mother herself spent most of the day at the hospital with the father.

Freddie now showed significant cognitive retardation, with an IQ of 66, confirmed by a mental age of 23 months when the Bayley Scales were given in addition. Although verbal items presented the greatest difficulty, there were also real deficits in perceptual organization, and his attention span was poor throughout. At the same time, examiners sensed that these scores did not reflect the child's true capacities. They spoke of an undeveloped potential and speculated that, given the opportunity, he could learn. Once again his responsiveness in the play session and during the separation experiment was age-appropriate. On the other hand, during procedures to assess Achievement Motivation he proved to be easily discouraged, to lack persistence even when interested in a task, and to accept help readily even with easy items. In short, his self-confidence was low, and we could see no sign whatever that he had begun to take pleasure in achieving goals through his own efforts. Also, unlike most other two-year-olds, he preferred that the cookie be given him although he had permission to climb the sofa to get it for himself. Last, the standard assessment of impulse control (based on behavior throughout the developmental test) took place during this visit. By our criteria he was scored as excitable, motorically active, showing strong (negative) affect with motor overflow, and seldom exhibiting modulation or inhibition. In short, impulse control was low in comparison to that of peers. Yet, it was after witnessing this session that the mother said, with wonder and sadness in her voice, that she had never seen him as friendly and biddable as he was with us.

The last visit, at 40 months, showed no major changes. His IQ had risen to 73, still in the retarded range. Two changes in the child's typical behavior were reported. One was that he was now as irritable and defiant with other people as he had long been with mother. In consequence, relatives were less willing to have him in their house, and his father needed the belt to control him. We found this easy to believe because, much as he enjoyed himself during the research sessions, he was more resistant and more easily driven to high anger than during any previous visit. In other ways his behavior had not changed. He still rocked himself to sleep. Most of the time he was as active and destructive, as impatient, and as much subject to explosive affect as he had been. The other behavior change reported to us can be interpreted as an effort on Freddie's part to cope with his own impulsivity. He now quite often withdrew to the bed- or bathroom, sometimes locking the door against intruders. As far as the mother could tell from his sounds, he played in a fairly calm and animated manner, talking away at a great rate. More strikingly, he had begun to replace disruptive outbursts of anger by stubborn passive resistance, as was described under the heading of impulse control.

Because of his general immaturity the testing and assessment procedures applicable at 34 months were administered again. During the play session his activity was somewhat less sustained and he seemed less involved than on previous occasions. As had been true before, he addressed himself to the examiner much more often than to his mother and this time remained entirely unruffled when his mother left. His response to the Achievement Motivation tasks was much as it had been at 34 months: he was easily discouraged, did not persist in the face of even minor difficulties, and was quite as pleased with the result when it was the examiner who accomplished it as when he had done it alone. He comprehended the Level of Aspiration situation as he had not before. Although he liked throwing the ball he remained cautious. After success in hitting the target four times in a row he finally increased the distance slightly and remained at the new level for three additional successes before he quit. The concept formation procedure (sorting like objects into boxes) showed that although he seemed to understand the task while it was being demonstrated and explained, he soon became confused, and his best effort consisted of placing three pairs of toy shoes into the same box.

Discussion

Freddie's life and development have been described in some detail because they illustrate the combined consequences of minor neurological complications often seen in premature infants and a grossly impoverished range of environmental support. Neurologic soft signs came and went though none was noted by 40 months. He made a poor start since for a large part of the first year he slept during much of the time that healthy babies spend in active engagement with the environment. When awake he often dulled his perceptions through prolonged rocking. This state of affairs is not uncommon among premature babies and is often followed by a fairly sudden shift to high irritability and activity, as occurred with Freddie. Under the best of circumstances this syndrome offers obstacles to harmonious development. (See the case of Gene for an example in which similar initial conditions found a more fortunate resolution.) At the hands of a minimally active or resourceful mother, in constant interaction with a rambunctious preschool-age brother, and somewhat haphazardly cared for also by the father and an assortment of relatives, Freddie lacked many of the props and comforts ordinarily available to toddlers. On the one hand he was rather helpless in the face of what must have been strong impulses and sensations, for otherwise they would not have led to so much crying, so much activity, so much rocking, and soon to more or less deliberate destructiveness. On the other hand, he grew well on a diet of milk, cereal, junk food, candy, and one meal a day. He developed a strong dependence on his mother's presence but subsequently learned to tolerate separation from her. It is perhaps noteworthy that during research visits he turned to the examiner rather than to his mother much more than did others at the same ages. Language as used in a social and concrete context was learned at a normal pace. Further, by the middle of the fourth year he had found some ways of at least partially protecting himself against affect storms and behavior disintegration.

The fact that at all times he functioned more effectively, and certainly more contentedly, during research visits than at home implies that he had the capacity to respond to novel objects and to people quite normally. It is true that this occurred in situations in which every effort was made to accommodate his momentary state and during which his motivation for purposive activity was roused and sustained by constant encouragement and attention. That cognitive development suffered greatly from the virtual absence of learning opportunities needs no discussion. It is impossible to know whether shortcomings in the realm of concept formation, verbal intelligence, and perceptual organization are based in part upon subtle neurologic deficits. For what it is worth, from observation of other premature children and from what is known about the plasticity of the nervous system we find it plausible to speculate that CNS weaknesses of this kind can be reduced and compensated for to some extent when the universal needs for stimulation, intimacy, and continuity are better met than they were for Freddie.

Postscript

Readers may wonder whether this mother was considered to have a psychiatric problem and whether Freddie should have remained in the intact group. As to the former, on only one occasion was the mother given a score of "psychiatric difficulty observed." This was early on, at a time when the mother had temporarily ceased nearly all housekeeping and caretaking activity and reported odd alterations in her state of consciousness that are not detailed here.

As to the latter, Freddie was one of quite a few children in the intact group whose development was troubled in the psychosocial sphere and impaired in the realm of cognition. He did not meet criteria for the presence of neuropathology, nor were his behavior problems sufficiently severe and atypical for his social milieu. No one in his family thought of him as anything but an unruly child. In addition, his behavior in the office and in some other situations was appropriate, suggesting that his difficulties were primarily tied to situational contexts rather than internalized to the degree required by our conservative definition of serious behavioral deviancy.

Gene: A Child Whose Extraordinary Needs Were Fully Met by an Extraordinary Family

Background

Gene was born into a large black family at a time when his next older sibling was already in fourth grade. Seven persons lived on the father's wages as an unskilled laborer and thus in near poverty. The mother was an unusually competent woman, and the family achieved an orderly and self-respecting way of life. They never applied for public assistance; to do so would have seemed demeaning to them. It is difficult to describe Gene's family without waxing lyrical. They clearly enjoyed one another; each person had to help by performing household chores that had been well defined by mother; and, by and large, all conformed to a set of well-defined rules of conduct. There were regular times for meals, for homework, for shopping, for church attendance, and the like. But—and this is what made this family unusual—fun and enjoyment were valued quite as much as duty. "They might as well enjoy themselves," the mother would say as she explained one or another of their domestic arrangements. Most sociability in the form of picnics, visits, and parties took place within the extended family, and if any one set of parents wanted a free evening, someone in the family took over. The single term that best describes the ambience of this mother is good will, which in her case was combined with practical good sense and impressive physical energy.

Ratings at 40 Months

Impulse control. Ill health accounted for great fluctuations in Gene's state and in the degree to which impulse control was present. By 40 months he had made considerable progress but, in comparison to peers, ego controls were still quite immature. Specifically, he found it exeedingly difficult to sit quietly even when he was interested in what he was doing. Temper outbursts occurred every day, most often when he attempted something that he could not accomplish easily. Gene's lack of composure, unlike that of most other excitable children, did not prevent perseverance in self-chosen tasks. He would scream, perhaps throw himself to the floor, and then return to the task still screaming loudly and angrily. He was motorically very active and also exceedingly impatient. Yet in his case the lack of modulation in all respects seldom led to serious conflict with other people (except peers). His family gauged their expectations to his state and were able to tolerate a great deal of troublesome behavior. The impulse control score was 2 (immature).

Structure. Gene spent six hours each weekday in the home of a sitter and was picked up by a teenage sister in midafternoon; soon thereafter his mother returned from work and took over. Although there was not a very rigid schedule, daily events succeeded one another with considerable regularity. Not only were sleep and mealtimes regular but outings and play times with mother, the bath, and many other things had to be carefully organized in a large family living in close quarters.

More important than the overall routines was the manner in which this home provided what we have called ministructure. This mother knew her child and saw to it that he was never left at loose ends. He did engage in solitary play with toys but always in the presence of older persons; one of the older siblings or the mother would intervene if he became restless or too wild. He was given ample opportunity for outdoor activity, reciprocal ball play being an all-out favorite. By design—that is, with the intention of teaching him to sit still—someone sat with him for such things as looking at picture books, block building, watching television, or singing songs but was careful to stop the moment he became restive. Mother spent a full hour each day letting him use crayons and scissors, materials that were kept from him at other times because on his own he would scribble on or cut whatever objects he encountered. He was taken along on errands to nearby stores (but not the weekly grocery shopping, as the supermarket was too much for him, or he for it). In many other ways, including swift punishment when he deliberately misbehaved, this highly animated and eventful household provided a predictable and stable environment. Within the home Gene's life had always been highly structured, and the rating for this EP had always been a 3. It is only because we knew less about his experience at the sitter's that a lower rating seemed a more prudent choice. The mother assured us that while in the sitter's care he was taken to the playground and otherwise well occupied. The EP rating for structure was 2 (present, not prominent).

Accommodation. This mother's way of dealing with her child served as a model to help us articulate what was meant by accommodation, and on all previous occasions the rating had been very prominent. Again, it was because of the shared caretaking arrangement that a lesser rating seemed more appropriate at 40 months. Some examples of the manner in which this child was accommodated have been mentioned—for instance, the recognition that frequent opportunity for "running around" was as necessary for him as providing carefully timed interludes of quiet activity—with the developmental goal always being to help him achieve better control. Mother directed the entire family to enforce those rules that she felt he could abide. That is, she accommodated his changing capacity and comprehension as she generated strategies for dealing with him. For instance, at this time temper tantrums were ignored unless they were aggressively directed at another person, in which case they were punished. Although she knew that outbursts might result, the mother decreed that when he tried to do something by himself he should not be helped at first request but encouraged to try again. As one last example, mother delayed toilet training until summer, when she could allow him to play without wearing pants. She thought that in this way he "could get there quickly" and therefore would be more successful. This account of a mother's deliberate style makes things sound less spontaneous than they were. This mother was a good observer of her children and had clear notions of how things ought to be. Almost everything flowed from this without much need for thought. We felt certain that her explanations of the reasons for how things were done were formulated in response to our questions and comments and that without the interviews she might not have become aware of them. The EP rating for accommodation was 2 (present, not prominent).

Focused attention. Most of the time a great deal was going on within this home so that there was continuous interaction among various members of the family, which included Gene but was not focused on him. Even on occasions when he was the center of attention—for instance, when his antics caused general amusement—this was far from the one-to-one encounters being rated. The mother as well as other family members, however, often devoted themselves entirely to the task of engaging him in an activity that he could not have sustained unaided. These times did involve mutual responsiveness of the focused variety. In addition, when the child was ill, troubled, or hurt this mother typically dropped whatever she was doing, and her efforts to make things right usually meant fairly prolonged and exclusive interchanges. By comparison to the majority of the children in our sample Gene received focused social attention that in frequency and intensity would fall near the upper extreme of the medium range. The EP rating for focused attention was 2 (present, not prominent).

Didacticism. It was only shortly before the 40-month visit that the family saw any point in trying to teach Gene things related to cognitive activity. Mother viewed his interest in playing cards as a chance to teach numbers. She and others now supplemented looking at picture books by getting him to name things and telling simple stories. Her choice of toys reflected educational goals. For instance, she chose wind-up toys to encourage fine motor coordination and small figures representing animals and various social roles (fireman, policeman, etc.) to acquaint him with things outside the home. It is not irrelevant that the entire troop visited the library once a week, and Gene also was invited to choose his own books. Gene was exposed to and participated in about as many didactically oriented activities as did most of our three-year-olds. Therefore the EP rating for didacticism was 2 (present, not prominent).

Frequency of conflict. Perhaps because the mother was so intent on stressing the positive and at the same time found it so difficult to view his angry outbursts as anything but comical, it was difficult to ascertain the actual frequency of conflict between Gene and his elders. Assuredly he became angry very easily, but more typically at inanimate objects than at people. We did hear of instances when he hit and yelled at mother and others. On most occasions, according to report, the adults either ignored these episodes or swiftly punished them. We were told that the siblings had to be admonished to be stricter; apparently they tended to indulge him. For lack of documentation, the EP rating for frequency of conflict was ? (unknown).

Intensity of maternal involvement. During the early years, when Gene was in precarious health, the baby and his well being were his mother's chief preoccupation, and a rating of high was then appropriate. At the time of this rating the mother remained devoted to her youngest, but her concern embraced the family as a whole. Now that he was older her interest in community affairs could be resumed. She told us that her return to work was dictated only in part by financial needs. She considered that it was not good for either her or for Gene if they spent all their days together. Home was more enjoyable to her now, as she returned to it, than before, when she had rarely left it. The EP rating for intensity of maternal involvement was 2 (present, not prominent).

Developmental Course

Gene was an intact child only in the sense that he showed neither definite neuropathology nor significant behavioral disorder during the preschool years. His medical problems were legion. He was slightly more than two months premature, and his pulmonary difficulties were so severe that he required several months on the respirator and could not be discharged from the ICU until his uncorrected age was 8 months. His mother became a familiar figure on the ward as she visited every single day and in time learned a good deal about how to care for a sick infant.

After he was taken home Gene slept most of the 24-hour day. Even when he was awake his physical vigor was minimal. He was held for feedings on a four-hour schedule and after each feeding was played with on someone's lap. This was possible only for a very few minutes as he soon showed discomfort. He was better off in his crib with toys, and mother made a point of coming close, speaking to him, and perhaps patting him very often, sometimes rousing him from drowsiness. The parents had been told that the prognosis for this baby was not good, but their attitude remained what a staff member called cautiously optimistic. Mother and others watched him carefully while he slept lest he experience respiratory troubles (which did occur off and on). Mother looked at her sickly baby and said, "He has a long way to go."

During the first research visit at the uncorrected age of eight-and-one-half months even the simplest items on the scale were difficult to administer and examiners were loath to tax this vulnerable infant. He was obviously retarded but a test score could not be obtained. We did see him immediately after feeding as he smiled and cooed responsively and was alert to visual and auditory stimuli for a few minutes.

When next we saw him, at 15 months, great changes had taken place. He still needed more sleep than healthy babies, but his waking time was mostly spent in energetic play. After he had learned to walk unsteadily at 13 months "there was no holding him." He busied himself toddling about, manipulating household objects, and trying to handfeed himself. He hugely enjoyed being played with as well as daily outings to the park, where he was removed from the stroller to encourage walking. By now he could tolerate weekly visits to fond relatives without undue fatigue. There were days, however, perhaps once a week, when he was irritable upon awakening and remained that way all day. On these occasions, he cried a good deal and was incapable of play. The only thing to do was to put him in his crib with a supply of toys and leave him there. On the whole his health had been fairly good during the interval, although he had had several febrile infections.

During the research visit he responded well to the testing situation and, to general amazement, achieved an MDI of 80. On the sensorimotor scales he proved to function at stage six for object permanence and at stage five for spatial comprehension. Both gross and fine motor coordination were rather poor, but his attention span and endurance during prolonged examination were satisfactory.

During the play session he stayed close to his mother and played only if she initiated the play action. He was content enough but not animated. Conventional communication signals were not yet in his repertoire; there seemed no need for him to communicate across a distance. This relative lack of distance (in the psychological sense) from the mother was confirmed during the open space experiment. He showed no interest in the expanse of space in front of him and stayed with his mother, a puzzled look on his face, presumably because, in compliance with our request, she neither said nor did anything at all.

As he was one of our especially vulnerable children, Gene was seen again at 22 months. During the interval he had gone through several infectious illnesses, typically accompanied by high fevers. Otherwise he had been well and quite active. He could now play with toys while his mother did her housework in the morning, even though after a while he became restless and discontent. Mother found that if she took him out of doors even briefly his spirits improved and he could entertain himself again. He preferred being out of doors so much that, with the help of siblings and even neighbors, it became the number one remedy whenever he became irritable or distressed. The mother tried to teach him a few rules of the "don't touch" variety but neither expected nor received obedience.

It required patience and ingenuity to administer the entire developmental scale as Gene's behavior was vigorous rather than coordinated. He obtained an MDI of 70. Clearly his comprehension and behavior organization had improved and he made good use of toys during the play session. He readily moved away from his mother though he remained aware of her and responsive to her. The self-chosen task of retrieving a piece of paper from a wastebasket (about his own height) engaged his attention for at least as long as play with toys.

When the open space procedure was administered this time he gleefully moved out to traverse the hall, glancing at his mother intermittently. When his mother left the room for the separation procedure he showed mild distress but soon resumed his play. When body awareness procedures were performed he proved able to point out two body parts on the doll but not on himself. During the symbolization experiment, which assesses prelanguage development and early speech, his behavior showed him to be impoverished rather than retarded in this respect. He was able to apply the tiny toy hairbrush to the doll's head and to seat the doll on the toy chair. Sensorimotor play nevertheless predominated. Overall we found that he had become more independent and self-directed and that his social responsiveness had matured but that his cognitive development progressed at a much slower pace.

By the age of 28 months Gene was, in a word, impossible. He had experienced several rather serious illnesses and one injury resulting from a fall. He was truly hyperactive, and for the first time several soft neurologic signs were noted. His mother, as well as everybody else, was worried about his excitability, impatience, frequent temper outbursts, and sheer inability to "stay put." Fortunately this difficult period occurred during the summer months, and the family relied on the one thing that seemed to content him, to let him run about outdoors. He liked active play with anybody, but it was only mother who could catch his attention for more quiet play. She said that at the most this could last for five minutes. As long as he was on the move he could participate in purposive and coordinated activity such as reciprocal ball play, a walk, or helping mother with cleaning chores. Mother recognized that he could not contain himself but sought to maintain a degree of discipline. When he became too unruly and disobedient he was spanked, more in sorrow than in anger.

During the developmental testing he was friendly enough but entirely unable to focus on most tasks. Some of the descriptive terms used about his test behavior were that the slightest impulse led to action and that he showed an urgent and exaggerated push to action. At the same time it was difficult for him to shift from one activity to another. The resulting MDI of 66 may not have been valid, but it was obvious that many of the age-appropriate items would have been beyond him even if his attention had been better. We were struck by the fact that although he did have rather severe tantrums when he had to wait or was made to sit still, other frustrating situations did not have that result. When a desired object was taken from his grasp or when he was forcibly removed from a dangerous position, he looked annoyed but soon found something else to do. Overall his behavior was explosive rather than angry or destructive.

The formal assessment of impulse control took place on this occasion and of course classified him as exceedingly low in this respect. When the open space procedure was repeated, once again he moved out into the hall, saw nothing to interest him there, and returned to the playroom, leaving his mother where she was. Thus this miniexperiment failed to serve its purpose on this occasion in that it did not elicit behavior directly related to the level of the mother-child relationship. This was not the case for the play session or the planned separation from the mother. For the first time, Gene was shy and self-conscious at the beginning of the play session. He was far more interested in social interaction with his mother than in the toys, and he remained somewhat tense throughout. When his mother left it caused great alarm, and he was totally unable to function until she returned. In both of these situations Gene showed one of the behavior patterns characteristic of the phase that Mahler called rapprochement, during which dependence upon the mother is temporarily increased.

As the concept formation (matching) task seemed incomprehensible to him, the body awareness procedure was repeated. He could now point to four body parts upon request and showed somewhat more mature behavior than some nonretarded peers by consistently pointing to the appropriate body part on his reflection in the mirror. The only thing that prevented him from doing so on his own body was self-consciousness which, following Zazzo we found to be associated with one phase in the development of a more mature sense of self. Shyness when attention was drawn to the child's mirror image also fits in nicely with what one would expect during the rapprochement phase in the individuation/separation process.

His hyperactivity had interfered with cognitive development and probably even with the application of such comprehension and skill as he possessed. In the psychosocial sphere his adaptation to the requirements of age-appropriate socialization demands had greatly suffered, but with respect to the pattern of the mother-child relationship his behavior was more or less on a par with that of most of his agemates.

At 34 months all indications were that cognitive development lagged by about as much as it had before, which means that he had progressed but not caught up. He was unable to cope with the Stanford-Binet test. The Bayley Scales yielded a mental age equivalent of 26 months (he was by now too old to permit the calculation of an MDI).

According to report he was still a very active child but had become somewhat easier to manage. In some situations he became so angry as to lose all control—for instance, when someone attempted to spoonfeed him or when he failed to accomplish something he had set out to do. The tantrums sometimes included hitting and yelling at mother. The fact that he responded to the spanking that he received on such occasions was cited as one of the ways in which he had improved. Others were that he lasted longer at sedentary play and that it was a great deal easier for him to wait for things. Active play continued to be a condition for his well being and was amply provided.

The impulse control assessment was given once again. Results confirmed the family's report in that control was still well below normal expectation but not to the degree observed at 28 months. When an unwelcome request was made he sometimes refused in a calm manner and sometimes "blew." Similarly, when asked to wait—for instance, for the examiner to complete setting out the test materials—he made visible efforts to comply, but often restlessness quickly turned into precipitate action.

In some other areas he had made considerable strides. He now pointed at any body part that was asked for and had no more difficulty with his own body than with a doll or the mirror. This time he was thoroughly pleased with the play session and used it well. On two occasions (within the ten-minute period) he displayed another one of Mahler's behavior indications for progress in the individuation-separation process, namely *refueling*. Having played for a while seemingly oblivious to mother and at a distance from her, he stopped, ran to her for a hug, and returned to his play almost immediately. Another indication of progress in the mother-child relationship was that he now tolerated separation with minimal disruption of his play and no overt distress.

At the 40-month visit the mother was finally able to report that he now "knows how to sit still." He remained an active child, but he now also enjoyed television programs, sitting with his elders as they were playing cards, or looking at pictures and listening to brief stories about them. He could sit and busy himself with crayons, paper, and scissors more independently than before, even though mother's watchful eye was still required. He accepted such restrictions as a time limit on play with a very noisy toy. On weekly visits to a physical therapist for a minor orthopedic problem he presented no special difficulties. He still had tantrums but they had become less frequent and he had also become more amenable to explanations and to disciplinary measures. All of what has been said applies to how things went at home. As described in connection with the experience pattern ratings, during the week he now spent half days at a sitter's home. The arrangement worked well for all concerned.

On this visit he was able to cooperate with the administration of the Stanford-Binet test and obtained an IQ of 72. The retardation was in large part accounted for by his failure to comprehend verbally mediated concepts. What especially impressed us was the change in his demeanor. He understood directions, worked willingly, tried hard to accomplish what was asked of him, and tolerated delays about as well as most peers. Yet during the pauses that were frequently provided he remained his usual active and exuberant self.

During the play session he showed more complex behavior organization than before. There were prolonged sequences involving cars and a good deal of collecting similar toys from the heterogeneous assembly. The concept formation tasks were attempted once again. Results were equivocal because the long delays involved became too much for him, and he started sorting while instructions were still in progress. He did understand the task and might have been able to complete it on his own. On this occasion the Achievement Motivation tasks were administered. His self-confidence was neither unusually high or low. He seldom persevered on difficult tasks without encouragement, but with it was highly persistent. Surprisingly, he welcomed help when it was offered, contrary to his typical behavior when help was offered on an action that Gene himself had initiated. It seemed to us that true achievement motivation as we defined it had not yet emerged. The end product of his endeavors seemed of little interest to him—it was performing the various activities that he seemed to value.

The Level of Aspiration experiment was something of a failure from our point of view, though not from his. He was delighted to throw balls toward the target and by and large increased his distance from it after success. However, he could not be persuaded to choose levels of difficulty (from colored stripes on the floor) before actually throwing the ball.

Discussion

We chose Gene for detailed presentation in part because the comparison to Freddie is instructive. Of the two, Gene had by far the more serious medical and biological problems. What they had in common was a history of drowsy inactivity during much of the first year, replaced by unusually high activity and irritability during the second. Both were reared in families whose socioeconomic status placed them in the lowest quartile. One could wish for no better illustration of the enormously varied styles of life experience that occur within this category.

During the preschool years neither child showed satisfactory cognitive development, yet Gene's early years are a success story and Freddie's are not. After 28 months, Gene progressed slowly but steadily, and although his verbal intelligence lagged the most, he did advance in all areas. More important, his high level of activity and the resulting attention deficit did not prevent for long the emergence of curiosity, pleasure in mastery, an urge to learn, and a desire to please. By the age of 40 months he was a friendly, enthusiastic, fairly self-confident, and distinctly communicative youngster. His relationships with members of the family were close and affectionate; with others they were amiable and cooperative.

He was one of the children who participated in the follow-up studies. When last seen, at the age of eight, he had gone through school in the usual way and was holding his own among his peers in the fourth grade. At this age our evaluation was focused on specific abilities rather than an IQ. He was below average in reading and received some tutoring in that area, but otherwise he did well in that his test scores in writing, spelling, and arithmetic fell at the center of the average range and his perceptual acumen was better than that. The family and the school, unbeknown to each other, reported that he was fidgety and still found sustained attention difficult. At the time of this evaluation multiple soft neurological signs were seen. One can feel reasonably certain that his attention deficit and the resulting cognitive difficulties were rooted in a mild neurological disorder.

By contrast, Freddie's activity level and impulsivity lessened only slightly during his third and fourth years. When he was 40 months old he spent most of his time and energy in endless battles against unwelcome demands from the outside and also against his own impulsivity. Although he did enjoy unhindered pursuit of those activities that offered no difficulty to him, there was little that attracted or pleased him in his daily life. He was attached to his mother but by all accounts friendly interchanges between the two, or between Freddie and anyone else, were rare, and we found ourselves believing his mother when she said that expressions of overt affection did not occur. Such words as fun, enjoyment, or a good time were never used or implied when Freddie was spoken of. At 40 months he was a tense, excitable, and often unhappy little boy who somehow conveyed a sense of distrustful vigilance. Regrettably, we shall never know how Freddie fared later on as we lost track of him. Nonetheless, he must have entered school ill equipped to meet its demands and his orientation toward people and the world about him was likely to interfere with his ability to make use of such pleasurable and constructive opportunities as might come his way.

Next we describe a little girl from an upper middle class home. The major features of her early life and development may strike the reader as extreme, but they were not atypical for her social milieu. Our small sample of children from affluent families contained several youngsters whose intellect flowered in a hothouse atmosphere and, we believe, at the expense of other facets of development.

Maria: A Gifted Child Who Was Expected to Excel in All Respects

Background

Maria's parents had wished to have children for many years, so that by the time she arrived she was welcomed as the fulfillment of everything for which they had hoped and prayed. Both parents were talented and well-educated people, ambitious, and successful at their lucrative jobs. They lived in a quasi-private community, within the city but not of it, so to speak. The houses were surrounded by large grounds, protected from city traffic, and entirely secure. This residence had been selected because it seemed to be ideally suited to raising children. The mother took a temporary leave from her job, though she maintained contact with her associates, and when Maria was about three her mother was more than ready to resume work on a part-time basis. The baby's grandparents lived in the adjacent house, and in many ways the two generations shared their daily life. The grandparents spent hours caring for the baby on most days. They were allowed to spoil the child and encouraged to cultivate her familiarity with the Italian language and culture.

Ratings at 40 Months

Impulse control. Maria was considered to be a remarkably well modulated and controlled child at all times. Like all toddlers, she had outbreaks of anger and impatience early in the third year, but she so seldom lost her temper and showed such patience and perseverance while engaged in tasks that at 28 months her IC rating was 4. Although her overall style had not altered, the period surrounding her third birthday was when she was her most impulsive. At 34 months she would scream and slam doors when she felt "insulted." At other times, which included some social conflict situations, she was described as calm, deliberate, persistent, able to wait, and on occasion resolutely stubborn. Thus her IC rating at 34 months was 3. By 40 months behavior storms were a thing of the past. She maintained tight control over movement impulses, vocal intensity, and affect display in general. When frustrated or otherwise annoyed she became tense, exceptionally quiet, and passively resistant. When she was especially pleased with something her expression was described as "radiating quiet but intense pleasure." Thus, she was considerably more controlled than most peers. The impulse control rating was 4.

Structure. Before the age of 40 months Maria's life had been very highly structured. Her mother, who was in full charge, was a methodical sort of person who devoted her considerable energy and ability to providing the very best opportunities for her daughter. To her this meant creating an atmosphere that encouraged learning as much as it promoted general well being. An inordinate amount of time was spent in teaching the child. In so doing the mother was ingenious, affectionate, imaginative, and skillful, with the result that Maria loved these occasions. Her life was structured in other ways as well. Mother planned each day so as to contain enjoyable and constructive experiences for her child, including outings of all sorts and many shared activities. A few months before the 40-month visit, however, the mother resumed her professional responsibilities. So as to not leave Maria with the grandparents for too long a time, she enrolled her in a morning nursery school. What could not have been anticipated was that no sooner had the mother resumed working than a major crisis arose in her organization which absorbed a great deal of mother's time and energy. Because of her mother's absence Maria spent most afternoons with her grandparents. Although most attentive, these relatives were bent on giving pleasure more than instruction so that, in their home, structure prevailed to a medium degree. The even tenor of Maria's life was disrupted in other ways as well. For the first time in her young life mealtimes and other routines became unpredictable. Overall a structure rating of 2 seemed to meet the case.

Accommodation. Accommodation had always been a prominent feature of Maria's experience and was only slightly less so at 40 months. By comparison to other children in the sample she was still accommodated more than most. Her mother was perceptive, and the manner in which we saw her adapt to the child's momentary state, to any sign of interest on the child's part, and to transient difficulties was not something that could have been performed for our benefit; it obviously reflected well-established patterns of interaction during which each partner understood the signals emanating from the other. As one observer summarized what was observed, "She [mother] supports, eases, and understands." Both parents realized that it was difficult for Maria to adapt to the changes that had occurred and spent considerable effort helping her over the rough patch. Not only were they tolerant of some defiant and even infantile behavior that normally would not have been allowed but they also consciously tried to maintain for her what they themselves called "continuity" in her life. For instance, they saw to it that Maria often saw her best friend although this child's family had moved away. Similarly, her mother worked at helping a reluctant Maria play with a new child on the block. At considerable inconvenience the customarily elaborate bedtime rituals were maintained. In short, not only was the mother's style accommodating on a moment-to-moment basis, but both parents felt that it was up to them to ease the stress under which Maria so obviously labored. In their own way the grandparents also felt that they needed to compensate Maria for what she had lost, which meant even greater indulgence than usual. For all we know, this may have yielded some additional sense of emotional support for the child. The accommodation rating was 3.

Focused attention. Maria was treated as a very important personage whose every utterance and action was responded to very fully. There were long conversations between Maria and each of her parents during which every effort was made to get her to verbalize her thoughts, wishes, and opinions. The last term is used advisedly because these parents went all out to include the child in all decision making, sometimes to a degree that might seem absurd. For instance, when new household furnishings had to be bought Maria went along and, if she did not like a sofa it was not purchased; her veto was enough. As her mother said, "She has to have a choice." All this was apart from hours of joint play with grandmother, father, and mother. As these play episodes were described to us, the adults usually devoted all of their attention to the child. To avoid exaggeration it should be said that independent play with her toys was welcomed and not interfered with, but at this period in time Maria was less willing to entertain herself than usual. The focused attention rating was 3.

Didacticism. Maria's cognitive development was fostered by all conceivable means. Educational toys and equipment abounded in the home of the grandparents as well as in her own. Both parents thoroughly enjoyed working with her (a term they used in distinction to playing with her) and found time for it every day. Conversations with her parents were geared to teaching language, concepts, and information. Stories were read to her, visits to the library were frequent, she was taken to museums and galleries and so forth. By the time she entered nursery school she knew the alphabet, had a concept of numbers equivalent to norms for six-year-olds (as judged by the 40-month Stanford-Binet), and could read a few simple words. She was well acquainted with puzzles, formboards, and the like and watched television shows designed for older children. The saving grace, from our point of view, was that play with other children, imaginative play with a huge array of toys, and outdoor activity were also cultivated. Withal, among the three-year-olds of our acquaintance within and beyond the research sample, there are none who received more concentrated teaching and very few who were taught as skillfully as Maria. The didacticism rating was 3.

Frequency of conflict. We were told that whenever open conflict with adults occurred in Maria's life it took the form of her refusal to "change her mind." Whether it was when she was asked to do something that she had decided not to do, or to refrain from something she intended to do, her response was to "go on strike," as the family called it. Her mother said that neither the withdrawal of privileges nor the promise of a treat nor persuasion was effective. Reasoning with her—giving a full explanation of all the pros and cons—would sometimes work. Maria's experience had always been and was now that by and large her wishes were respected and sometimes responded to as though they were commands. This may explain her dismay when this was not the case, but it may also have contributed to her becoming a reasonable child who became antagonistic to her elders infrequently, though then with a vengeance. The frequency of conflict rating was 2.

Intensity of maternal involvement. Maria was and always had been a primary focus in mother's life. The family's life and their dreams for the future revolved around the child. The mother's professional and social interests remained important to her, however. One might say that an exeedingly strong emotional investment in the child was assimilated to and became a part of her broader scheme of values and goals. We attached a question mark to the rating because at the time of the 40-month visit mother was concerned and anxious about her daughter's difficulties in adapting to the recent changes and preoccupied by the problem of how to undo the damage caused by her necessary absences from home. For this reason a rating of high had been considered. The final involvement rating was 2(?).

Developmental Course

Maria was moderately premature but, except for her birthweight, she was a healthy, normal infant. Her brief stay in the ICU was uneventful. She continued to be a healthy child, suffering no more of the usual childhood ailments than do most full-term babies.

Under the anxious eye of a devoted mother the baby settled in nicely once she was at home. Regular rhythms of sleeping and eating were soon established, and altogether she was an easy baby to take care of. No one but the parents and grandparents had direct contact with her. All four of them played with the baby whenever they had a chance and Maria had "every toy there is." At 7 months she was an alert, active youngster who enjoyed all the procedures provided that her mother stayed very close. When the examiner's face came too near she sobered, but when he kept his distance she smiled and cooed responsively. Her MDI was 103 and, when the *Object Permanence* scale was administered, she proved to be a perfect illustration of stage four behavior in that she kept searching for the hidden toy beneath the pad where she had found it before, no matter how often she observed it to be placed beneath a second pad.

When Maria came in for the 15-month visit we were told that all manner of new skills had come in all at once, beginning at 8 months. Crawling, pulling herself to standing, and walking followed one another in quick succession. She walked unaided on her first birthday and since then would not allow anyone to hold her hand as she walked about. According to the mother she had learned to say quite a few words and knew their equivalent in Italian. During observation and testing it appeared that she did have a specific sound to indicate "I want" and knew and used the names of some people and a few objects. Her mother tended to interpret Maria's utterances liberally, crediting the child with greater maturity than she possessed. This is a pattern we have observed repeatedly in children who later showed superior verbal skills. It begins with consistent labeling long before the child can comprehend, followed by enthusiastic reception and overinterpretation of early utterances, and later changes to very exacting standards for accuracy and syntax in language use. Maria might well have shown superior verbal skills in any case, but the fact remains that this proclivity was fostered at a very early age. Object permanence was now unshakably at the stage six level, and she had moved into that range with respect to spatial relationships as well.

During the play session Maria used all the toys but in a very sociable way. That is, she maintained continuous contact with both her mother and the staff member. Toddlerlike, her favorite activity was to empty and fill containers. Two conventional communication signals were observed, pointing and showing an object. The open space experiment led to behavior prototypical of Mahler's hatching stage. She marched right out into the hall, roamed widely, and had to be retrieved (in this situation she never once turned to look at her mother). Thus, with the exception of some isolated test items, Maria's behavior and capacities were very much like those of most other 15-month-olds. This stood in marked contrast to the fact that her mother treated her much as one would a two-year-old, in the choice of toys, games, and television shows as well as in the type of outing thought appropriate. The grandparents, on the other hand, still viewed her as a babe in arms and treated her accordingly.

At 28 months Maria had clearly entered into a much more mature and dependent relationship with her mother and, at the same time, her intellectual development had progressed apace. She worked very hard during the developmental testing and obtained an IQ of 127. Her approach to tasks was extraordinarily mature (this may have been a kind of pseudomaturity) in that, when dubious about her ability she might say "I will try it;" when she recognized her failure she used a stock phrase indicating that she would be able to do it once she was three. (We could hear mother's intonation as these words were spoken by the child.)

On the body awareness assessment she could not only name any body part one might ask for on herself, pictures, and dolls but went beyond standards for her age group by referring to the mirror image by her own name. She was also one of the few children in the sample who was able to put together a puzzle of a human figure (an item from the Merrill-Palmer Scale intended for older preschool children). During the play session she became involved in fairly complex play with dolls, interspersed with such age-typical maneuvers as heaping toys on her mother's lap, only to carry most of them away again. Although her contact with her mother was sporadic, she could not tolerate separation. As her mother was about to leave, after due explanation, Maria protested loudly and ran to her. This told us all we needed to know, and the mother never left the room. The child's behavior during the open space procedure reflected the same change in the mother-child relationship in that on this occasion Maria took a few tentative steps, turned back to her mother, and remained close to her.

The assessment of impulse control showed her to be one of the most controlled children in the sample. When asked to wait she visibly suppressed the urge to move but always succeeded in withdrawing her hand again until the "now" sign was given. She worked with seemingly endless patience, and there were no outward signs of annoyance on difficult tasks or when she was mildly frustrated. Her voice and movements remained well modulated and contained throughout. Although her behavior was less spontaneous and colorful than that of most two-year-olds, she did show some animation. For instance, some of her successes and especially praise pleased her greatly. Some of the tasks elicited intense concentration and a few others bored her but were carried out good-naturedly. This pattern conformed precisely to what her mother had told us, before the testing, as typical of Maria when she was "at work."

According to very credible reports, we saw only one aspect of what this little girl was like at home. The first thing mentioned when we asked the family if Maria had changed in any way was that she now often lost her temper. Specifically, she would scream and perhaps throw objects when she was denied something. If she saw a toy, a dress, or any other thing she liked, she asked that it be bought at once. If this did not occur she turned into a holy terror. It should be mentioned that, until her desires became excessive, Maria's experience had been that whatever she asked for *was* bought for her, if not by her mother then by the grandparents. Actually she did not so much ask for things as demand them, in full expectation of compliance. A second new behavior characteristic was that she had developed a number of fears. These were much like those of other two-year-olds. She became terrified during medical examinations and was afraid of moving machinery such as motorized lawnmowers and cranes. Last, her imaginative play with dolls had become intense. It usually reenacted personal experiences such as visits to doctors, to restaurants, or to her parents' offices. In short, Maria had left toddlerhood behind and had become a little girl with a rich inner life. Her behavior now reflected the tensions, the conflictual feelings, the new anxieties, and the new coping mechanisms that this entails.

When Maria was seen again shortly before her third birthday, at 34 months, she was somewhat precociously involved with the oedipal dilemma. She declared that she would marry her father or else a much admired boy from the neighborhood. Also, she wished for a baby sister, and this imagined baby, who was talked about to all and sundry, was very vivid to her although not quite on the level of an imaginary companion. Her play with dolls now featured domesticity, and the care of this fantasy baby sister was a prominent theme. Another telling symbolic gesture consisted of the fact that she had cut out a picture of a crying girl from a magazine and, when she was dissatisfied or angry, she silently presented it to her mother. This mute appeal had the virtue of avoiding open conflict and yet accusing mother where she was most vulnerable by saying, in effect, "you are making me unhappy."

The mother had just returned to work on a part-time schedule, and Maria led a curious double life. At least half of her day was spent with the grandparents, who still persisted in dressing and feeding her as though she were a baby and treated her with great indulgence in all other ways. When her mother took over, things went to the opposite extreme. Mother—in fact, both parents—treated her as a companion and as a partner in all their doings. Thus Maria became a connoisseur of fine restaurants and stores; during visits with her parents' friends she joined in the conversation and was listened to even on matters of which she knew nothing; and her decision to stay in diapers a while longer was accepted without demur. With all this, the ample and variegated teaching continued unabated, as did carefully planned play periods with somewhat older children (she did not get along with her agemates) and long sessions with her father, who shared his interest in music with the child. Maria gave every sign of knowing herself to be somehow "special," and she also gave a good deal of evidence of being troubled. Primarily this showed itself in what her mother considered to be a lack of zest and a tendency to cling to her mother. She did not fuss at her mother's leaving but upon her return seldom left her side. Mother thought that Maria was not nearly as happy as she used to be. Her fears now were of hairy, man-like creatures about whom she dreamt, and of small animals that she thought might bite her.

Her intellectual development continued to flourish throughout all this; her IQ was 129. Though verbal concepts and language use were the most advanced, her performance was superior in all other areas as well. Similarly, she coped with the Achievement Motivation tasks in a competent and deliberate manner. Each task was approached with perseverance, mild pleasure at well-earned success, and unusual clarity about what she could and could not accomplish. During the developmental test it took a while before Maria overcame her initial shyness. Even after she was able to converse and cooperate with the (male) examiner she remained somewhat tense and distant in her manner. During the play session she did not become involved in play. Instead she engaged her mother in conversation, made requests of her, and did not leave her side. Throughout the visit Maria stayed so close to her mother that separation was not attempted. The demands of the Level of Aspiration experiment were met in a rigid manner. She chose to throw the ball from the most difficult position and kept throwing from that distance whether or not she was successful.

At the time of the 40-month visit Maria had become used to daily attendance at a morning nursery school. Because her mother needed to be away from home a great deal more than she had planned, nursery school did not serve its original purpose of reducing the time Maria spent with her grandparents. It was said that Maria coped much better than before with the constant shift between two different caretaking environments, that she no longer had angry outbursts when something was denied her, and that the previous fears seemed to have disappeared. Yet her mother did not feel that all was well with her daughter. Maria now misbehaved in a manner that was entirely uncharacteristic. In her parents' absence she would do such things as creating havoc in her room or deliberately tracking dirt to a spotless area in the house. We shared the mother's belief that to this overly meticulous little girl such deeds must have seemed like serious crimes. At any rate, the family understood such episodes as silent protests at the mother's relative unavailability. Even in her mother's presence she was subdued, sitting quietly until someone enticed her into some sort of shared activity. Otherwise, things went on much as before, including long sessions with father during which he "worked on" music and hours during which mother "worked on" learning as these parents saw it. The child was still included in adult activities, and the mother tried to compensate Maria for what was lacking by giving even more weight to her preferences than before. Details about her daily life at 40 months are given in the documentation of experience pattern ratings.

What we saw at the 40-month visit was a pretty, intellectually precocious little girl so dutiful that it hurt to watch. Her IQ had risen to 136. To begin with she was shy with the examiner and, much as at 34 months, remained distant and somber in her dealings with him, although she was entirely cooperative. She dealt with the Achievement Motivation tasks much as she had before. There was no doubt that she placed a high value on accomplishing difficult tasks. On the rare occasions when she accepted help, her response to praise showed that she did not feel she deserved much credit. During the Level of Aspiration experiment she again managed to evade specific acknowledgment of success or failure. She invented a system of moving up and down the scale of difficulty and stuck to it regardless of whether or not the ball hit the target (thereby often doing the easier thing after success at a more difficult level).

The World Test brought forth behavior which reflected the combination of high ability and marked inhibition that was characteristic of her at that time. This test presents the child with a very large array of miniature toys so attractive that, as a rule, no child (and, for that matter, few adults) can resist them. Tight-lipped and largely silent, Maria concentrated on building a construction using every single toy—something we had not seen before because so much ingenuity is required to find space for them all without piling up the toys. In spite of her obvious recognition of each toy object she used them as though they were geometric forms and created an orderly design representing nothing. Having watched other children using the enchanting toys, knowing that imaginative play once was one of Maria's strengths, and observing her strained facial expression, all observers were agreed that the material must have provoked fantasies or play ideas that aroused anxiety and that therefore she bent every effort toward literal compliance with the request to build something in a manner that spared her unpleasurable feelings. All adults expressed their genuine admiration for her achievement, and a photograph of her structure was offered in appreciation. Yet this child, who so enjoyed acknowledgment of her abilities, showed nothing but mild relief to have done with the whole thing.

Discussion

Our reflections on some of the forces shaping the development of this girl have been expressed or implied in the recounting of Maria's story. It remains only to say that when we met her again at six years of age, both our positive expectations and our concerns for her well-being proved justified. At that time her IQ was 121; it would probably have been higher were it not for her extreme fear of failure. The tester, who was not familiar with Maria's history, thought she behaved as though giving a wrong answer was a catastrophe. No amount of reassurance made any impression; the child could not be persuaded to say anything unless she was absolutely certain of the answer. As might be expected, she was the best student in her class, and she was also a participant in additional enrichment classes. Her mother described her as exceedingly ambitious and competitive. Much could be added to round out the picture of a rigidly controlled, generally obedient child who greatly valued her many possessions and felt more comfortable with her old friends from preschool days than with schoolmates. To a clinician, her drawings reflected the presence of strong aggressive feelings, yet everything we learned indicated that open aggressiveness was altogether foreign to her nature.

Last we describe something of a miracle, a case that (in greater detail than can be presented here) ought to be required reading for social workers, psychologists, and all professionals in the field of child mental health.

Lenore: Normal Development In An Atypical Setting

Background

The arrival of this baby coincided with a major turning point in her mother's life. Very shortly before the baby's birth the mother experienced a religious conversion. For her, the new life in her care and her own new life as a Christian were inextricably merged. Previously the mother had led a somewhat dissipated existence ever since she had left the parental home. She was at odds with her relatives, had no close friends, and was attuned to street life. She described herself as having had and still experiencing severe depressions. Various short-lived contacts with psychiatrists had left her with a scornful attitude toward that profession, an attitude she also maintained toward all social institutions except the church. She attributed her emotional difficulties to an extremely unhappy childhood and was resolved to protect her daughter from a similar fate. Withal, she was an articulate, intelligent, and likable young woman.

Throughout the time we knew them this family lived on welfare and in undesirable quarters. With respect to all externals their life was disordered, ill managed, and unsatisfactory. But a kind of consistency and cohesiveness was achieved because the mother never deviated from certain overriding principles. These included ruthless honesty and the conviction that children should never be coerced.

Ratings at 40 Months

Impulse control. Lenore presented herself as a child who combined lively spontaneity with good control. Like most young children she was subject to impatience and excitement but she was usually able to subdue overt manifestation of these states. It should perhaps be mentioned that on infrequent occasions Lenore was capable of mustering unusually high levels of control while in some rare situations she went to pieces and altogether lost control. The impulse control score was 3 (age-adequate).

Structure. This three-year-old's daily routine was not regular except for the fact that she attended a daycare center nearly every weekday. She awakened at variable hours (her mother did not believe in waking her) so that after breakfast and the morning toilette she might reach the center as early as nine or as late as twelve. About once a week she was unwilling to go at all and was allowed to stay home. Although details of life at the daycare center are not available, we do know that such things as counting and the ABCs were practiced and that there were toys, games, and books, so that some structure was almost certainly provided. Upon returning home late in the afternoon mother and child did everything together. This included joint preparation and consumption of meals and also long and complicated conversations in which the mother not only gave very full answers to all questions but also talked to the child about her own concerns. She said that Lenore was not like other children; one could talk to her as to another woman. On days when they did not attend church in the evening, as they did about twice a week, a male friend of the mother came to visit. He played with and talked to the youngster a great deal and tried to teach her things. Even on weekends some sort of directed and purposive activity was always going on. Mother and child shopped together, went to McDonalds, or visited friends. In short, Lenore participated in organized children's groups or else in activities that had meaning to her during most of her waking day. The EP rating for structure was 2 (present, not dominant).

Accommodation. To an unusual degree, the mother's way of dealing with her child was intentionally geared to achieve certain goals. She wanted to make sure that her daughter became a good Christian, which meant, among other things, that everyday concerns were decided and talked about in terms of religious precepts. It also meant that the child must be given no cause to hate, distrust, or fear other people. In some ways this rather rigid style led to actions that were in fact accommodating. For instance, the mother did not believe in hitting children and by and large lived up to her conviction that children are to be treated with respect. Therefore she explained the reasons for requests or commands, allowed the child access to all objects because she wanted her to know that the home was as much hers as her mother's, and, further, she did not hesitate to apologize if she felt she had been in the wrong. In other ways the same ideals led to a failure of accommodation, at least in our judgment. The child was required to cope with information beyond her comprehension in relation to sexuality, religion, all sorts of evil in the world, and financial dilemmas. Something else also led to accommodating as well as unaccommodating components of the mother's style. She considered Lenore to be special because of her prematurity and also because she was to be the agent for the mother's spiritual salvation, and therefore she made allowances for Lenore's likes and dislikes in areas where most parents do not. What may well be more important is that, for this same reason, everything the child did and said was responded to by the mother as important, which itself implies some accommodation.

Last, mother considered that Lenore had reached a stage in which she wanted to learn everything. Her choice of toys, or of books and magazines to share, was intended to advance Lenore's learning and may have done so. The degree to which Lenore was accommodated was neither more nor less than we saw in the majority of other children. Yet much of it struck us as a byproduct of the mother's preconceived beliefs based on her own childhood rather than on characteristics of Lenore's behavior. The EP rating for accommodation was 2 (present, not dominant).

Focused attention. In her own home at 40 months, Lenore received a great deal more concentrated social attention than most preschoolers do, specifically in the form of frequent and prolonged conversations with her mother, episodes of joint play or looking at books together, and the nearly daily play sessions with a friend of the family. This pattern would have been assessed as 3 (very prominent) except for the fact that Lenore spent so much time at the daycare center. Since details of that setting remained unknown to us, the EP rating for focused attention was 2 (present, not prominent).

Didacticism. As already mentioned, Lenore was encouraged to use suitable play equipment, books, crayons, and the like both at the daycare center and in her home. At the center she was taught numbers, letters, and similar preacademic content. In view of her nearly full-time attendance at a child care facility a rating of high could have been considered. However, there was so much going on by way of outings, imaginative play, and involvement in household affairs that learning, or rather being taught, was not a really dominant feature of her experience. The EP rating for didacticism was 2 (present, not prominent).

Frequency of conflict. By all accounts Lenore and her mother had developed patterns of interaction that made open conflict between them a rare event (the same could not be said of Lenore's fairly stormy toddlerhood). The final score was mandated by the fact that we had no idea how things went at the center in this respect. The EP rating for frequency of conflict was 2 (present, not prominent).

Intensity of maternal involvement. At this time, and always before, Lenore was the primary focus of her mother's thoughts, feelings, and actions. As is characteristic of this pair, the form that this closeness took and the reasons for it were entirely atypical.

The mother literally saw herself in the child. She was certain that they possessed the same personality characteristics and interpreted everything about the child in terms of her own experience. This went so far that she felt in her own body when Lenore needed sleep or food and arranged these matters in terms of her own state. On the same basis she thought she could anticipate how the child would react to events and situations and—at least with respect to minor occurrences during the research sessions—she was usually correct. This was a matter of overidentification, not of symbiotic closeness. At no time had the mother been reluctant to have the child spend time with others provided that she approved of them, and she expected more independence and general maturity from the child than do most mothers. However much this was dictated by grave concerns about her own vulnerability, the mother behaved in such a way that Lenore knew herself as a person vital to her mother's well being. The EP rating for intensity of maternal involvement was 3 (very prominent).

Developmental Course

Lenore was only slightly premature, but her birthweight of just below 1500 grams necessitated placement in the ICU. In spite of this marked fetal growth retardation she did well and was discharged after less than two weeks. She was an alert, well-functioning infant from the outset. And in spite of numerous infectious illnesses, her physical and psychological development was entirely normal throughout.

She was a source of wonder and delight to her young mother, and this mother-baby pair soon became the object of solicitude and affection for numerous members of the church community. Mother and baby spent every weekday evening at the church, where the baby was passed from lap to lap. Although she presented a self-sufficient air, the mother at first knew nothing about baby care and willingly accepted help. A woman who became the baby's godmother played a central role. Not only did she teach the mother such things as how to bathe a tiny infant, but she also babysat when needed and took the infant into her own home at times when the mother became too tense and depressed. Other friends and neighbors also stepped in to help as needed.

At 7 months Lenore obtained an MDI score of 115 and showed unusual persistence and behavior integration as she sought to obtain and manipulate test objects. Her sunny social responsiveness to all and sundry was notable.

At 15 months her performance was somewhat uneven, but she received an MDI score of 101 nonetheless. Her fine motor coordination was relatively poor, but she succeeded with some items that do not become normative until 18 months. She was a most sociable youngster who spoke several words and was very good at initiating and prolonging reciprocal games of the peek-a-boo variety. During the play session she approached the toys at once and stayed with them while maintaining visual contact with her mother. She was seen to employ five different conventional communication signals, including pointing, showing, the negation headshake, and the word *no*. In the open space experiment she illustrated perfectly what we had come to expect at this age; she gleefully entered the large corridor and roamed about without a backward glance at her mother; she finally had to be retrieved.

Between the 7- and 15-month visits Lenore had become an active and somewhat mischievous child who tested her mother's patience and endurance. Her urge to move about, to get into things and inadvertently destroy objects, brought her to grief, as did her tendency to become angry. At such times she screamed and sometimes threw things, but all-out tantrums were not reported (of course, we asked). The mother thought Lenore had become moody; there were times when nothing pleased her. We have every reason to believe that, during the same time span, the mother herself often felt deeply angry and/or depressed so that nothing would please *her*. They lived in abject poverty, and life was even less regulated than before. Mother and baby tended to get up very late, to eat at odd times, and to alternate between rushing about on errands and staying home doing nothing in particular. Church attendance had dropped to twice a week. What saved the day was continued interest and support from the godmother and others. According to the mother these friends came to visit, played with the baby, took her out, and sometimes kept the baby in their own homes for a few days—we don't know how often. The mother's sense of connectedness with the baby continued unabated. Her greatest fear was that she herself might become seriously upset because she believed that whatever she felt would be felt by the child as well. It is difficult to convey the contrast between what clinicians would expect to see in a child who lived with a mother as distraught as Lenore's mother was and under conditions that alarmed social agencies, and the friendly, well developed, and to all appearances contented little girl we met at 15 months.

An important change in Lenore's life had taken place some time before the 28-month visit. During the interval, the mother had "gone under," meaning that she had become so depressed as to be unable to eat or do much of anything. Church members were instrumental in placing the child in a daycare center where she now spent practically all day except on weekends. Things so arranged themselves (this mother had a talent for making people want to help her) that other mothers picked up and returned the child to her home. This arrangement probably lessened the stress on mother. At any rate, she was again able to function rather well in relation to Lenore and in general. Her religious fervor had returned, and nearly every evening was spent in church, where Lenore slept at least as much as she played. The mother's mood was anxious rather than angry. To her the task of dealing with a willful two-year-old was a test imposed by God; she had to prove to herself and Him that she could be both strict and understanding with the child and—above all—honest with her.

The mother-daughter relationship was intense. The mother's ability to report on the behavior of her child in minute detail (some of it confirmable) testified to her availability and responsiveness, as did the youngster's trusting and affectionate behavior with her mother. Surrogate grandparents and other friendly persons were still amply present, as was mother's friend, who spent a great deal of time with the child. Lenore was actually used as a guidepost to mother's actions, but whether or not she had any way of sensing this we do not know. If the child liked a new acquaintance that person was made welcome. If not, further contact was discouraged because "children know."

During the testing situation we had occasion to observe behavior similar to what had been described to us. At first Lenore was as friendly and cooperative as we had always known her. Then she became frightened of a camera which was masked behind a cloth so that only the photographer's shoes were visible. She paled, looked anxious, said the word "camera," and refused all proffered test items and toys. The apparatus was huriedly removed, but she remained negativistic and actively resistant. After an interruption, testing was resumed in a different room, and she took delight in participating with all items. (A full year later she pointed to the corner where the camera had been and said "feet" at a moment when she had become anxious over a broken toy.) Her IQ was 88 and would have been a good deal higher were it not for her lack of familiarity with objects that most two-year-olds can name.

In the play session she used the toys in a constructive and fairly well-organized manner. Throughout she maintained contact with the mother, telling her what she was up to, but she did not physically approach her. For reasons we could not discern, there were a few brief episodes during which Lenore looked tense and uncomfortable. The separation procedure had a strong impact in that she looked troubled and ceased all play, waiting for her mother to return. The body awareness inventory posed no difficulty for her. She easily named more than the expected number of body parts, and it made no difference to her whether it was her own body, the doll, or the mirror reflection. She surpassed most agemates by referring to the mirror image by her own name. Her demeanor during the open space procedure suggested a relatively mature style of interaction with the mother. With neutral affect she moved quite far into the hallway and after a while turned around and urged her mother to come and join her, all in a relaxed and good-natured manner. The matching task (concept formation) proved her able to classify and sort objects, though toward the end some landed in the wrong box although they had been named correctly. The impulse control assessment confirmed both our impressions and the mother's report: Lenore was scored as a well-modulated and contained youngster who seldom lost control. It was not that she was pliant; rather, her refusals to cooperate or obey were usually calm and resolute; if anything, her voice was lower and her activity decreased at such times. A few times, under pressure, she did raise her voice to shouting and physically resisted. She was very good about waiting although this was difficult for her, and she also persevered on tasks that taxed her patience.

We have little information about the period between 28 and 34 months. On the day of the 34-month visit the mother was deeply depressed and spoke chiefly about her disappointments and resentments. She now seldom went to church, feeling that her friends there were unwilling to help her. At the same time she made it clear that religion was as important to her as before. She was willing to talk about her daughter, whom she described as utterly lovable, mature for her age, and her only solace. In particular, she stressed that the child sensed her mother's moods and did what she could to comfort her. She would pet her, try to entertain and distract her by bringing books or toys, and in general made the mother feel that the child was "taking care of me." The only other thing we were told was that Lenore was now eager to learn and to do things. She continued to attend the daycare center, where, at times when mother was not up to caring for her, it was arranged for Lenore to stay overnight with neighbors.

Lenore herself was in fine fettle when we saw her. She was sociable and enthusiastic during testing and obtained an IQ of 95. Her language use was extraordinarily good. She spoke in long, syntactically correct sentences that expressed complex meaning with clarity. For instance, "I let others play with my toys . . . I don't like to share." During the play session she was absorbed, paying little attention to the adults. Most of her play was of a simple imaginary sort, as in serving meals to dolls. The separation procedure did momentarily disconcert her, but she soon turned to the examiner as a play partner. On this occasion the concept formation tasks were solved easily. The assessment of Achievement Motivation was made for the first time. Lenore worked diligently at the various tasks (which are selected for their high interest value to young children) and appreciated the result of her labors with a good deal of pride. Pleasure in accomplishing something difficult was great, whereas success with easy tasks elicited no particular affective response. In keeping with our definition of achievement motivation, Lenore consistently refused help on tasks she could master but accepted help some of the time on items she found too difficult. Overall, the child's easy spontaneity, good mood, adequate cognitive functioning, and fairly good health led us to conclude that between the daycare center and a devoted but gravely troubled mother she led a life that offered what she needed to grow and thrive.

By the time of the 40-month visit a great improvement in the mother's state and some changes in their lifestyle had occurred. This time we heard more about mother, child, and their life circumstances than ever before, which is saying a good deal. Much of the information about the family's life at this time has already been described as part of the documentation of the 40-month experience pattern ratings and will not be repeated here. The mother had become affiliated with another church of the same persuasion, and her religious fervor had returned to its previous high pitch. She was far less depressed and much more active socially and domestically than before. Although Lenore continued to attend the daycare center, her mother spent more time in direct caretaking (bathing, grooming, preparing meals) and busied herself providing nice clothes, good toys and books, and a pleasant home. There were casual visits with friends and neighbors, including the godmother, and the male family friend was again a daily visitor. The mother continued to talk about her daughter in glowing terms, believing her to be very bright, possessed of an excellent memory, easily hurt in her feelings, and unusually mature. We learned that Lenore had developed a fear of any visible bodily injury and of any sight that could remind her of possible injury, such as the color red, which reminded her of blood. We were able confirm this by the child's response to a toy that had one bright red part. Less intense but also new were fears of having her hair washed and of the shower; reportedly, she cried thinking she might be drowned. Otherwise she was described as a generally happy and responsive child. And so she proved to be.

On this occasion her IQ was 92 and the pattern of her performance had not changed. Vocabulary and syntax were excellent, she could tell complex stories in response to pictures, and perceptual acumen and integration were also very good for her age. What she largely lacked was the ability to deal with words and percepts that had no concrete or socially imbedded meaning. Thus pointing out the larger of two lines or geometric shapes was beyond her, even though objects and meaningful pictures were readily classified by size; nor could she specify similarities though her response to the material was relevant and coherent.

When the Achievement Motivation series was carried out again nothing had changed except that her skills had grown. She rose to challenges, enjoyed success, persevered, and accepted help reluctantly and rarely. Much the same picture emerged when the Level of Aspiration experiment was performed. After success she increased her distance from the target, temporarily decreased it after failure, and she enjoyed herself. She was able to deal with the World Test and became absorbed in building a structure representing animals, which were appropriately grouped with fences and trees, and she also built something resembling a landscape containing houses, persons, trees, and vehicles. (The majority of children in our sample were unable to do more than sort and align the miniature objects.)

Discussion

At three and a half years Lenore was a healthy, well-adapted, and cognitively able child. Professionals who had come into contact with this mother-child pair, including ourselves, had felt grave concern on the child's behalf. This small family lived under the pressure of chronic poverty, and the mother seemed so beset by inner problems and so incompetent to fend for herself that it was feared she might lack the capacity to provide constant and conscientious care. As to the effects of poverty, the mother's way of coping may have served self-preservation and immediate adaptation, even if it was open to criticism on other grounds. She spent what money there was on things that were important to her, including pretty clothes for both of them, trips to the movies and to restaurants, and books and toys. At the same time, bills were in arrears, necessary furnishings were not available, and the cupboard was often bare. Thus many necessities were provided by friends and neighbors who brought food and cash. As to the effects of the mother's personal problems, all one can say is that in some respects they did leave their mark upon the child. For example, even though the nature of her fears as a two-year-old was typical for her age, her pervasive fear of injury was unusually intense.

Beginning early in the third year she was precocious with respect to what might be called social sophistication. She comprehended and later spoke of her mother's feelings and perplexities, was hypersensitive to emotional nuances (a characteristic also shown in the brief contacts with staff members), and was independent with respect to practical self-help very early. Her favorite play theme of reversing roles with mother also had an element of precocity. We think that Lenore's ability to cope with and gain from an overly close relationship with her mother may have been possible only because she spent a large portion of her waking day in another and less demanding setting.

PART III Results for The Deviant Group

Our report on the development of children who had conspicuous behavior difficulties (the behavior group) and of those who had suffered neurological impairment (the neuro group) consists largely of a comparison of each of these deviant groups with each other and with the intact group. It will be possible to be fairly brief because the reader is now familiar with the variables we looked at and how we report results. All of the analyses and descriptive accounts mentioned for the intact group were performed for the deviant groups and in exactly the same manner, many of them well before the research population had been divided into three groups. In some respects the deviant groups did not differ from the intact. Where such similarity contributed no new information, as was true, for instance, of many socioeconomic background characteristics, we limit ourselves to a mere statement of the fact without documentation. In contexts where the similarity was an important finding—for instance, that among the deviant children impulse control and IQ related to each other in much the same way as in the intact group—results are reported and discussed in full.

We begin with a description of the background characteristics of the deviant groups and then give an account of cognitive development, impulse control, and the degree to which each of these was associated with social class. Thereafter, experience patterns found in the deviant groups will be described along with the interrelationships between experience patterns and the other variables.

Chapter 7

Socioeconomic Background, Cognitive Development, and Impulse Control

The process of identifying some of our subjects as manifesting more than ordinary behavior difficulties and others as neurologically impaired was described in chapter 2. In table 7.1 we summarize the composition of the two deviant groups. As would be expected, boys outnumbered girls in the neuro group while in the behavior group the sexes were evenly divided. Whether by chance or otherwise, socioeconomic status was not related to the frequency of behavioral maladaptation or to the incidence of neurologic deficit. For our immediate purpose this is fortunate: the deviant groups can be compared directly with each other without having to take social-class effects into account.

Although the deviant groups were evenly distributed over the SES quartiles it is possible that some of the background features associated with social class were different for the deviant groups from what has been described in chapter 3 for the intact. We scrutinized the demographic data and found that in most respects the life circumstances of families with deviant children conformed completely to those reported for the intact group. That is, social-class differences were of the same kind and of the same order. Specifically, the ethnic composition, age of mothers at the time the baby was born, marital status, head of household, and similar items together reproduced, on a smaller scale, the patterns found in the larger group.

Only one of the background variables differed for the deviant groups—the arrangements made for the primary care of the child. Since SES differences in the primary-care pattern were found in the intact group, figure 7.1 depicts these as well. Because the number of children is so small we combined the two lower and the two upper SES quartiles into a low and a high group. In figure 7.1 we show that the child's daily care was shared by two persons more often among the intact than the deviant children. In the deviant families caretaking patterns differed but little as a function of SES; one exception occurred for the lower SES group only at the age of 40 months, when publicly supported daycare centers became more readily available. The reasons that more of the children with special problems were cared for exclusively by the mothers are not difficult to recognize. The interview material was unequivocal on this issue. Many mothers of children with behavior difficulties told us that he or she was "so bad" that neither relatives nor sitters

Table 7.1: Composition of Behavior and Neuro Groups by Sex and SES

Neuro				*Behavior*			
SES	*N Cases*			*SES*	*N Cases*		
	M	*F*	*Combined*		*M*	*F*	*Combined*
I	3	1	4	I	3	3	6
II	5	1	6	II	4	2	6
III	3	2	5	III	3	4	7
IV	3	3	6	IV	2	4	6
	14	7	21		12	13	25

Figure 7.1 Shared Primary Caretaking in the Intact, Neuro, and Behavior Groups by SES Quartile (By Age, in Percentage)

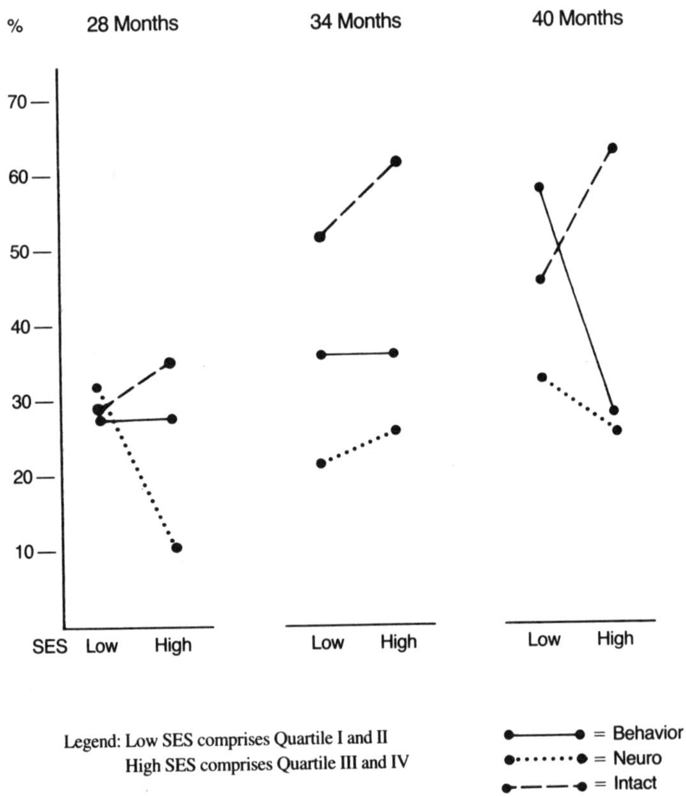

Legend: Low SES comprises Quartile I and II
High SES comprises Quartile III and IV

Figure 7.2 Reported and Observed Psychiatric Problems or Feeling of Isolation in Mothers for Three Groups

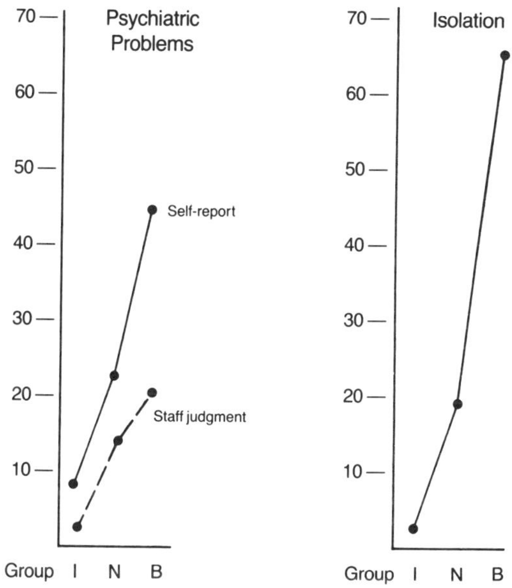

I = Intact (N = 36)
N = Neuro (N = 21)
B = Behavior (N = 25)

Note: Staff judgments of psychiatric problems refer only to mothers who had not themselves reported such problems.

were willing to take them on. The mothers of neurologically impaired children more typically expressed unwillingness to entrust the child's care to anybody else. Often they said that they alone had the necessary patience and knew the child's "ways" well enough to meet his or her needs.

In addition to demographic facts, chapter 3 reported some items that concerned maternal attitudes and behavior characteristics. In some of these areas we found sharp differences between the mothers of deviant children and those of intact ones. In figure 7.2 we show for all three groups the proportion of mothers who reported or exhibited psychiatric problems, as well as the proportion who described themselves as isolated.[1] As mentioned earlier, a mother's spontaneous report of psychi-

1. Perhaps it should be mentioned that, unlike most of our other calculations, the percentages in figure 7.2 are based not on the frequency of scores but on the number of mothers who reported the relevant information or who clearly manifested behavior that justified a staff judgment. Thus, whether a mother spoke about her problems often or very rarely, she was counted only once, and the presence of psychopathology received a single score whether the condition was transient or chronic.

atric illness and the staff's judgment that psychopathology was present even though the mother made no mention of it were scored separately. From figure 7.2 we learn that both acknowledged and unacknowledged psychiatric problems were very rare among mothers of intact children.

Among the twenty-five mothers of children who had major behavior difficulties, however, sixteen (64%) reported and/or displayed psychiatric problems of their own. Few mothers of children in the neuro group thought of themselves as suffering from psychiatric difficulty, or perhaps they were unwilling to divulge concerns about themselves. Yet five (24%) of the twenty-one mothers in this group manifested symptoms (chiefly depression and anxiety) much like those that other equally afflicted mothers referred to as mental health problems.

Several questions must be asked in connection with these findings. One of them concerns the relatively high incidence of acknowledged, or else very overt, psychological disturbance among our mothers. In the entire research population, intact, neuro, and behavior groups combined, 20% of the mothers considered themselves to be emotionally disturbed or, as they were apt to think of it, as suffering from severe nervous troubles. Our coding scores were not based on any sort of psychiatric evaluation. All we knew for certain was that these women described themselves as suffering from such difficulties as sleeplessness, crying spells, inability to eat, feelings of extreme tension and agitation, fearfulness, and uncontrollable rages. If these and similar states meant that periodically these mothers could not cook or clean house, or had to withdraw from their children for fear of hurting them in anger, or felt so anxious away from home that they could neither shop nor visit relatives, or stayed in bed most of the day, then we considered the difficulty severe enough to merit scoring.[2] Such disruptions of at least fairly adequate functioning tended to be transient. Some of these mothers had recurrent episodes, but between times could manage well enough. In some we witnessed a single episode in response to an acute life crisis, such as an unexpected divorce. It should be mentioned that symptoms of lesser magnitude were reported by a great many of our mothers who were never considered for the psychiatric difficulty category. Mild depressions, low-level anxiety, tension headaches, and irascible tempers were often described to us.

For the population at large the incidence of moderately severe though time-limited psychological disturbance and of subclinical yet distressing symptoms is not known. The little information that has surfaced comes primarily from social casework, from clinical records, more recently from descriptive accounts emanating from the women's liberation movement, and, last but not least, from published autobiographies. Such sources suggest that the incidence of psychopathology in our research group is no larger than might be found in any unselected sample. As

2. The research population contained a few psychotic women who required periodic hospitalization and also a few drug addicts. These more gravely impaired individuals, however, seldom assumed primary caretaking responsibility for their child, and thus most were excluded from our coding procedure.

yet the consequences of this kind of stress reaction among mothers for the children in their care have been explored by novelists, not by psychologists or social scientists.

None of this would be important in connection with our study of premature infants were it not for the striking association between the presence of such maternal upsets and the occurrence of behavior difficulties in the children at toddler ages. That maladjustment should occur more often in the children of mothers who are themselves beset by emotional distress would be expected. But the magnitude of the difference between mothers in the intact and behavior groups exceeds expectation. Clinicians, social workers, and early childhood educators know from first-hand experience how often children cope and develop rather well in spite of the fact that they live in families where manifest psychopathology exists. Conversely, among the behaviorally maladapted children whom professionals come to know, a goodly proportion are reared in families who, by ordinary standards, function quite as well as most other families.

That so large a number of children in the behavior group had mothers suffering from serious difficulties of their own is out of step with what clinical experience would lead us to anticipate. We wondered whether some characteristics of our research children made them especially vulnerable to less than optimal conditions of childrearing. Two tentative suggestions can be made. One has to do with the age at which our children were observed. It is only within recent years that developmental difficulties in very young children have aroused much professional concern. Such concern is most often focused on learning difficulties rather than on other behavior problems that may precede or accompany them. Thus nobody knows how many toddlers go through phases of disequilibrium during which they function so maladaptively as to arrest or distort developmental processes, at least temporarily. It is more than likely that many behaviorally deviant children return to normal patterns of adaptive functioning in the course of further growth and development.

Although the follow-up studies are not completed, more than half of our research population is participating in a study that follows them into school age. Those from the behavior group who were seen again at the age of 6 years were, for the most part, not characterized as overtly and significantly maladapted at the later age. Yet only a very few functioned well in all areas. In other words, the fact that 64% of the toddlers with behavior problems were cared for by mothers suffering from a degree of psychopathology does not mean that the incidence of maladjustment would be equally high at school age or beyond. The upshot of all these considerations is that perhaps at toddler age, when the relationship to the mother is at the fulcrum of all development, children are more vulnerable to the disruptive or unsatisfying consequences of maternal emotional disturbance than will be true at somewhat later ages. Whether or not very early behavior disorders of the kind we observed exert a limiting or otherwise detrimental influence upon subsequent development is a completely open question.

The second suggestion, entirely compatible with what has been said already, is the possibility that prematurity has a bearing on the issue. The literature on prematures suggests, and our own observations tend to confirm, that low-birth-weight infants are less resilient in the face of stress and deprivation than are full-term babies. This may also apply to the toddler's capacity to cope with a family atmosphere made less gratifying and more disruptive than is usually the case by emotional problems on mother's part. We think the notion worthy of consideration, though on the basis of our observations we can do no more than speculate.

In figure 7.2 we also show the large proportion of mothers in the behavior group who felt themselves to be, and by description were, isolated. By isolation we mean not only that there was no other adult to share the home, but also that the mother was not connected to a social network of any kind. In these mothers social isolation appears to have been largely a consequence of their own psychopathology. Of the women who were isolated at one time or another during the study period, all but

Figure 7.3 Overt Delight and Overt Negative Affect toward Child in Mothers of Three Groups (Ages Combined, in Percentage)

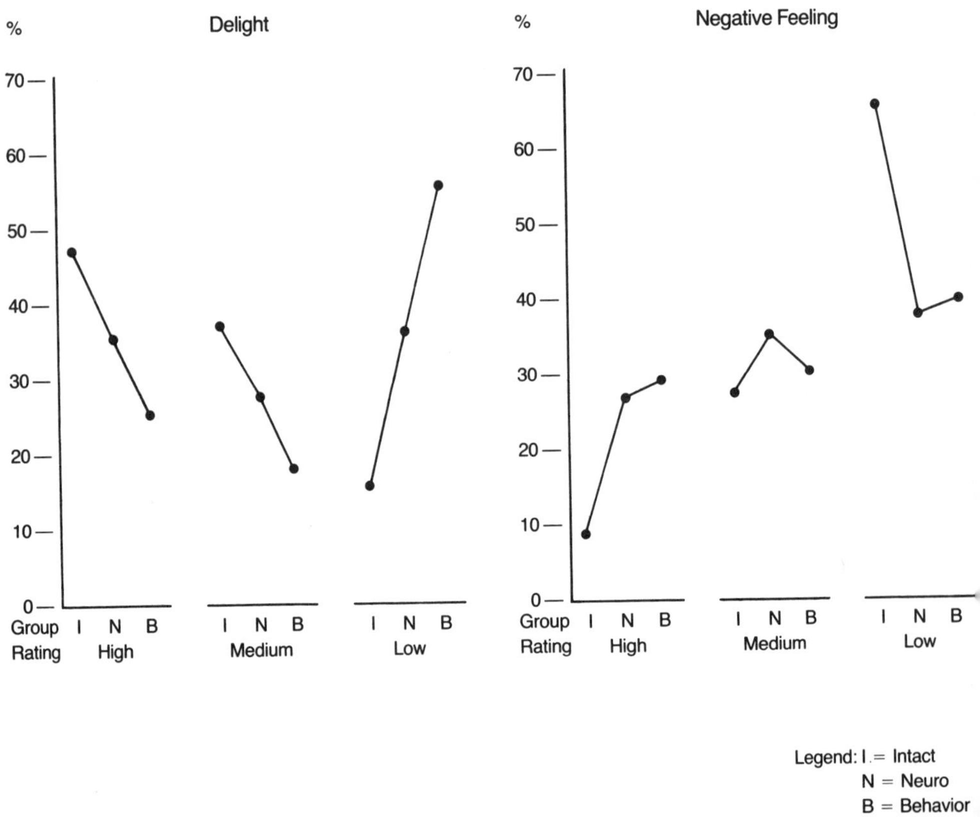

two also reported or manifested psychiatric difficulties. In our research group, the circumstances associated with the emergence of fairly serious behavioral disturbances in the children at preschool age include both maternal psychopathology and temporary isolation of the mothers.

One other background characteristic differentiated between the intact and the behavior group. This was the extent to which mothers tended to express overt delight and, conversely, openly negative feelings in relation to the child. In figure 7.3 we show how many mothers in each group received each of the three possible ratings on these dimensions. Mothers of behaviorally disturbed children showed delight in the child far less often than did those of intact children. In fact, a good half of the mothers in the behavior group were not observed to show pleasure or pride in the child as compared to only 16% in the intact group.

Predominantly negative feelings about the child were expressed by many more of the behavior and also of the neuro mothers than by those of intact children. Correspondingly, the virtual absence of the display of negative feelings was by far more typical of the intact group. These are not two different ways of recording the same state of affairs. It is quite possible, and was indeed observed that a mother seldom if ever expressed delight in relation to the child but, at the same time, did not express negative feelings either. As far as the conspicuous display of negative feelings about the baby was concerned, the neuro and behavior groups were similar to one another. Because of our definition of negative feeling, this similarity is more apparent than real. At the negative pole we scored strong annoyance, anger, and something akin to dislike, but we also scored the expression of worry and concern when it was of such pervasiveness and intensity as to be painful, leaving little room for enjoyment of the baby. In the neuro group negative feelings were almost always of the last-mentioned sort. In the behavior group worry and concern occurred quite often, but so did anger and irritable dislike.

Clinician members of the research team were fascinated to observe that all but one of the maladjusted children (and he had strong autistic features) whose mothers credibly reported that the child was nothing but a burden to them and/or seemed unable to show approval or affection openly nonetheless developed a strong and dependent relationship with the mother. They clung to her, protested separation from her and some sought to please and beguile her persistently, but without notable success. The quality of these relationships was of course tenuous and typically ambivalent and almost certainly lay at the core of the behavior difficulties that the children had developed. Yet observations such as this again confirm what other clinical experience also taught us: that an intense attachment to the mothering person is not always based on previous or current gratifying contact with her. It may also arise from strong needs for intimacy and security that remain largely unfulfilled while, at the same time, mother remains a centrally important person in the baby's life.

The next thing we needed to know was how our atypical children fared with respect to cognitive development, and to what extent the connections among SES, IQ, and IC held true for them. In figure 7.4 we show the mean IQ for each of the

Figure 7.4 Mean IQ for Intact, Neuro, and Behavior Groups by Age

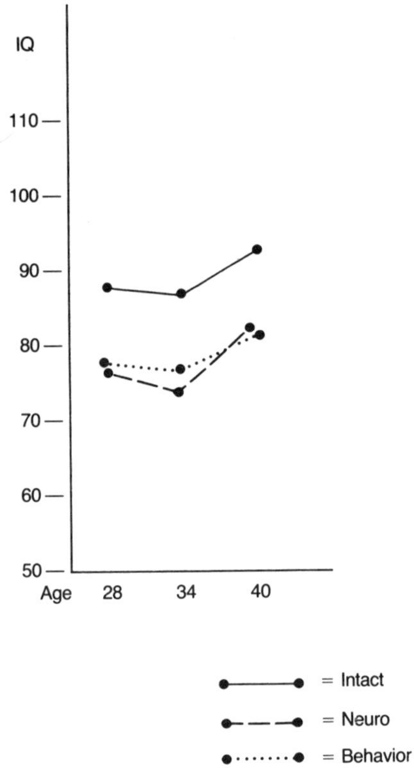

three groups at the ages of most concern to us. As one would expect, both of the deviant groups had mean IQs below that for the intact one. But, contrary to expectation, there was next to no difference in mean IQ between the neuro and behavior groups. The former included children of high intelligence who suffered from mild or moderate deficits in the sensory or motor areas, yet it also included cortically damaged children who were severely retarded. As shown in Figure 7.5, similar mean IQs resulted from very different patterns of performance. Most of the behaviorally disturbed children had IQs in the borderline or dull normal range (70 to 89); very few of the Neuro children fell within that range. Instead, they tended to be either markedly retarded or well within the normal range. Specifically, among the neurologically impaired, 62% (at 34 months) to 88% (at 28 months) attained IQ scores either below 70 or above 90.

We then wondered whether the effect of socioeconomic status of the family upon the cognitive development of the offspring was as pronounced in the deviant groups as we found it to be in the intact one. In table 7.2 we show that a correlation

Figure 7.5 IQ Distribution for Neuro and Behavior Groups at Three Ages

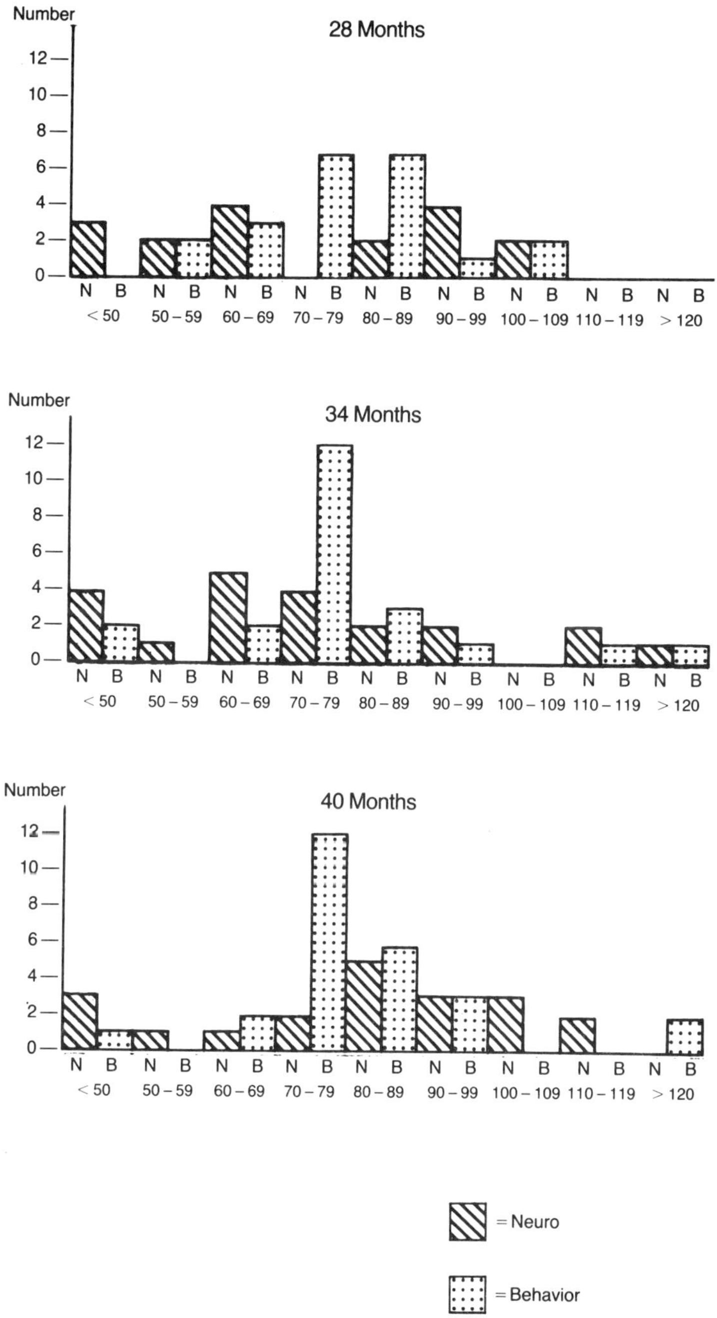

Table 7.2: Pearson Correlation between SES Index and IQ (Deviant Group, by Age)

Age (in months)	*r*	*S*
7*	.0122	.468
15*	.0861	.287
28	.3197	.021
34	.4972	.000
40	.3873	.004

*At age 7 and 15 months MDI scores were calculated on the basis of age corrected for prematurity.

exists between the SES index and IQ for the entire deviant group. Much as we found among the intact children, this correlation is significant between the ages of 28 and 40 months, but not earlier. In table 7.3 we give the mean IQ for each SES quartile in all three groups. In the deviant groups, the number of children in each quartile is very small, yet a consistent pattern does emerge. In figure 7.6, which is based on the same data, we show more clearly that there is a massive difference in cognitive development between children in quartile I and those in quartile IV. This discrepancy is quite as large as that reported for the intact children. Although the intact group shows an orderly increase in mean IQ from one SES quartile to the next, this cannot be said for either of the deviant groups. In the behavior group, the mean IQs for quartiles I, II, and III barely differ from one another. In the neuro group, the

Table 7.3: Mean IQ by SES for Intact, Neuro, Behavior, and Total Deviant Groups by Age

	Intact			*Deviant*			*Neuro*			*Behavior*		
	Age			*Age*			*Age*			*Age*		
SES I	28	34	40	28	34	40	28	34	40	28	34	40
N	11	14	16	9	10	10	3	4	4	6	6	6
IQ	76.2	71.5	78.0	69.4	67.0	72.9	65.6	67.2	67.2	71.3	68.6	76.6
St.D	15.8	19.7	15.3									
SES II												
N	12	11	12	10	12	11	5	6	5	5	6	6
IQ	82.5	82.6	88.3	76.6	69.7	79.8	78.4	70.3	85.2	74.8	69.1	75.3
St.D	14.2	13.1	13.1									
SES III												
N	15	13	15	11	11	12	5	5	5	6	6	7
IQ	93.2	93.7	95.6	76.5	73.7	79.6	70.6	69.2	77.0	81.5	77.5	81.4
St.D	11.8	16.2	12.7									
SES IV												
N	14	13	14	10	10	12	5	6	6	5	4	6
IQ	97.8	99.1	106.3	83.4	92.5	91.7	85.8	89.3	92.5	81.0	97.2	91.0
St.D	11.8	14.7	13.8									

Figure 7.6 Mean IQ by SES Quartile for Three Groups by Age

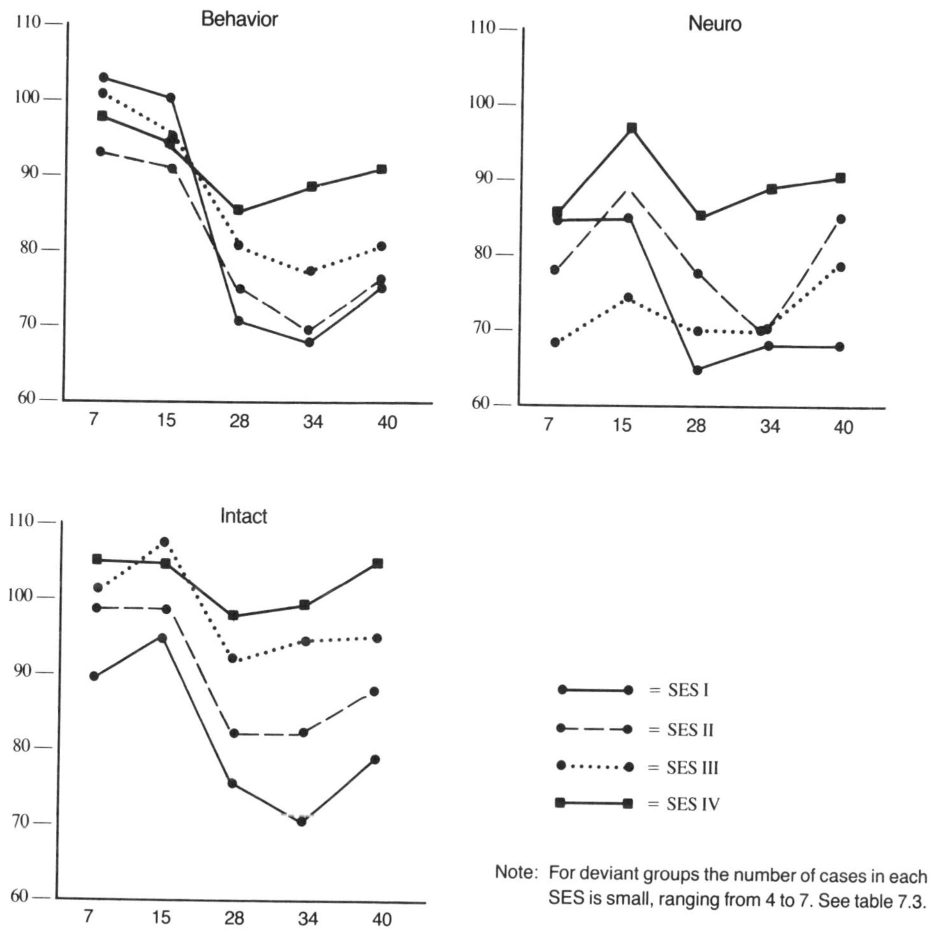

Note: For deviant groups the number of cases in each SES is small, ranging from 4 to 7. See table 7.3.

mean for quartile II floats above that for Q-III throughout. This apparent anomaly is easily explained. It so happened that the Q-III children, as a group, were more severely damaged than those in Q-II. (Figure 7.6 shows that, even at 7 months of age, the mean MDI for Q-III Neuro children was 68, while that for the other quartiles ranged from 78 to 87.)

A somewhat more discriminating measure of SES effects upon the early development of the deviant children shows the relationship between the distribution of IQ scores and social class (figure 7.7). The number of cases within each IQ range is so small that we thought it best to combine adjacent SES quartiles and thus to compare

Figure 7.7 Distribution of IQ Scores by SES for Neuro and Behavior Groups (Ages Combined, in Percentage)

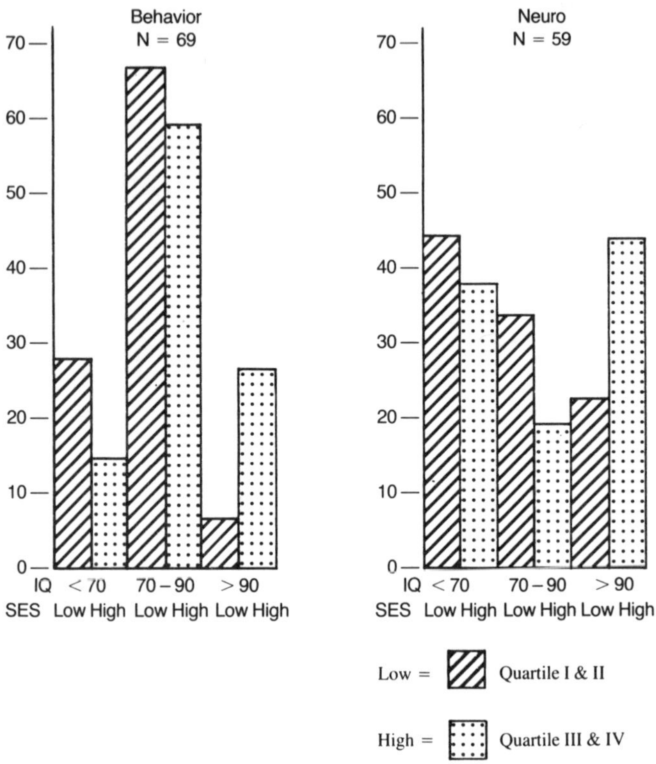

a high with a low socioeconomic group. For the same reason, scores obtained at the three age levels were combined. Clearly, the low SES group contained a larger proportion of retarded children while the high group contributed by far the largest proportion of those with IQs above 90. In this respect, there are practically no differences between the intact and the behaviorally deviant groups.

The neuro children showed a more limited but definite relationship between social class and cognitive status. The high SES group contained many more children who had IQs above 90, but SES did not affect how many children fell into the retarded range. Clinically, this makes good sense. Children who have suffered cortical damage respond well to favorable environmental settings but are not likely to reach normal levels of cognitive functioning. Children whose neurological impairment did not significantly involve the cortex are expected to respond to learning opportunities in much the same manner as do healthy children. In short, socioeconomic background is related to cognitive development in children who showed pronounced behavior difficulties as well as in those who were neurologically impaired. Yet in both deviant groups, factors other than social class affected the learning process to a considerable extent, more so than was the case for the intact group.

If impulse control is as important for overall development and for cognitive development as we have proposed, there should be great differences in this respect between the intact and the deviant groups. In fact, we found radical differences between the two deviant groups; in addition, we also found that both deviant groups differ sharply from the intact one (figure 7.8). The distribution of IC scores in the intact group took the form of a steep normal curve. More or less by definition, the large majority of children were held to manifest an age-appropriate balance between control and impulsivity (a score of 3). A degree of undercontrol and unusually strong control were seen in a comparatively small number. For the behavior group, we show in figure 7.8 that most children were undercontrolled, with only 22% receiving the age-appropriate score of 3. The few instances of simultaneous over- and undercontrol, which also indicates a special problem with impulse control, occurred only in the behavior group. Overall, the level and distribution of impulse-control scores were radically different in the behavior and intact groups.

Figure 7.8 Distribution of IC Scores for Neuro and Behavior Groups (Ages Combined, in Percentage)

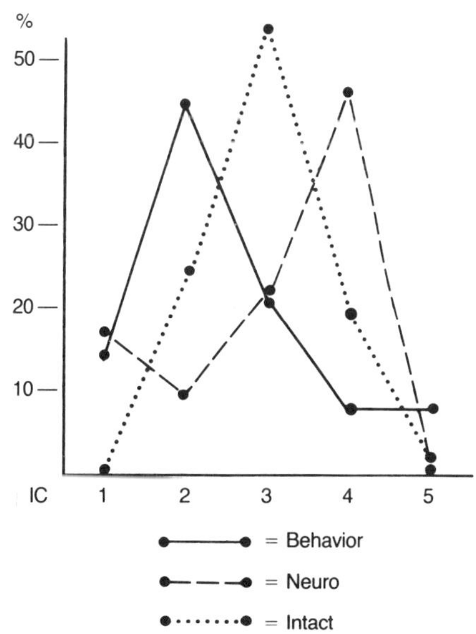

The comparable data for the neuro group are at first glance surprising. As a function of brain damage we might expect a large proportion of these children to suffer from a lack of impulse control. Instead we find that undercontrol, especially at the more moderate level corresponding to an IC score of 2, was quite rare. Pervasive overcontrol (4) was the most common, though a near-absence of control, as reflected in a score of 1, was also seen. Among the neurologically impaired children who found their way into our research population, impulse control tended to be a matter of either/or. There were those who could not muster even low levels of control, yet many more learned to defend themselves against threatening impulsivity by suppressing overt response to excitatory states to an unusual degree. The term *learned* is used advisedly. Not only did we have the chance to see some of these children literally struggle for control, becoming tense and sometimes tremulous as they held their voices at low volume, moved restlessly, and showed autonomic signs of effort such as labored breathing or changes in skin color, but we also observed that the proportion of neuro children who exerted greater control than most agemates rose from 36% at 28 months to 46% at 34 and 54% at 40 months. In short, the distribution of impulse-control scores was vastly different in the deviant and intact groups, and only a small proportion in either deviant group conformed to normal expectation. While the behavior group tended to be undercontrolled, the neuro group was distinguished by the prominence of overcontrol.

It would seem that the nature of the developmental deficit in the deviant groups accounts for much of the variation in impulse control. For this reason it is possible that there is no direct link between social class and the rate at which these children developed ego control. In figure 7.9, where we show the frequency with which each IC score occurred within each SES quartile, it is clear that social class has a limiting but by no means determining effect on the distribution of IC scores. Once again we used the combined scores from all age groups. In the behavior group the very lowest level (IC 1) was most frequent in quartile I while the only children who were judged to be overcontrolled were members of quartile IV. Otherwise, levels of impulse control did not systematically vary with the socioeconomic setting in which these children lived. Among the neuro children only one SES effect is discernible: overcontrol was the more frequent the higher the social class.

Having found definite but limited associations between socioeconomic status and cognitive development, as well as between SES and the development of ego control, we now address our central theme. That is, we can now explore whether or not less than appropriate degrees of impulse control lead to less than age-appropriate cognitive development in children who show neurological impairment and in those with fairly severe behavior problems. If the theoretical considerations advanced before are correct, the relative lack of impulse control should tend to delay or retard cognitive development (in our age group), whether this is due to a deficit in the central nervous system (CNS), to emotional difficulties, or to experience that fails to promote the development of impulse control. In table 7.4, the mean IQ is given for each IC score for the deviant groups. For convenience we have

Figure 7.9 SES Distribution for Each IC Score for Neuro and Behavior Groups (Ages Combined)

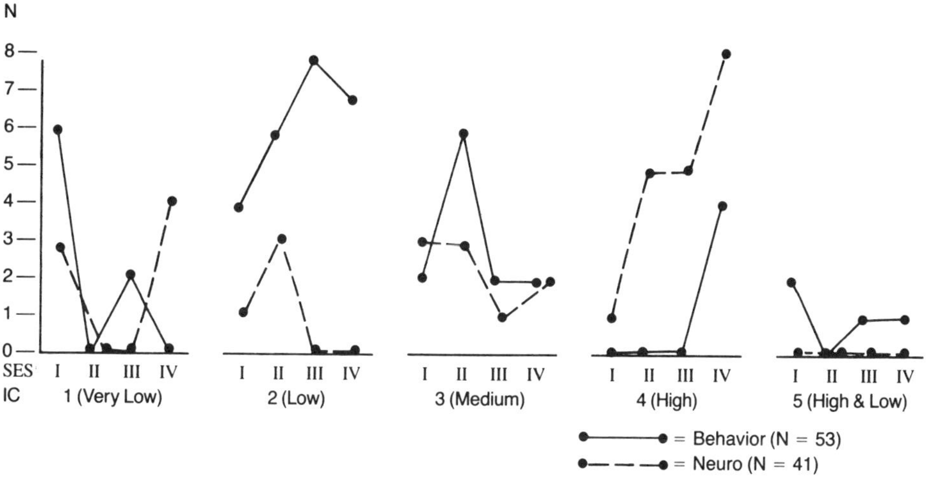

added the corresponding values for the intact group, although they have already been reported in chapter 4. These means are a bit difficult to interpret because the number of children in some IC categories is so small. Unfortunately, it was precisely in the deviant groups that it was often impossible to obtain a valid IC score. Small as the numbers are, the pattern is much the same at each age level, so

Table 7.4: Mean IQ for Each IC Scores for Intact, Behavior, and Neuro Groups by Age

	IC Score										
Age	*1*		*2*		*3*		*4*		*5*		*N*
Intact Group	N	IQ	N	IQ	N	IQ	N	IQ	N	IQ	
28	1	66.0	12	77.1	23	94.1	10	100.2	0		46
34	0		10	74.9	19	93.8	9	97.9	1	62.0	39
40	0		11	86.0	25	94.6	9	105.8	1	73.0	46
Total	1		33	79.3	67	94.1	28	102.3	2	67.5	131
Behavior Group											
28	3	70.3	8	77.2	4	87.5	2	84.5	2	76.5	19
34	2	78.5	8	71.2	5	79.2	1	125.0	0		16
40	3	80.3	9	83.8	4	75.7	1	126.0	1	81.0	18
Total	8	76.1	25	77.7	13	80.7	4	105.0	3	78.0	53
Neuro Group											
28	3	57.3	1	61.0	3	96.3	4	97.0	0		11
34	2	49.5	1	67.5	4	77.0	7	98.0	0		14
40	2	49.5	2	72.5	2	89.0	8	99.1	0		14
Total	7	52.8	4	67.5	9	86.1	19	98.2	0		39

that mean IQs for each IC score, when ages are combined, can be accepted as a reasonable index of the underlying relationship. In table 7.4 we show that relatively low IQs prevail among the behaviorally disturbed children so that it made little difference whether controls were poor or adequate. The single behavior group child who was overcontrolled at each age (and contributed three of the four scores in that column) showed accelerated cognitive development. Among the neurologically impaired children we do find the anticipated positive association between level of impulse control and mean IQ.

More important than mean IQ is the question of the degree to which the risk of mental retardation is indexed by the presence of poor control even in maladjusted or neurologically impaired children. In figure 7.10 we compare the distribution of IQ scores for children whose control was inadequate (scores of 1, 2, or 5) with the distribution for those with adequate controls (scores of 3 or 4). In both the behavior

Figure 7.10 Distribution of IQ Scores for Well-Controlled and Ill-Controlled Children in Neuro and Behavior Groups (Ages Combined, in Percentage)

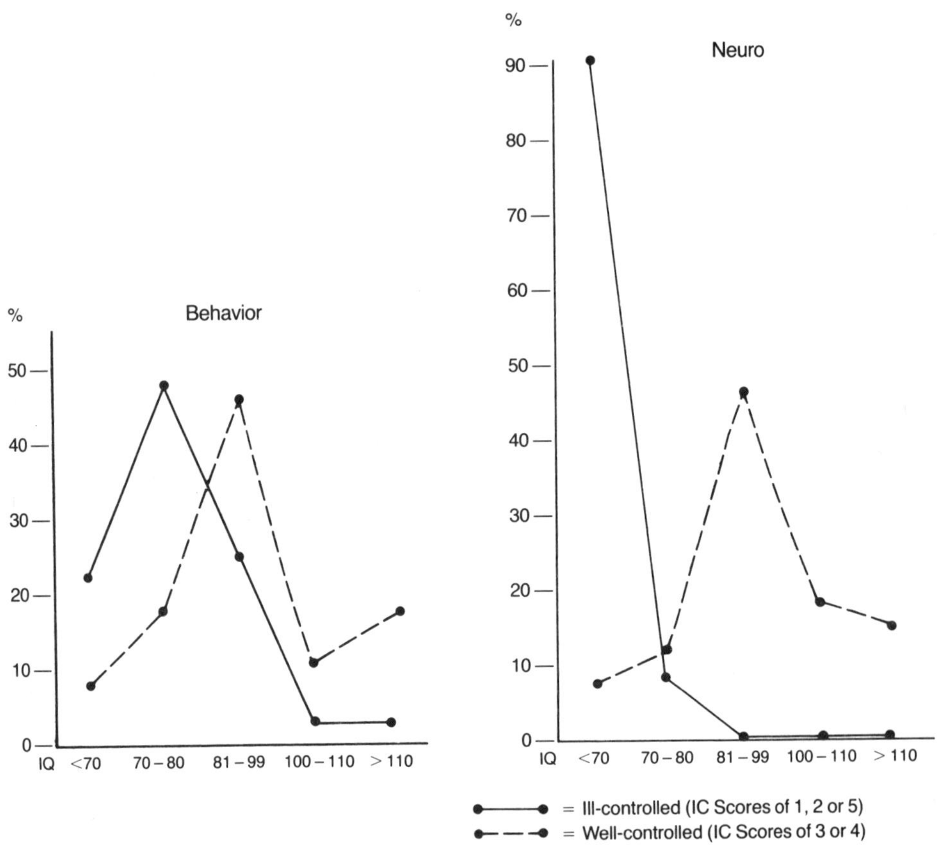

and the neuro group low IQs were found chiefly in children whose IC was low for age whereas, with one exception, IQs at or above 100 were observed only in children with adequate control. Average IQ scores for these children, ranging from 81 to 99, also occurred more often when control was adequate. For the neuro group the dependence of IQ upon IC is more dramatic than for either the behavior or the intact group. Here impulse control played a decisive role in determining whether or not intellectual development could proceed in a fairly normal fashion. All the neuro children who lacked to some extent impulse control had IQs below 80. Only two of the children with adequate impulse control (contributing five scores between them) fell below the 80 level. In summary, all the data concerned with cognitive test scores and impulse control in deviant children confirm what had already been found for the intact group: impoverished or impaired cognitive development is found predominantly when impulse control is less than age-appropriate. In our consideration of the issue for the intact group, we stressed that good ego control does not necessarily lead to good cognitive development, but that a lack of such control is an impediment to cognitive advance, at least during the toddler years. The comparisons given in Figure 7.10 are wholly compatible with this formulation.

For the intact children it was possible to demonstrate a correspondence between cognitive status, SES, and impulse control. Figure 7.11 is designed to do the same

Figure 7.11 Mean IQ and Mean IC by SES Quartiles for Three Groups (Ages Combined)

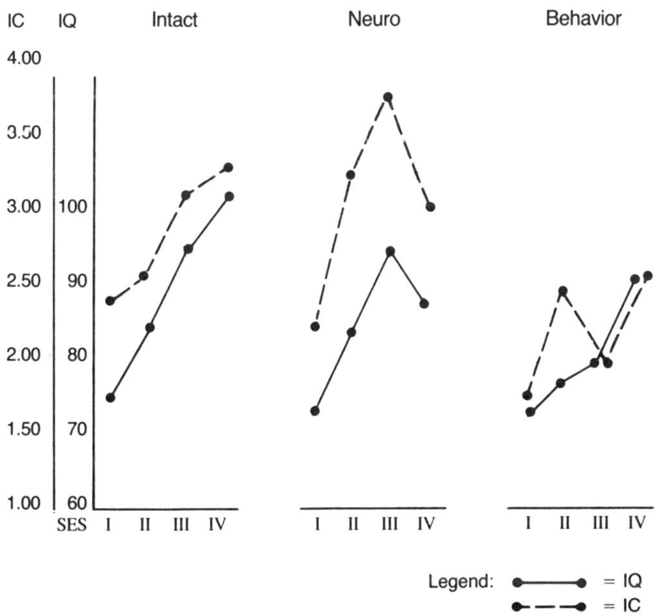

for our neuro and behavior groups. For the intact group it had been possible to report mean IQs for the well controlled, as compared to the poorly controlled, children within each quartile. For our deviant groups this would have been unsatisfactory because the lower quartiles contained very few children whose ego control was adequate. Therefore, in figure 7.11 we show the mean IQ as well as the mean IC for each quartile. It demonstrates that there is an upward drift from one SES quartile to the next both in IQ and in IC scores. In the behavior group, however, impulse control was less than age-adequate in all quartiles, which accounts for the fact that increases in mean IQ are very small except for the jump from Q-III to Q-IV. As we have seen from other ways of looking at the same material, the rise and fall in IC and IQ run closely parallel in the neuro group. The coordination to social class is nevertheless inconsistent because the fourth quartile contained some more severely brain-injured children, which lowered mean scores for IQ and IC.

In summary, for the neurologically impaired and behaviorally disturbed children we found the same network of interrelationships noted in the intact group, albeit with some exceptions. In both deviant groups cognitive scores tended to rise with ascending SES, as did the levels of impulse control that the children managed to achieve. In both deviant groups relatively poor impulse control went with relatively low cognitive test scores, and relatively high IQs were typically attained by children whose impulse control was unusually tight. There were also differences between the two deviant groups, chiefly that a degree of undercontrol was prevalent among the maladjusted children whereas overcontrol was predominant among the neurologically impaired.

Chapter 8

Experience Patterns and Developmental Outcome

We have seen that test scores and levels of impulse control in both of our deviant groups differed greatly from those observed in the intact group, and also that cognitive development and impulse control scores for behaviorally disturbed children showed altogether different distributions from those for the neuro group. We now want to see whether the experience patterns characteristic of each of the two deviant groups show equally sharp differences when compared to those of the intact group.

In figure 8.1 we show the distribution of ratings for each experience pattern for the behavior and the neuro groups. To facilitate the comparisons to be made we have added the distribution curves for the intact group as well. For the deviant children we are dealing with exeedingly small numbers at each age level; therefore figure 8.1 combines the ratings for the three ages.

Two aspects of experience, the intensity of maternal involvement and focused attention, received much the same ratings in the deviant and intact groups. One might note, however, that minimal involvement with the baby on the mother's part occurred only a few times among the behaviorally disturbed children and not at all in the other groups. The fact that all of our youngsters received about the same amount of focused attention obscures very real differences in this respect. We had defined this variable very broadly, and the nature of the interactions that took place while an adult's attention was wholly focused on the child was typically somewhat different in each of these groups. For the behavior group intense disciplinary encounters as well as vigorous and at times provocative play episodes loomed large. In the neuro group, mothers often needed to concentrate on the child if routine chores such as dressing and feeding were to be accomplished with some efficiency. These kinds of episodes also occurred among the intact children but other varieties, such as sustained reciprocal play and shared activity (for example, looking at picture books), contributed to the final rating for these children far more often.

For structure, accommodation, and didacticism, differences between the deviant and intact groups are very striking. The absence or minimal presence of behavioral events that fell into one of these patterns was noted in a great many of the behaviorally disturbed children while among the intact ones this was a fairly rare state of affairs. The neurologically impaired children fell in between the other

Figure 8.1 Distribution of EP Ratings for Three Groups (Ages Combined, in Percentage)

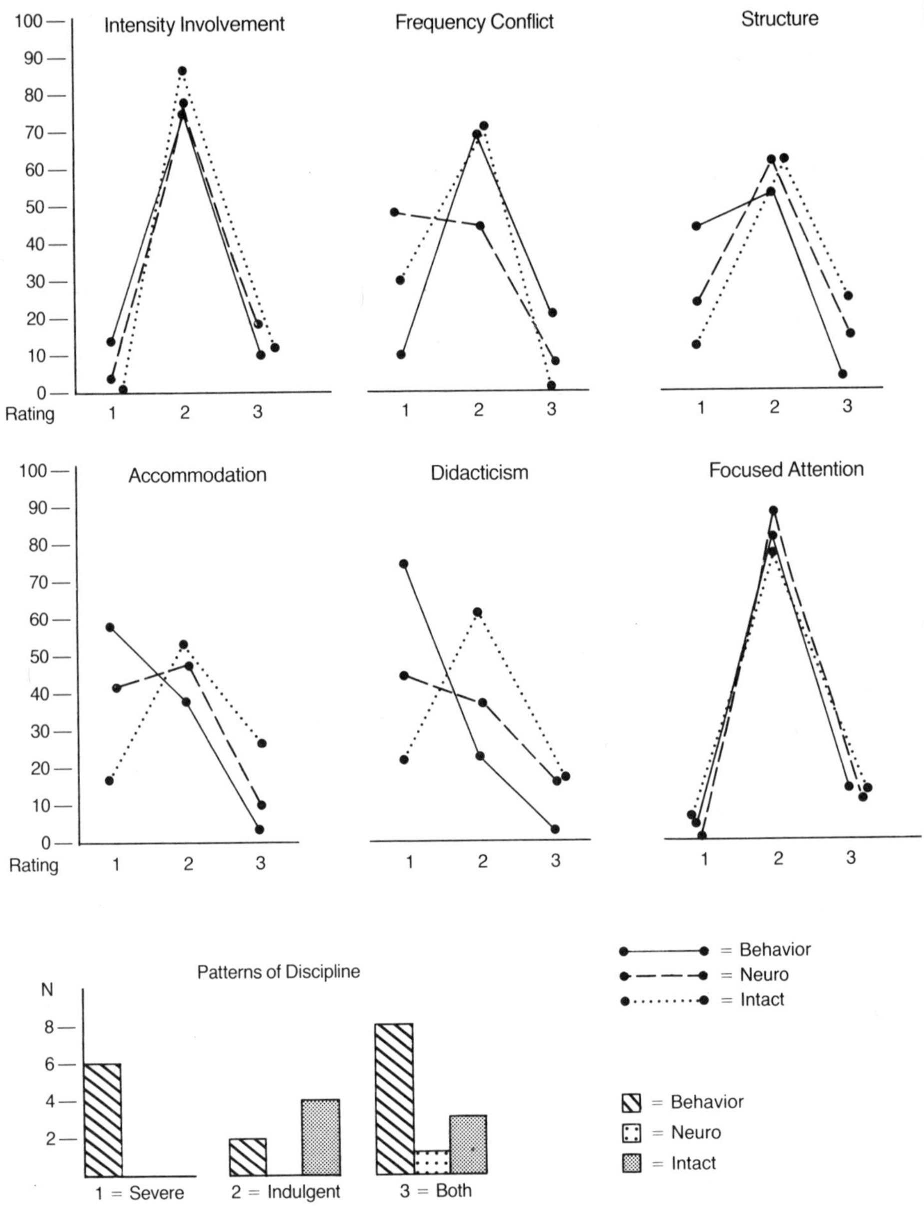

two groups: they lacked these varieties of experience more frequently than intact children, but not to the extent noted in the behavior group. At the same time, a very high prominence of these experience patterns was almost never seen in the deviant children. In consequence the medium score of 2, characteristic for the majority of children in the intact group, was by no means the most frequent for the behavior group in the areas of accommodation and didacticism, and barely so with respect to structure. The three groups also differed substantially in the relative frequency of conflict with adults. The rating of absent or minimally present was seen in almost a third of the intact children but was very rare among the deviant ones. Conversely, the rating of prominent or very frequent occurred almost exclusively in the behavior and neuro groups, though even there it was not common. In figure 8.1 we also report on selected patterns of discipline (by number of ratings rather than percent); we find that unremitting severity and the combination of marked severity and marked indulgence were most frequent in the behavior group. The one remaining pattern, pervasive and consistent indulgence, was very rare and then applied mostly to intact children. Overall, it is apparent that those experience patterns that in intact children bear a strong and positive association with both impulse control and cognitive advance are often lacking in the lives of children whose development was impeded for one reason or another.

We already know that social-class differences existed in relation to cognitive development among the deviant children, though they were not so marked or so consistent as in the intact group. Critical questions to be examined are: (a) do differences in daily life experience (EP ratings) correspond to differences in the rate of cognitive development, and (b) are differences in EP ratings largely accounted for by social class, or is it the quality of responsiveness on the part of these somewhat atypical children that yields a relative lack of supportive life experience? As a first step in that direction we turn to an inspection of the direct relationship between SES and patterns of experience. To be consistent with what has gone before, the distribution of EP ratings should vary somewhat with social class but not so decisively as was true for the intact group. For our deviant group we present the relevant information in figure 8.2. The format of this figure is like that of figure 6.2, but it will be best again to describe briefly how to read it. The columns represent EP ratings from high (3) to low (1) in descending order. The rows represent SES quartiles from low (I) to high (IV), and we report the number of ratings rather than proportions. In figure 8.2 we show that neither intensity of maternal involvement nor frequency of conflict seem to depend on social class. (The possible exception is that in the neuro group it was only in quartile IV that unusually little conflict was observed.) These two aspects of experience were found to be independent of SES for the intact group as well.

With respect to the degree of structure in the child's life, our expectation was fulfilled, although within limits. In the neuro group a virtual absence of structure could be found in every quartile, but very highly structured daily life was seen only in children from the upper groups. It is worth noting in passing that a lack of

Figure 8.2 Distribution of EP Ratings by SES for Neuro and Behavior Groups (Ages Combined)

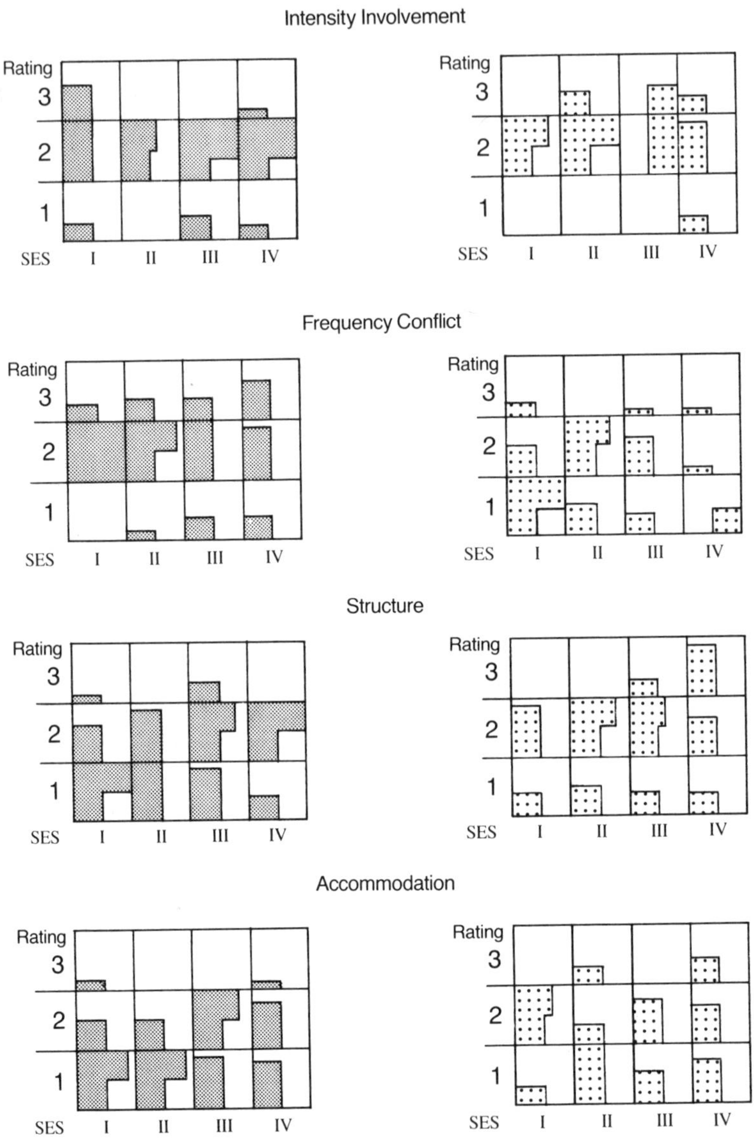

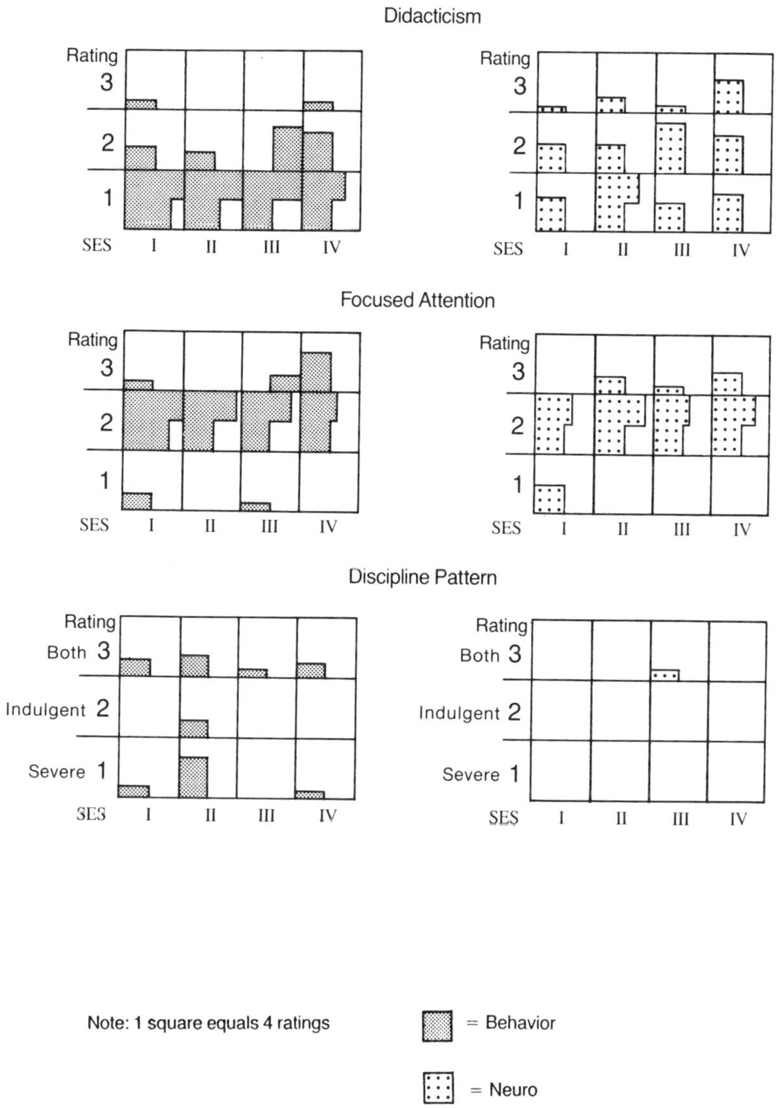
Didacticism
Rating
3
2
1
SES I II III IV
Focused Attention
Discipline Pattern
Both 3
Indulgent 2
Severe 1
Note: 1 square equals 4 ratings
= Behavior
= Neuro

structure was especially conspicuous in quartile II. This is surprising when we recall that this was the very quartile for which we reported mean IQs higher than those for quartile III. In general, low structure is associated with low IQ, but, unless the means should prove misleading, this does not appear to hold true for the neurologically-impaired children in that quartile. We shall attempt to solve that puzzle when we discuss impulse control and the consequences of (certain kinds of) neurologic deficits for the texture of experience.

The situation for the behavior group is rather different. The relative absence of structured life experience is very largely a function of SES. A rating of next to no structure was assigned in twelve of eighteen instances in quartile I. The frequency of this low rating decreased from one quartile to the next; only three of fifteen such ratings were given in quartile IV. This implies that the social circumstances which accounted for relatively low degrees of structure among the poorer intact children also often counteracted structuring among the behaviorally disturbed youngsters.

Accommodation varied as a function of social class to a lesser degree among the deviant children than among the intact ones. For the neuro group socioeconomic standing had no bearing whatsoever on the degree to which the children were accommodated. In the behavior group a lack of accommodation was fairly widespread in all social groups. A virtual lack of accommodation was more frequent, however, in the two lower quartiles (69% and 73% in Q-I and Q-II *vs.* 41% and 46% in Q-III and Q-IV).

In the deviant groups the potential influence of socioeconomic status upon didacticism was overshadowed by the fact that in all social groups so many of the children received a score of minimally present, presumably because they could not or would not participate when teaching was attempted. In the neuro group medium and high levels of didacticism occurred somewhat more often in the upper than the lower quartiles. Among the behaviorally deviant children, medium amounts of didactic experience were observed more often in the two upper quartiles.

Focused attention was provided for all the children as a regularly recurrent but not especially prominent aspect of daily life. SES-related differences were not apparent. Last, the somewhat unusual disciplinary patterns we had selected occurred in the behavior but not the neuro group. It may or may not be important that of the seven instances of unrelieved severity, six were contributed by the lower SES groups.

Thus, for the deviant children the effect of social class upon the distribution of experience patterns was limited. In the behavior group a near-absence of structure was closely linked to low SES, and didactic experience was provided somewhat more often in the upper two quartiles. Among the neurologically impaired children high ratings for structure and low ratings for frequency of conflict were limited to the upper SES groups. The fact that SES had a large impact upon experience patterns in the intact group and a lesser impact in the deviant groups confirms the commonsense assumption that the experience of deviant children is shaped by their perception of life situations and by their inherent reaction characteristics to a greater extent than is seen among others. This being the case, the degree to which environmental circumstances (here SES) lead to similar experiential consequences is necessarily reduced.

Theoretically, patterns of experience, regardless of how they come about, should be related systematically to the readiness to develop impulse control at the appropriate ages. We already know that in the deviant groups impulse control covaries with cognitive development in much the same manner as in the intact group, but we have yet to establish a direct link between experience patterns and the emergence of impulse control. The necessary information is conveyed in figure 8.3. We show for each experience pattern rating the distribution of IC scores. In addition, the mean IC for each rating is entered in a column at the extreme left-hand side of figure 8.3.

Our constant struggle with unwieldy data is especially acute in relation to this portion of the data. The number of children receiving any one of the EP ratings ranges from zero to thirty-eight, and much the same unevenness applies to the IC scores, for which the *N* ranged from zero to eighteen. The mean IC for each EP rating is the most straightforward index of an association between the degree to which a particular aspect of experience is associated with impulse control. Unfortunately, some of these means are based on very few scores and thus might be fortuitous. Although it is more cumbersome, the distribution of such IC scores as were available within each EP rating gives a more accurate picture of the relationships involved. Yet to make the IC score distribution comparable in all EP categories, the frequencies had to be transformed into percentages. These percentages, in turn, are the less telling the fewer the number of scores on which they are based. As there is no way out of this dilemma, we decided to enter the appropriate number of ratings beneath each distribution curve. For example, only two neuro children received an EP rating of 3 (frequent, prominent) for frequency of conflict. Both of these children—thus 100%—had exceedingly poor control (IC of 1).

As has been stressed before, we view these numerical comparisons as condensed descriptions that can be useful even when they are meaningless as a statistic. Our thinking has been guided by the principle that quantitative statements based on very small numbers should be given next to no weight if and when they conform to expectation. In such a perspective, the fact that in two children high levels of conflict went with low impulse control is best regarded as a noncontributary item. On the other hand, when even a few instances run counter to our understanding of the matter they should be taken seriously. When we earlier reported that some children with relatively low control nonetheless obtained relatively high IQs, for example, it was worthwhile to examine these exceptions in some detail in order to discover how the unusual or unexpected result came about.

The material brought together in figure 8.3 does not contain surprises of this sort. Those aspects of experience that for the intact group bore a positive relationship to impulse control showed the same relationship for the deviant groups: the mean IC in the areas of structure, accommodation, didacticism, and focused

Figure 8.3 Mean IC and Distribution of IC Scores for Each EP Rating for Behavior and Neuro Groups (Ages Combined, in Percentage)

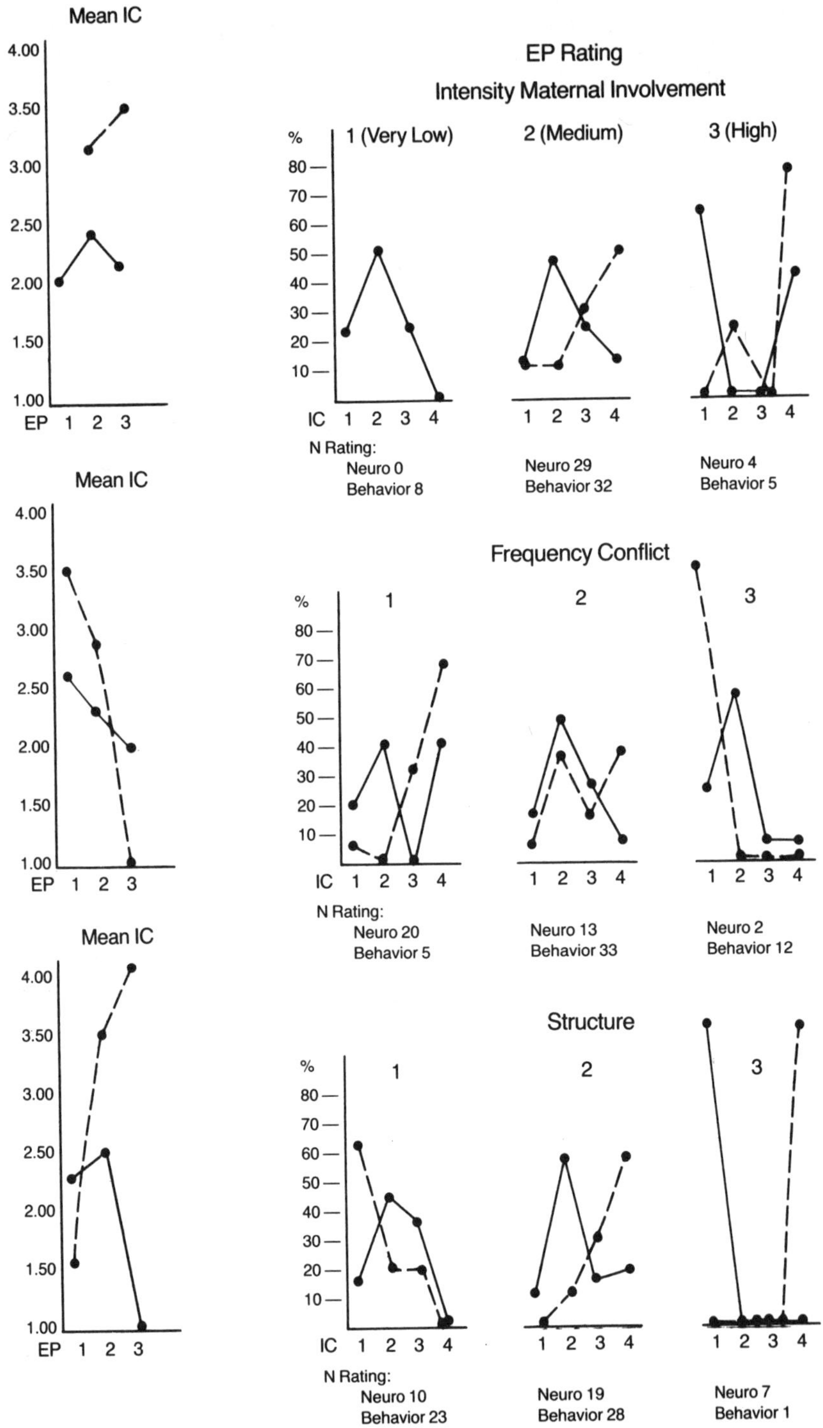

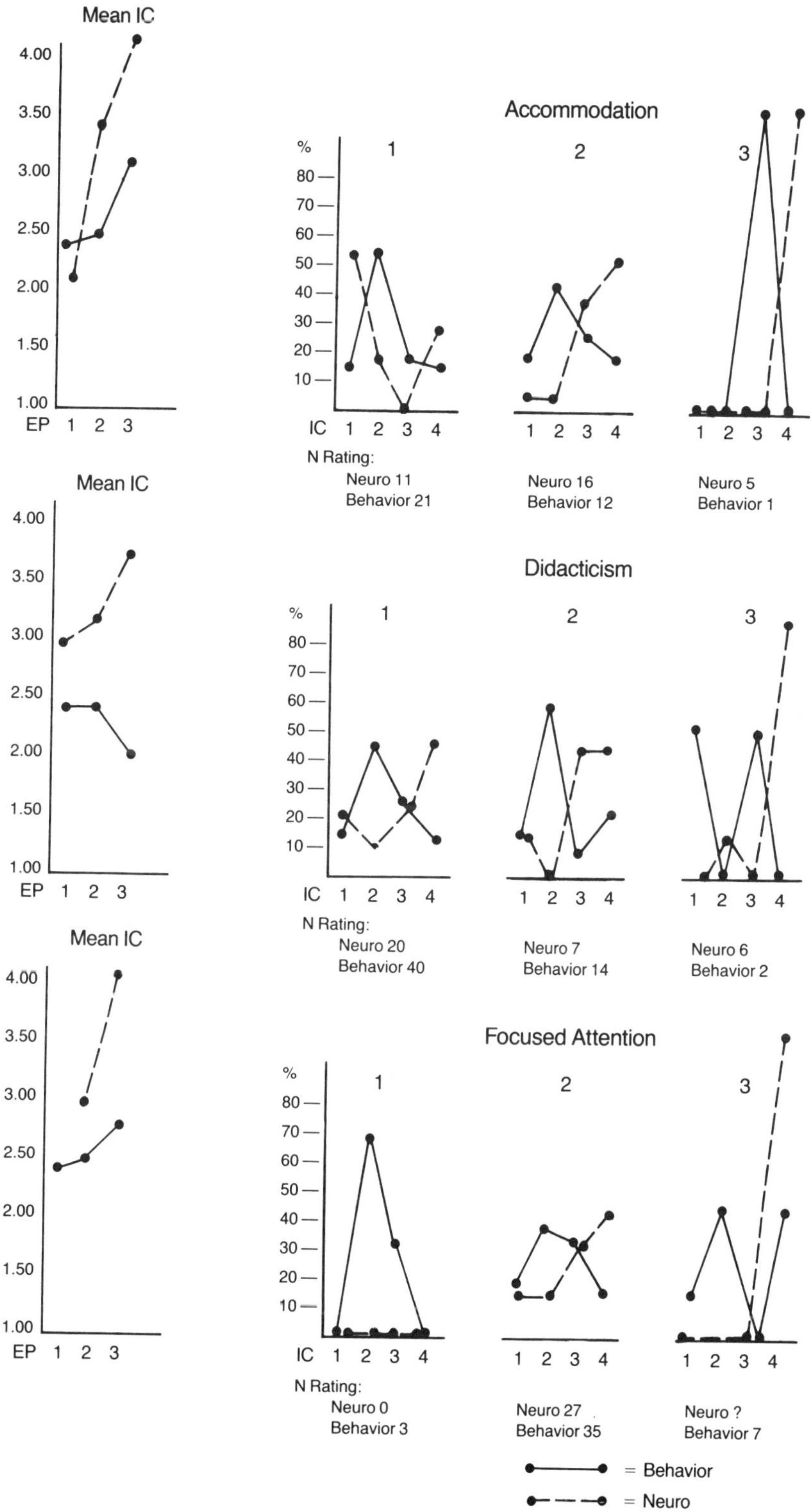

Mean IC
4.00
3.50
3.00
2.50
2.00
1.50
1.00
EP 1 2 3
Accommodation
%
80
70
60
50
40
30
20
10
1
2
3
IC 1 2 3 4
N Rating:
Neuro 11
Behavior 21
Neuro 16
Behavior 12
Neuro 5
Behavior 1
Mean IC
EP 1 2 3
Didacticism
N Rating:
Neuro 20
Behavior 40
Neuro 7
Behavior 14
Neuro 6
Behavior 2
Mean IC
EP 1 2 3
Focused Attention
N Rating:
Neuro 0
Behavior 3
Neuro 27
Behavior 35
Neuro ?
Behavior 7
= Behavior
= Neuro

attention was always low when these experiences were minimally present and a good deal higher when they were a regular though not an especially prominent feature in the children's lives. Among the behaviorally disturbed children these domains of experience were almost never rated as unusually frequent; hence the isolated instances when mean IC was still higher with the shift to a rating of 3 fall into the category of result that we have decided to consider trivial. Some five or six of the neuro children did receive high ratings for these experience patterns, and that this was invariably associated with strong ego control is of some importance, especially because with one exception (didacticism) all of the children with an EP rating of 3 were overly controlled (IC score of 4). The descending mean IC scores as frequency of conflict rises from minimal to high reflects the circumstance that on this experience variable a rating of 3 denotes maximal prominence of a disruptive rather than supportive aspect of experience. We commented earlier that frequent conflict with adults is likely to be a behavioral manifestation of fairly low impulse control, although it could be mitigated or accentuated by whatever caretaking style was prevalent in the home.

The distribution curve of IC scores on the right-hand side of figure 8.3 serves much the same purpose as a scattergram. It allows the reader to judge the degree to which differences in mean IC scores correspond to manifestly different patterns in the raw data. For all ratings except didacticism, the distribution curves confirm the relationship between IC and the EPS, as indicated by the mean values for each. For two children in the behavior group the decrease in mean IC with the transition from medium to massive didactic teaching is an artifact since one had poor impulse control and the other did not, yielding a "mean IC" of 2.00. One is reminded of the fact that for the intact children the level of impulse control was much the same whether didacticism was medium or very great.

Nevertheless, for didacticism, the behavior group differs from the others. The degree of impulse control shown by the behaviorally disturbed children who received no teaching was very much the same as that shown by children who were taught about as much and as often as most peers. This is in sharp contrast to the neuro group and also the intact children, who showed much higher levels of control when there was a moderate amount of teaching than when there was almost none. In general it would seem that those children with behavior problems who were able to participate in teaching or learning situations enjoyed receiving a friendly variety of attention, and their problems with control arose chiefly when they felt thwarted or coerced. These are children who were equally content and composed in other situations that made no unwelcome demands on them. Although the experience of being taught did result in better test scores than the scores of those who were not offered or failed to cooperate with teaching efforts, the fact that learning did take place did not in and by itself aid these children in achieving more adequate levels of control in stressful situations.

Next we turn to the question of the degree to which a direct link exists between patterns of experience and the rate of cognitive development. A rather strong

Figure 8.4 Mean IQ by EP Rating for Neuro and Behavior Groups by Age

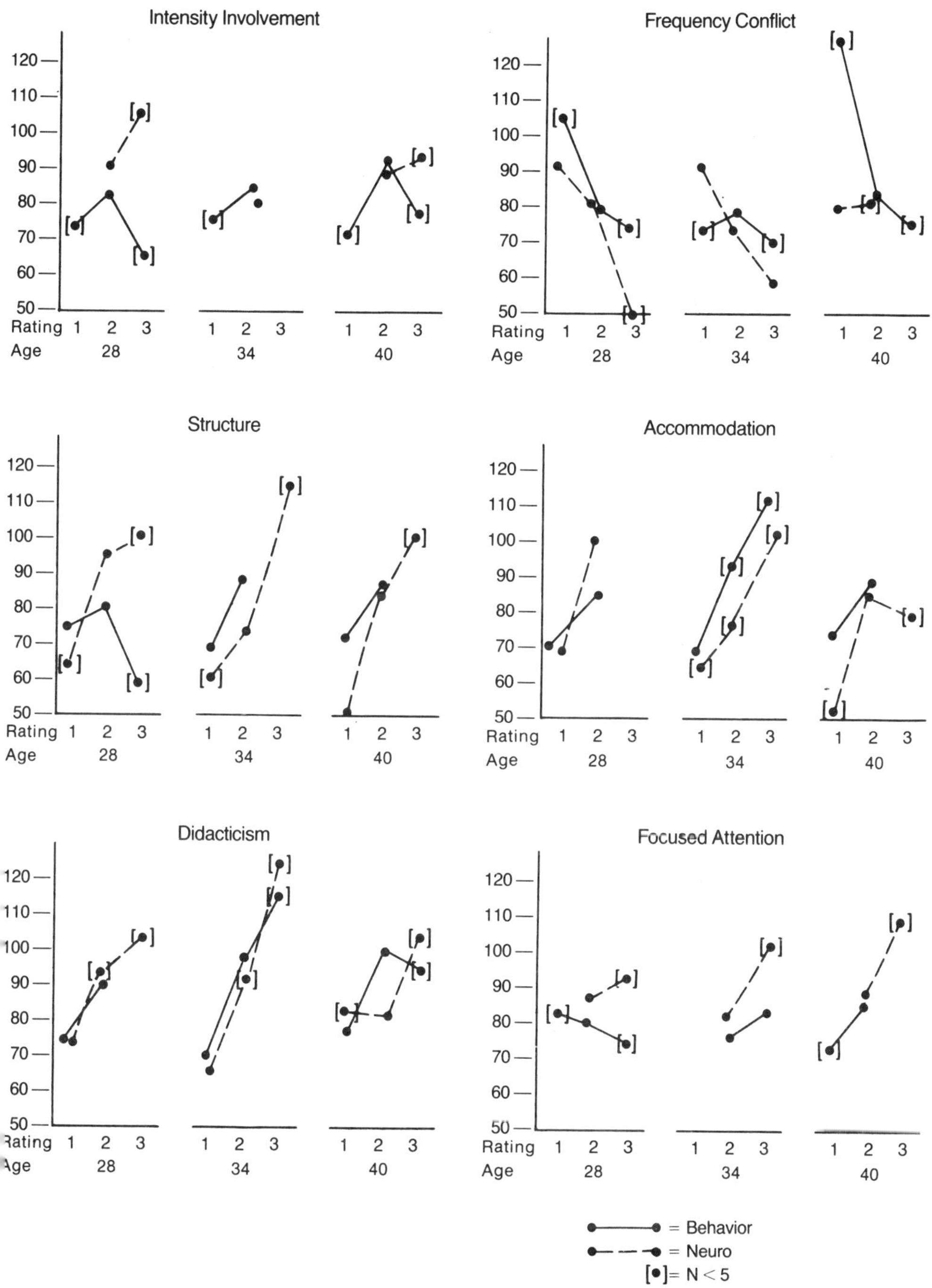

positive relationship between IQ and the presence of most of these varieties of experience (all but intensity of maternal involvement) was demonstrated for the intact group. In figure 8.4 we show the mean IQ for each experience-pattern rating for the neuro and the behavior group at three age levels. For both groups it is apparent that structure, accommodation, didacticism, and frequency of conflict are related to IQ. As was mentioned earlier, a rating of 3, indicating that the dimension of experience in question was very prominent in the child's life, was very rare indeed. Therefore the means for extreme ratings are often based on very few scores. In order to alert the reader to those mean IQ values that may well be spurious we bracketed the IQ notation whenever the number of cases was less than five. Once these presumably trivial results were disregarded the relationship between EP ratings and IQ was essentially the same at 40 months as it had been at 34 and 28 months. Cognitive development was more advanced when structure, accommodation, and direct teaching were regularly present in the child's life, and when frequency of conflict was comparatively low. This association was as clear-cut and consistent for the neuro as for the behavior group.

A lawful relationship between these particular aspects of experience and cognitive development during the toddler years is plausible only if it can be shown to be of the same kind whether the children function well or ill, and regardless of the nature and the probable cause of malfunctioning. In figure 8.5 we combine the two deviant groups and compare the mean IQ for each experience pattern thus obtained with the corresponding mean IQ values for the intact group. The curves depicting mean IQs for these two groups rise and fall in striking parallel. There is good reason to believe that the degree to which the deviant children could respond appropriately to structure, accommodation, direct teaching, and focused attention has a great deal to do with their cognitive development.

To complete documentation of our central thesis we need to establish a connection among all three of the major variables: experience pattern ratings, impulse control, and cognitive test scores. We have already reported that for the neuro group low IC and low IQ invariably went together. In the behavior group IQ and IC also covaried systematically, although there were some exceptions. What we do not yet know is whether the variations in IQ and IC are coordinated to the ratings these children received with respect to each dimension of experience. In figure 8.6 we show that this is the case. Mean IC and mean IQ scores rise and fall together, and these changes are consistently related to ratings received for the experience pattern. The one exception—the high IQ and fairly low IC for behaviorally disturbed children who received a great deal of teaching—was shown earlier to be an artifact.

As part of reporting the results for intact children we explored the degree to which there was an overlap between the ratings any one child received on the different patterns of experience. On the basis of tables reflecting congruence among ratings, we decided that there were enough discrepancies to justify the conclusion that the ratings are not so closely interwoven as to imply one another.

Figure 8.5 Mean IQ by EP Rating for the Intact and Combined Deviant Groups by Age

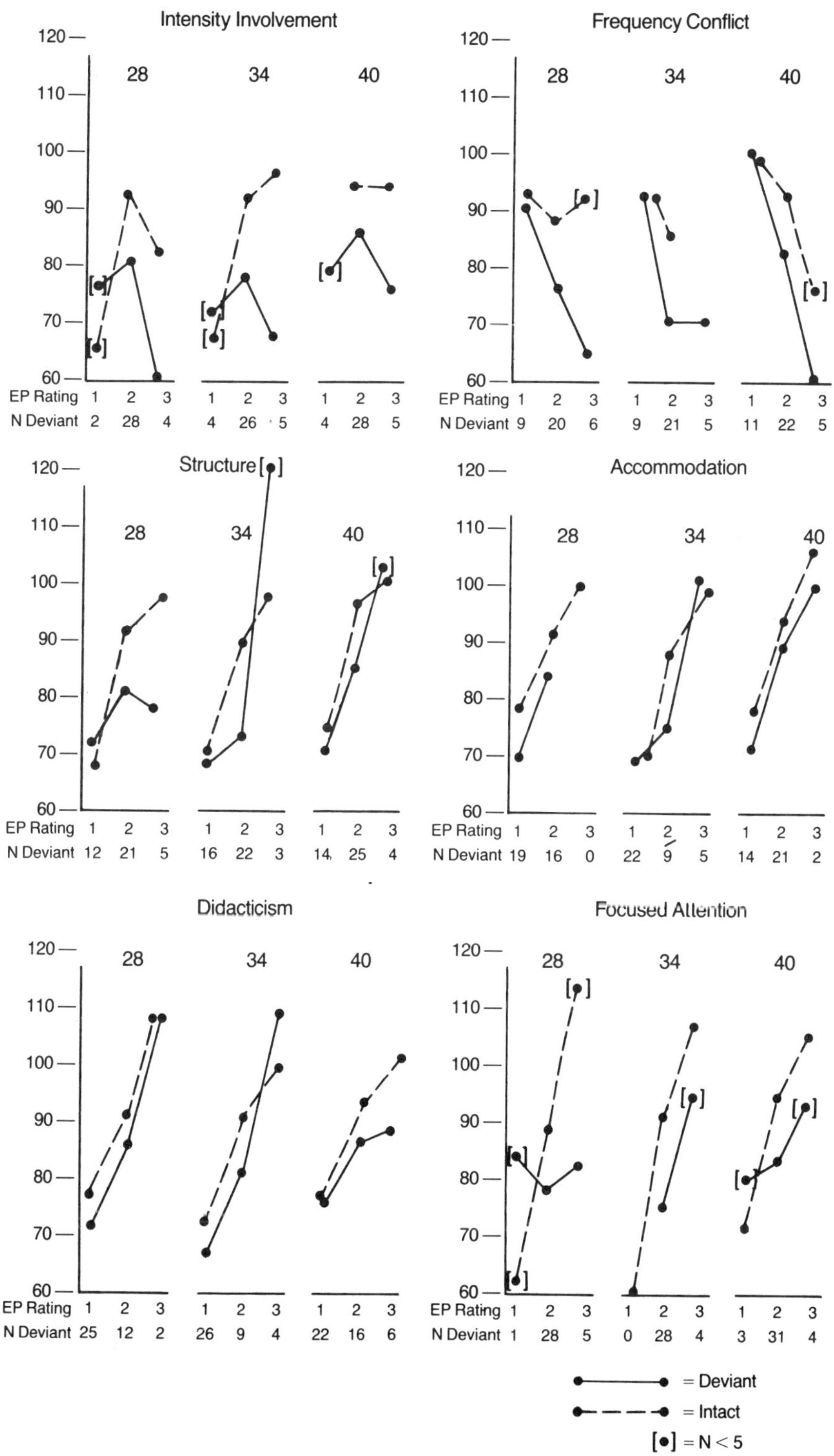

Figure 8.6 Mean IQ and Mean IC for Each EP Rating for Neuro and Behavior Groups (Ages Combined)

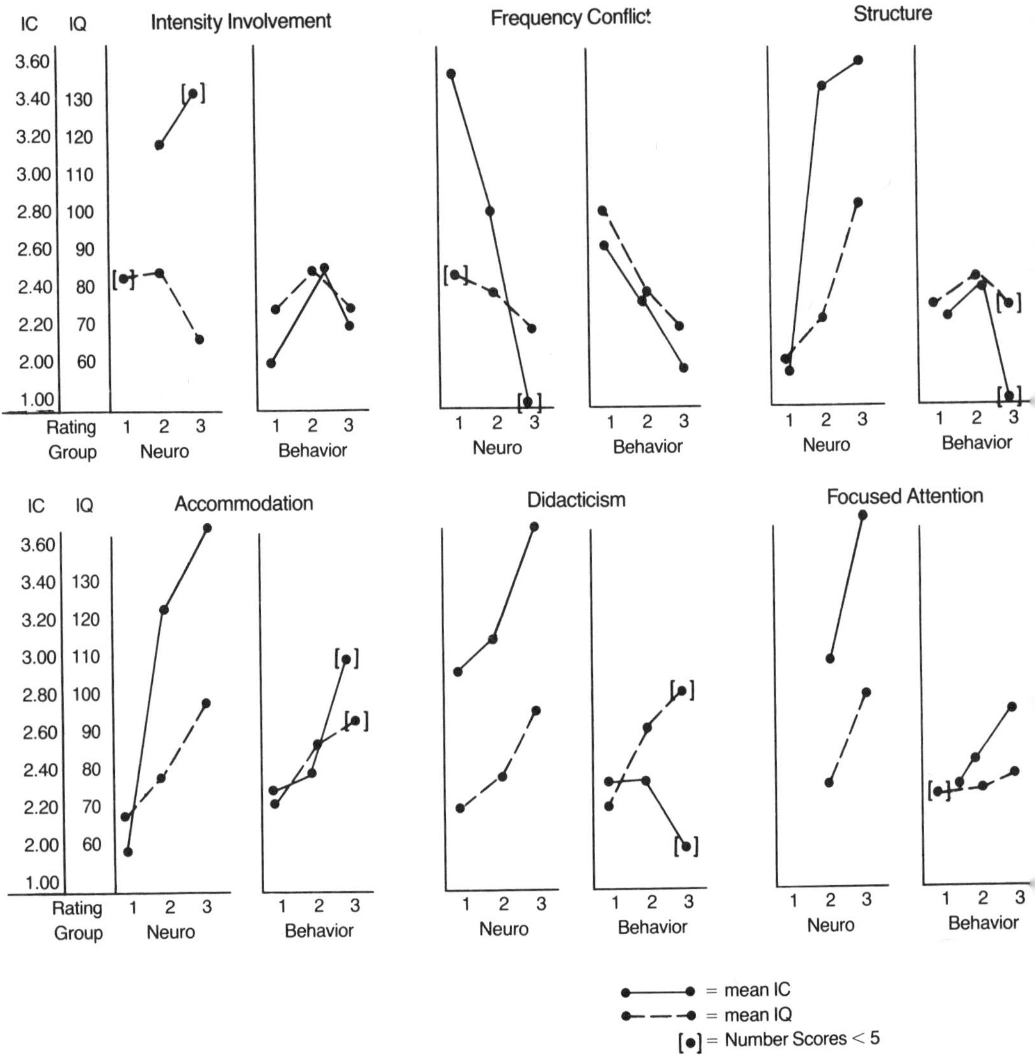

That is, the various EP ratings do tap separable components of daily experience. However, since children quite often received the same rating on different dimensions of experience, and also on the basis of psychological considerations, we recognized that there are some overlaps and that an intrinsic affinity almost certainly exists between several of our categories of experience. Some—for instance structure and accommodation—were closely allied to each other. Others, such as structure and focused attention, showed marked disparity. The same analysis carried out for the two deviant groups led to identical conclusions. It adds no new information and is therefore excluded from further discussion.

For the intact group we pursued the possibility that relatively ample experience in some aspects of life experience may compensate for distinctly meager representation of others among the developmentally supportive areas. Composite ratings representing the entire set of experience-pattern ratings for a single child were constructed. They fell naturally into three groups: those with exceptionally rich experience backgrounds, those who had very sparse supportive experiences, and the middle group in this respect. We demonstrated that the interrelationships among IQ, IC, EP ratings, and social class held when the aggregate of EP ratings was used rather than each rating in its own right. The same analysis was also made for the deviant groups. Once again the results were so similar to those for the intact children, and also so similar to what was shown for the separate patterns of experience, that we decided not to report on it in detail.

At this point we have gone as far as possible to demonstrate that for this group of children socioeconomic status, stable patterns of experience, impulse control, and cognitive development show consistent relationships to one another. This completes the primary task we had set for ourselves. Once more, this time in relation to the deviant children, we shall present some vignettes in order to put flesh on the skeleton, so to speak. We hope that the reader will then be in a position to know and to imagine the concrete and individualized reality that of necessity is masked by all the labels and the numbers we employed.

Second Interlude:
Vignettes of Two Neuro and Three Behavior Group Children

When it comes to the selection of illustrative case material for the development of deviant children, there is no such thing as a typical case. We chose to present typical problems or biologic deficits and a variety of ways in which children and families coped or failed to cope.

The first two vignettes, about Robert and Isabella, describe children whose developmental difficulties arose from mild but definite pathology. Both families made special efforts to accommodate the child's needs, although Isabella's parents were inclined to deny her intrinsic deficit. Robert's handicap was visible and too conspicuous to be denied, as his parents at first tried to do, and the adult members of the family struggled hard to acknowledge and understand his difficulties.

Robert: A Very Small Boy in a Very Large Family

Background

Robert's parents were obviously in earnest when they spoke of wanting a large family, for he was the eighth child born to them within a ten-year period (his siblings included one set of twins). They were resourceful in adapting a five-room apartment to the requirements of so large a brood and somehow managed to find space for pets as well. For this family, their own home and the housing project in which it was located were a safe haven in a hostile world, primarily because the neighbors were congenial and helpful to each other. The surrounding streets were felt to be dangerous and were in fact part of a crime-ridden area. The father was the only member of the family to venture out of doors after dark and was in the habit of calling home several times a day just to make sure that all was well. Both parents dreamed of some day being able to live where there was ample space indoors and out.

The father's wages were reasonably good but could not support such a large family, especially as Robert was not the only child who required special medical attention. With the help of Medicaid and food stamps the family managed to live in a very simple but moderately comfortable style.

Robert was born six weeks prematurely and his birthweight was close to 1200 grams, which meant that he was also small for his gestational age. He was not only tiny but also very ill and remained in the ICU for a full three months—much of this time on the respirator. From the beginning he was considered to be at grave risk for neurological and pulmonary illness, and he was expected to be mentally retarded. The parents knew all this when they took him home but were skeptical of the prognosis. Later, when she had come to know us, his mother told us that her determination and belief had saved the life of one of the older children and that she could will (her word) Robert to do much better than was predicted.

Ratings at 40 Months

Impulse Control. At nearly three and a half years Robert was more patient, more persistent in the pursuit of difficult goals, and more restrained in the expression of anger and joy than the majority of his peers. Yet he was anything but listless or apathetic. He showed enthusiasm, zest, stubbornness, mischievousness, and annoyance openly though mostly at moderate levels of intensity. The impulse control score was 4 (more control than most).

Structure. Robert's life was structured in part because family routines, such as bed- and playtimes, were very regular and in part because he always found himself in social situations that directed or compelled his activity. For instance, his place at the family table was fixed as was the sequence in which the children were served at mealtimes, as was the custom for the youngest children to join the older ones for homework after supper, equipped with their own pencils and notebooks. Whether he was "helping" his mother with household chores, playing football (of sorts) with father, or being shown picture books, he knew what was expected of him. He also spent a good deal of time playing with a group of neighbors' children under the supervision of one of the mothers. There he did his best to imitate the actions of the other youngsters. Fortunately they accepted and even protected him to some extent. It was precisely because of his visible handicap, combined with his outgoing friendliness, that a special role was assigned to him, and he was seldom at a loss. The EP rating for structure was 2 (present, not prominent).

Accommodation. An accommodative style of childrearing was natural for Robert's mother and governed her behavior with all her children. A combination of experience, intelligence, and goodwill enabled her to forestall difficulties and attune her expectations to developmental changes in the child. For example, when Robert showed reluctance to remain in his own bed, his mother tried a variety of methods to no avail and finally solved the problem by installing a nightlight. Also, this boy was painfully awkward in his attempts to dress himself, yet unwilling to have it done for him. This extremely busy mother gave him inordinate amounts of time and helped only when he agreed to it. Again, breakfast for the whole family coincided with Robert's favorite television show, yet, when he watched, his food intake was poor. It involved additional labor to serve his breakfast at a later time, but this is what was done. Last, with good reason, this mother was afraid that her boy would hurt himself during one of his many falls as he manfully attacked the slides and bars in the playground. She had to force herself not to interfere, thinking that he might become discouraged if he felt that his mother did not trust him. Much could be added in support of our judgment that the appropriate EP rating for accommodation was 3 (very prominent).

Didacticism. Both parents were more than eager to see their son learn and would have been glad to teach him more if he had been able to absorb it. As it was, they provided paper and pencil and praised his scribbles. They showed him picture books and invited him to listen to stories, and they encouraged him to watch educational television programs. His progress, most notably in language, was appreciated fully. The EP rating for didacticism was 2 (present, not prominent).

Frequency of conflict. Little Robert was described as a goodnatured, friendly, easy-going child, far less rambunctious than any of his siblings. His mother said, "He is not mischievous, he just talks too much." He did get angry, as would any child, but this did not lead to overt conflict. He would pout, sulk, and look defiant in a manner that struck the adults as so comical that such episodes often ended in hugs and laughter. The EP rating for frequency of conflict was 1 (minimally present).

Intensity of maternal involvement. This mother felt very close to her fragile child and, in speaking of him, showed strong affect as she emphasized how lovable he was. A rating of 3 might have been appropriate were it not for the fact that her inner life and her actions were dictated by her intense commitment to the well being of the entire family. The EP rating for the intensity of maternal involvement was 2 (present, not prominent).

Developmental Course

When Robert was discharged from the ICU he was a tiny baby, frail, weak, and markedly unresponsive. His mother could not always hear his soft cry and therefore kept him by her side or else went to his crib to check on him every few minutes. It was not until the uncorrected age of six months, when his gestational age was four months, that he "woke up," as his mother put it. His behavior changed suddenly in that he moved more, smiled and cooed responsively, stretched his arms toward toys and people, and soon seemed to prefer his mother to all others. Relatives and friends were eager to help care for the baby but the mother considered that only she knew how to shield him and yet provide constant gentle stimulation.

At the time of the 7-month visit Robert looked and behaved much like a normal and alert 3-month-old. His test performance was very uneven. Motor coordination, both gross and fine, was poor, and this accounted for the low MDI of 58. Yet the *scales of sensorimotor intelligence* showed that he functioned predominantly at the stage three level with respect to prehension and object permanence—in other words, by this measure his behavior resembled that of a normal 7-month-old infant. The exception was that, unlike healthy children, he lacked some of the more primitive coordinations (stage two) in his repertoire. Throughout the session observers noted that his behavior was well integrated, that he used such skills as he possessed zestfully, and that his attention span was excellent. The summary of the developmental evaluation ended on a note of cautious optimism: "it may be that his potential is greater than that suggested by the MDI . . . unless deterioration should set in" (a course that was initially thought likely by some of the medical staff).

When he returned at 15 months Robert's progress exceeded all expectations. Physically there had been no major change; his weight, height, and head circumference all were well below the first percentile of the normal distribution, and only recently had he begun to creep. However, his MDI, which at this age taps chiefly perceptual discrimination, comprehension, attention span, and fine coordination, was 90 and thus well within the normal range. He demonstrated stage six behavior with respect to object permanence whereas spatial relationships were dealt with at stage four and five levels. His social behavior was also in keeping with normal expectation. He required about fifteen minutes to overcome initial shyness but thereafter he enjoyed playful interaction with the examiner and became interested in every task presented to him. Yet, in order for him to function with optimal spontaneity, it was necessary that he remain in the close vicinity of his mother. During the play session he was hesitant and clung to his mother to begin with, although he then began to play contentedly. Conventional communication signals were not observed or reported. The open space procedure was of course omitted as he had not yet begun to walk. What impressed us more than his test performance was that Robert's behavior was well organized, nicely attuned to changing circumstances, and notable for its verve and for a friendly receptivity toward the social and physical environment.

The next research visit had to be postponed so that Robert was 32 months old when he was brought for what should have been the 28-month visit. Once again, all of us were struck by the contrast between his odd appearance and obvious handicap, on the one hand, and the confident, alert, and resourceful quality of his behavior, on the other. In addition to microcephaly and small body size Robert now manifested orthopedic difficulties. He walked stiffly, tripped and fell often, was altogether awkward, and we also noted a number of other soft neurological signs. Once again observers marvelled at his alertness, social responsiveness, attention span, and the degree to which all of his behavior was well integrated and appropriate. In these respects his functioning was, if anything, superior to that of many healthy peers.

Another child had been born into the family some months previously. We were told that Robert found it difficult to relinquish the role of the baby in the home. To begin with he showed jealousy and resentment quite openly. The mother had known what to expect and jokingly commented that his small size made it easy to carry one of her two babies on each arm. She demonstrated how she would hold and rock both of them and enact a little drama during which she addressed Robert as "my big baby" and the infant as the little one in rhythmic sing-song. After a while Robert's attitude "turned around" and he became very affectionate and possessive toward the baby. We thought that his ability to master hostile feelings by means of this well-known maneuver (reaction formation, in psychoanalytic parlance) was yet another sign that the ego development of this handicapped child was healthy and age-appropriate.

On the Stanford-Binet test Robert attained an IQ of 73. In part, the retardation consisted of motoric awkwardness and poor speech articulation. For the first time, however, we observed a marked immaturity also in the areas of perceptual acumen and comprehension. As before, he made excellent use of the abilities that he possessed, leading the examiner to predict that later on he might well function within the normal range. The formal assessment of impulse control described him as well modulated and well organized, in keeping with what we were told about his typical behavior at home. Robert now showed strong concern in relation to the issues of separateness from the mother and of individuation generally. When the open space procedure was administered and he found himself confronted by the large hallway space he took a few steps, noticed that his mother had not moved, and remained immobile by her side. In other words, his behavior was much like that of the majority of 28-month-olds. During the assessment of body awareness he was fine until he was asked to identify his reflection in the mirror, whereupon he became painfully embarrassed and remained mute. The mother volunteered that at home, when he unexpectedly caught sight of his reflection, he did not like it and became self-conscious. He enjoyed the play session, during which he managed to involve both his mother and the examiner in his play with toys. The overall impression gained on this visit was that Robert now showed moderate delay in the development of most cognitive functions, although to a lesser degree than would have been expected on medical grounds. His social and emotional development impressed us as entirely normal—we had rarely if ever seen a severely handicapped preschoolage child who seemed as well organized and mature as Robert was.

When he came back at the age of 42 months Robert was still tiny (by now his height and weight were entirely off the curve), his orthopedic difficulties had not improved, and his articulation was so poor that quite often we failed to understand him. Yet, as before, he was a friendly, lively child, interested in everything we had to offer. Although language use and fine coordination were not good, he now achieved an IQ of 80. His comprehension of verbally-mediated concepts, his fairly good memory and perceptual discrimination, and his excellent attention span compensated for his weaknesses. On the concept formation tasks he understood the basic requirement but had difficulty when pictures rather than objects had to be sorted. A good many of the 40-month-olds in our group had the same problem. From his behavior in response to the achievement motivation procedure and the level of aspiration experiment we learned that Robert now evaluated his own performance by objective standards. He accepted help somewhat reluctantly on tasks he found difficult and was most pleased when he was able to manage on his own on such items. When deciding upon the distance from which to throw a ball into a target, he lowered his standards after failure but chose to increase the difficulty of the task after success. In his case the materials used in the world test invited imaginative play more than structure building, but with encouragement he did produce an end product, which was more decorative than representational in nature.

About his life at home we learned that he had become somewhat more independent of his mother and now "adored" his father. He regularly played with children of approximately his own age, usually in their home or out-of-doors and under the supervision of one of the other mothers. The other children accepted him in spite of his physical shortcomings. His mother thought that they liked him because he tried so hard and hardly ever cried. Robert had become a devotee of certain television programs and knew the times when they were scheduled. In general, it seemed, he led a busy, sociable, and apparently contented life. The one thing he truly feared was the family cat. He was not agile enough to outrun it or strong enough to repel it, and he cried for help when the animal approached him.

When he was six years old we saw Robert again. He had remained very small, was motorically impaired, and tended to slur speech sounds. A diagnosis of spastic dysplasia had since been made. He was still a friendly, curious, and loquacious youngster. His IQ on the WISC was 76, and the pattern of performance was little changed. His strong areas—that is, those in which he was not retarded—were comprehension of verbal concepts, memory, and attention span. Visual-motor integration was markedly impaired, and he could not cope with the demands of a standard scale measuring prereading skills. The latter was in spite of the fact that he had attended a Headstart program and that the family worked with him every day, trying to prepare him for school attendance. With all his physical and cognitive limitations, he led a very normal and satisfying life. He was learning slowly but surely, he performed his assigned chores and abided by household rules exactly as his siblings did, he had many friends with whom he played daily, and there could be no doubt that he was liked by those who knew him and loved within the family.

Discussion

There is no accounting for the fact that reasonably solid cognitive development and entirely satisfactory socioemotional development occurred in a child for whom the prognosis had been very grim indeed. It must be relevant that Robert was a cherished member of a stable family and that both parents from the beginning expected him to be slow to learn but were confident that in the end he would be "all right." Family standards entailed the expectation that all members must abide by established rules and must help to maintain the home, and little Robert was no exception. In this setting the child was able to fit into a niche provided for him, not only in the flow of events in a large family but also in the neighborhood. It seems likely that a favorable developmental outcome was aided by more than the fact that he received loving attention throughout his life. Beyond this, he lived in an orderly and comprehensible world; there was seldom any doubt as to what was expected of him, and there was always a physical and social locus where he belonged. He was constantly exposed to adaptive demands and challenges which, fortunately, were of a kind that, for the most part, he could meet.

Isabella: A Child With Typical Signs of Minor Neuropathology

Background

Isabella's parents were hard-working, deeply religious, and in some ways ambitious people who had planned on having a large family (they wanted at least six children). The mother, however, had a chronic health problem which became life-threatening during her first pregnancy (with Isabella). A Caesarian section had to be performed when the baby's gestational age was just beyond 5 months. At first both mother and baby were gravely ill, but both made good recoveries. Before Isabella was discharged from the ICU the parents were advised that some CNS injury had taken place and that Isabella's physical and mental development might be impaired. These parents believed that divine providence saw to it that they were strong enough to bear whatever burdens were placed on them.

Supported by father's steady wages, the family lived in crowded quarters in one of the safer neighborhoods of the city. Both parents were active members of a local sectarian church. Weekday evenings and much of the weekend were spent in church-related activities, from attendance at service to teaching Bible school, missionary work, and social events. Isabella's family differed from others with equally strong religious commitments in one respect: they were extremely tolerant. They assumed that errors and evildoing were the result of weakness rather than wickedness and that there was good in everyone.

Ratings at 40 Months

Impulse control. Isabella was an exceedingly well controlled little girl. She sat quietly through long services each evening, well supplied with crayons. By all criteria—patience, frustration, tolerance, perseverance in the face of difficulty, voice quality, and style of affect expression—she conformed to our definition of unusually strong impulse control. At the same time, she was a lively child who enjoyed physical activity such as running and dancing. Her face registered annoyance, discomfort, fearfulness, amusement, mischievousness, curiosity, and what was described as "quietly radiating joy." In short, in her case unusually strong control existed side by side with considerable spontaneity and zest. The impulse control score was 4 (unusually strong).

Structure. Basic routines were very regular in this household. Because the family did not return from evening church until late at night, Isabella slept until about noon. After lunch there was a long play period, followed by supper and a nap until it was time to leave for church again. On weekends Isabella lived in the home of her maternal grandmother so that the parents could devote time to church affairs. Family meals and "free time" took place in the grandmother's home.

No matter where she was, Isabella's day was filled with goal-directed activity. She played well-organized games with her dolls, danced to radio music, "read" her books with and without adult participation, used crayons and paint, and was taught letters and numbers, always under the watchful eye of adults. The mother and father observed, commented on, and at times participated in the child's play. They did not usually direct it except in one respect. When Isabella departed from their standard of good behavior—that is, when they thought that she was noisy, assertive, or wild—the adults regularly intervened. In a gentle, soft-spoken, serious manner they chided or instructed the child. Thus ministructure was nearly always present and was consistent and friendly but also inexorable. The EP rating for structure was 2 (present, not prominent).

Accommodation. At this particular time in the life of the family the parents had occasion to make deliberate and seemingly successful efforts to accommodate Isabella more than they had earlier when accommodation seemed less necessary to them. The child was upset by the arrival of a baby sister and had begun to use babytalk, to want to be cuddled, and constantly to ask for reassurance that her parents still loved her. Through participation in a comprehensive health program the parents learned about sibling rivalry and did their best to include Isabella when they attended to the baby, to demonstrate their affection for her, and to permit Isabella to express negative feelings about the baby. In all other ways Isabella was expected to adapt herself to parental standards as she had before. The EP rating for accommodation was 2 (present, not prominent).

Focused attention. Isabella was listened to when she spoke, carefully watched and guided, and never ignored. She experienced focused attention as moral precepts were explained to her and at times when her mother taught her simple skills. Most of the time, however, social exchanges between Isabella and her parents were brief and did not meet our criteria for this variable. The EP rating for focused attention was 2 (present, not prominent).

Didacticism. Education was valued highly in this home. Once Isabella had reached the age of three years, the family began to teach her letters, numbers, colors, and shapes. This was done casually, as much to keep her busy as to instruct her, and remained subordinated to the teaching of moral values. That the mother tended to give detailed explanations and that all adults engaged in more than casual conversations with the youngster probably served to teach language use and comprehension. The EP rating for didacticism was 2 (present, not prominent).

Frequency of conflict. Isabella's parents abhorred conflict and the overt display of anger or hostility. Long before the child had reached the age of 40 months they had taught their little girl to adopt the gentle, courteous, and cooperative manner that they themselves habitually employed. Interestingly, she was permitted to disagree or to refuse requests made of her, provided she did so in a polite and modulated manner. The EP rating for frequency of conflict was 1 (absent or rare).

Intensity of maternal involvement. The facts that the childbearing had been so dangerous to the mother's health and that Isabella's prognosis had initially been guarded certainly intensified this mother's feeling for her child. On the other hand, her affection and concern embraced the entire family, and therefore her strong emotional investment in the child did not overshadow equally strong feelings in relation to some others. The EP rating for intensity of maternal involvement was 2 (present, not prominent).

Developmental Course

The mother was so pleased to have the baby home, and so determined to be optimistic, that she spoke of Isabella as a healthy, normal infant. Indeed, the baby slept well, liked to be played with, but was also content in crib and playpen, and the early developmental milestones emerged more or less at the expected times. The mother was less concerned than anybody else about the fact that Isabella never cried when hungry and needed to be coaxed whenever food was offered.

At the time of the first visit (7-month) Isabella was so extremely small that she was diagnosed as a failure-to-thrive baby. Pediatricians who had not met the family before suspected that the baby was neglected. A good many obvious stigmata and a variety of soft neurological signs added to the overall impression of an abnormal infant. During the developmental examination Isabella functioned much as her mother had described her. She was excited by the toys, moved a good deal in tense, darting motions, was undisturbed by contact with the examiners, who were strangers to her, and her physiognomic and vocal responsiveness was limited. She obtained an MDI of 91 and functioned at stage three with respect to object permanence and prehension (sensorimotor scales).

At 15 months Isabella had made good progress in spite of a number of minor illnesses. Her MDI was 107 and she exhibited some stage four behaviors with respect to object permanence and spatial relationships (sensorimotor scales). During the play session she used most of the toys and tended to remain in her mother's vicinity. She made visual and vocal contact not only with the mother but, even more frequently, with the staff member. Her most conspicuous conventional communication signal was to point at an object and say "that" while looking at the other person and clearly expecting some acknowledgment. When she was confronted with the open space situation she proceeded to march out into the hall, roamed for a minute or two, then returned to the playroom—all without overt attention to her mother or anybody else.

We were told that she had begun to walk before she was 12 months old and that since that time walking about the apartment and climbing furniture had become her preferred occupation. She apparently hugely enjoyed the father's vigorous play with her and was equally contented and busy at the home of the maternal grandmother, where she spent the weekends. (Much of the time the parents and other relatives were there as well.)

The mother had become concerned about Isabella's poor appetite and had introduced an extra meal as well as snacks. It seemed to us that the child's food intake should have been sufficient, but her height and weight at this time still fell below the first percentile of the expected distribution. Altogether, the discrepancy between Isabella's appearance—several stigmata, tremulous, tiny, and active in small, darting movements—and her entirely normal and age-appropriate behavior impressed all of us.

For the next year, up to the 28-month visit, Isabella developed well, and the rhythm of family life remained unaltered. The whole family still spent two to three hours at church every weekday evening, enjoyed a snack and some family sociability thereafter, and all went to sleep some time after midnight. Isabella played indoors under her mother's close supervision, was given four meals a day, and took a nap before it was time to go to church again. As before, all weekends were spent in the apartment of the maternal grandmother. From description and observation it was apparent that, by ordinary standards, Isabella was a rather quiet and almost docile child, yet her mother thought her to be extrordinarily active. In support of this assertion she pointed to Isabella's fidgeting during the testing session and her occasional attention to something other than the task at hand. At such times Isabella was corrected: in a very kind and gentle, but relentless manner, she was told to sit up straight, to stop tapping her foot, to speak softly, to be careful, and the like. The grandmother's report confirmed the impression that the child was never free from restraint except, perhaps, during vigorous play with her father. As far as we could ascertain, Isabella did not mind at all, perhaps in part because she was permitted to express opposition if she preserved good manners while so doing.

The developmental evaluation at 28 months showed that Isabella functioned in accordance with average expectations, both intellectually and socially. Her IQ was now 98. She had no difficulty in naming body parts on herself, on the doll, or on pictures but could not do so on her reflection in the mirror; being asked to do so made her too self-conscious (body awareness procedure). The play session, the separation procedure, and the open space experiment all indicated considerable progression in the development of the mother-child relationship. Specifically, much of the play session was spent in transporting toys to and from her mother's lap; separation disrupted her play activity, and when confronted with the large floor space (open space) she took a few steps, looked anxious as she returned to her mother, and then remained close to her. The issue of distance from and dependence upon the mother had gained new importance for her, as would be expected at this age. The formal assessment of impulse control took place during this visit, and of course rating scores described her as very well modulated, contained, and controlled.

The 34-month visit coincided with a difficult time in the life of this family. The mother was pregnant, and grave complications had developed. She required hospitalization but attended the research session in a wheelchair, as her ward and our quarters were located in the same building. All procedures were carried out although the family (father and grandmother) viewed the research session as an opportunity for a leisurely visit with the mother.

On this occasion Isabella was obviously worried by her mother's illness. She was more timid and subdued than we had known her previously but otherwise remained her pleasant and cooperative self. She was able to interest herself in everything we offered and obtained an IQ of 99. On the Achievement Motivation tasks, Isabella proved to be easily discouraged but responsive to encouragement. She always welcomed help but thoroughly appreciated her success when she was able to accomplish a task by her own effort. Achievement motivation, in the sense of taking greater pleasure in achieving difficult goals than easy ones, was clearly present though she was cautious rather than confident in her approach. A relative lack of self-confidence combined with a keen dislike of failure was shown still more clearly during the Level of Aspiration experiment. She began at the easiest level, remained there through several successes, and made sure of avoiding a last-minute failure simply by dropping the ball into the basket before declaring herself finished. In the play session Isabella was busy and content. She organized her play in such a way that all four adults became involved, if only to acknowledge her communications.

The entire family, including the grandmother and baby sister, was present for the 40-month visit. The mother was no longer acutely ill, and the family had resumed its customary style of living, to which the needs of the infant had been assimilated. During this visit Isabella was quiet, graciously cooperative, and friendly. Her IQ was now 103, and the concept formation scale offered no special difficulty to her. On the World Test she became absorbed in building a well-organized structure utilizing every single object. Although she must have known that the adults were pleased with her performance, her general approach to tasks and her self-confidence remained true to pattern. To the Achievement Motivation tasks she responded as she had before in that she was interested, enjoyed success when it came her way, accepted whatever help was offered, and needed encouragement to persevere. During the Level of Aspiration experiment she combined token compliance with instructions with an avoidance of the risk of failure by adopting a rigid system. She began at the most difficult level and moved downward step by step whether or not she had succeeded. Overall, her cognitive and social development had continued at much the same pace and in entirely the same style as before. She was seen as a well-functioning child of average competence who was somewhat more compliant, more controlled, and more timid than the majority.

The family had much to say about some notable changes in her behavior at home. Her response to the arrival of the baby sister had been negative and—for her—extreme. As mentioned in the discussion of experience patterns, she demanded to be fed and cuddled, spoke babytalk, and constantly asked for reassurance about her parents' continued love. She also verbalized her dislike of the baby but was gentle when she spoke to the baby or touched her. The second major change was that her imaginative play had become intense and pervasive. Her make-believe games incorporated certain impressive figures from the television screen (such as Wonder Woman) as well as a sizable number of imaginary companions. The family had come to know several of these imaginary figures, whose names and personality characteristics remained the same for weeks at a time. For instance, certain girlfriends went along to keep her company at church, and it was not unusual for one of the make-believe friends to join her at the dinner table. It seemed to us that the strong and conflicted feelings she experienced in relation to the sibling must have intensified her fantasy life in a way that helped her cope with such resentment as she felt.

Discussion

Isabella's development was described in some detail for two reasons: she was one of a number of children who developed well during the preschool years in the presence of minor neuropathology of the same sort that, in other instances, led to behavioral or developmental difficulties. We speculate that the quality of experience during the early years can be a decisive factor in determining whether or not biologically vulnerable infants develop without disruption. Isabella, however, also furnished an example for the well-documented fact that sound development during the early years does not provide protection against later difficulties.

When we met Isabella again at the age of six years she and her family were very troubled. Since the beginning of the school year—that is, for more than four months—the child had fiercely resisted school attendance. Every morning she cried bitterly, resisted physically, and often vomited. She freely answered questions about why she did not want to go by saying that her mother might be hurt or might die while she was at school (the mother's illness was neither worse nor better than it had been before). As is often the case with school phobias, she settled down once in the classroom. There and in general, however, she exhibited signs of tension and some immaturity. She sucked her thumb during the daytime, had become very restless and fidgety, and when angry she stiffened her body, became red in the face, and refused to talk. Intellectually she functioned well (IQ 105). Verbal ability and abstract reasoning were superior although arithmetic and early reading skills lagged behind.

The next evaluation took place when Isabella was almost nine years old and in fourth grade. By this time she had again become a quiet, cooperative, and apparently contented little girl. Nonetheless, the mother thought her immature and told us that the child clung to her, was easily intimidated, and was still given to thumb- and fingersucking. Her test performance reflected below-average competence in most areas, especially arithmetic and reading. Educational tutoring was recommended because it was thought that her mild scholastic difficulties could easily deteriorate to academic failure if she continued to feel discouraged.

With the next three vignettes, those for Betty, George, and Caroline, we turn to the description of children who had unusual difficulties that could not be linked demonstrably to biologic vulnerability or deficit. The circumstances of the families and the way in which the adults dealt with life's exigencies and with their children are unusual as well. By and large, the children with behavior difficulties grew up in families beset by physical, emotional, and social stresses more severe than those seen in the majority of families in the intact group. These three vignettes are typical in another way as well. Each family, and certainly each mother, was totally committed to the children. No effort was spared in trying to provide what was held to be the essential and the best possible care for the children, and all were remarkably persistent in pursuit of this goal. A more casual and almost diffident acceptance of the child and of conditions of existence was sometimes observed in some of the other families whose children fell into the neuro or intact group, but never in the mothers of the most seriously troubled children in the research group.

Betty: A Very Troubled Child

Background

Betty's parents were of Hispanic origin but both had grown up in New York City. They had been reared in poverty, and each had worked hard to achieve an education and a comfortable middle-class existence. The mother suffered from a chronic disease and required close medical supervision. She was a warm, responsible, and articulate person in her midtwenties who did not hesitate to tell us that during adolescence her behavior problems had been so severe as to require regular contact with a psychiatrist over a period of years. As to her present status, she thought of herself as extremely nervous and subject to emotional problems (her words), but, to her as to us, it was her physical frailty that caused concern.

In addition to Betty, the family consisted of the parents, a preschool-age daughter, and an elderly aunt who was too ill to live alone. They were a stable and harmonious family group that strove to live by a well-articulated set of values which included altruism (a word they would not have known), respect for authority and religion, but also enjoyment of whatever good things life has to offer. As will become apparent, it was difficult for these parents to combine cultural and family traditions from the old country with their more recently acquired and more liberal middle-class orientation.

Ratings at 40 Months

Impulse Control. How to deal with excitement and impulsivity lay at the core of Betty's problems, yet, probably for that very reason, her behavior patterns did not conform to our rating criteria. At home she was lively and responsive in her mother's company and rather quiet and tense in her absence. At all times she was described as very stubborn. When told to do something she did not want to do she typically froze into mute inactivity, although once in a great while she exploded into a massive tantrum. Tantrum-like behavior could also occur when her mother left her even with her father or the aunt, to both of whom she was greatly attached. The most disturbing aspect of her behavior was that when her mother took her out of the home (to visit friends, stores, or offices) she became mute and subdued, seldom looked at anybody, and barely moved. Thus, depending on the situation, she could show severe generalized inhibition, normal spontaneity, or the abandonment of all control. The impulse control score was: ? (unscorable).

Structure. Daily routines in this home were very regular. Meals, bedtimes, outdoor play in the backyard, hours spent with her sister in the father's workshop—all were regular and predictable occurrences. Betty spent much time with her sister, and we were told that at times they ran around or watched television peaceably enough, but at other times they quarreled as they competed for the same toy. There were playful rituals connected with some household routines. For instance, the afternoon bath was an occasion given over to fun and games that involved much splashing, in which the parents often joined. Seldom was Betty left to her own devices. She was played with, told stories and sung to, and taught simple skills such as reciting her full name. If Betty's experience was not as orderly and structured as such a background would suggest, it was because of her extreme willfulness, which led to frequent punishment and to disruption of ongoing activity. Also, she had little interest in play with toys—of which there were many—but rather sought to involve the adults in active social interchanges. The rating for structure was 2 (present, but not prominent).

Accommodation. The difficulty with this rating was that the mother's attitude and intentions were accommodating, but the nature of her efforts and therefore the results were not. Primarily this was because her judgment of what could be expected of a three-year-old was faulty and her methods of controlling behavior were inept and especially unsuited to this little girl. These parents took it for granted that the way to train a child to be obedient was to proceed from a warning to a threat of punishment with the belt to the use of this enforcer. On lesser occasions a few slaps by hand were administered. The mother recognized that Betty was terrified of the belt and attributed the child's timidity and fearfulness to its use. Also, not once but many times, she wondered aloud how it could be that neither Betty nor her sister was at all obedient although the rod had not been spared.

A small but very typical example of failure in accommodation is worth citing. The child was seldom hungry at breakfast time, but the mother enforced a full meal by bringing out the belt (the sight of it was usually sufficient as Betty knew from past experience that it might well be used). At lunch time Betty *was* hungry, but the mother considered this an unimportant meal and offered less than the child was ready to consume. We also thought that the mother's failure to recognize that Betty's shyness was excessive led to a lack of accommodation. If anything, this mother was rather pleased by the girl's dependence upon her which meant that she saw no reason to help Betty to overcome it and in fact encouraged it in many subtle ways. Some of the mother's efforts at accommodation were appropriate. For instance, she presented the father with an ultimatum by saying that if he was going to be strict with Betty he would have to spend ample time in pleasurable play with her as well. The rationale was that children cannot love their parents unless the pain of discipline is counterbalanced by enjoyable companionship. To have assigned a low rating for accommodation might have been misleading, and therefore the EP rating for accommodation was ? (unknown).

Focused attention. For the most part, Betty experienced focused attention from her mother. This came about because the little girl did more than constantly seek social interaction with her mother; she was apt to become angry and distressed unless *all* her mother's attention was concentrated upon her. In peaceable situations this might mean play in which the mother was an active participant, conversations, shared household activities, and also being read or sung to. Quite as often it was a matter of conflict between the two during which Betty's explosiveness or passive resistance commanded her mother's full attention. The aunt and father also spent time in close interaction with the little girl, but with them Betty was more tolerant of social situations in which she was merely a participant. The high rating we assigned does not mean that most of Betty's social interactions were of the focused variety; it merely means that by comparison to most peers in the research sample this experience came her way relatively often. The EP rating for focused social attention was 3 (very prominent).

Didacticism. Betty was taught occasionally by her elders, but no one in this family was aware that even three-year-olds can learn things other than little tricks (like uttering her full name on request) or the basics of obedience and propriety. She had a very large number of toys but did not seem to be familiar with blocks, puzzles, formboards, or the use of crayons; nor did the mother mention such materials. The older sister had a blackboard which Betty disregarded. Even her dolls, battery-operated toys, and other playthings found little use; she was more likely to carry one of them about than to play with it. The EP rating for didacticism was 1 (minimally present).

Frequency of Conflict. When Betty reached the age of 40 months it was difficult to decide upon a rating, as the frequency of conflict fell between the upper extreme of the score of 2 and the lower end of the range of 3. Certainly, conflicts between Betty and her parents, especially her mother, occurred a good many times each day, but such conflicts tended to be fairly frequent among many of our three-year-olds. The lower rating was selected because Betty spent considerable portions of each day in a peaceful state so that conflict was no longer a dominant feature of her transactions with caretaking adults. The EP rating for frequency of conflict was 2 (present, not prominent).

Intensity of maternal involvement. The mother's life centered on her family, very much including her own parents, and she maintained intense emotional bonds with all of them. It is true that at first Betty's prematurity and later her unusual behavior did cause her mother to invest especially strong feelings in her younger child; yet it was her strong belief that the needs and feelings of everyone should receive equal consideration. The mother was an intensely emotional person, and by comparison to those of other mothers in our sample her feelings about Betty could be described as unusually strong. There were daily episodes of almost lover-like interchanges during which they hugged and cuddled and verbalized how much they loved each other. Her investment also took the form of shaping family life in such a way that Betty's needs often took precedence over those of others, and certainly over the mother's own. One reason for her faithfulness to the research program surely was that she valued talking about the child endlessly, and we were the most receptive audience she was likely to have. The decisive reason for settling on the lesser rating was that, contrary to our definition of this variable, her interest in other people and her investment in them were also very high. The EP rating for intensity of involvement was 2 (present, not prominent).

Developmental Course

Betty was born six weeks ahead of time. To begin with her medical condition caused concern in spite of an age-appropriate birthweight. She responded very well to care on the ICU and was essentially symptom-free when she was discharged three weeks later. At 7 months of age there were some neurological residuals in the form of fine tremors and hypertonicity, but thereafter her medical history was uneventful. The mother's own health was far from good when she took Betty home, which increased her anxiety about taking care of a tiny baby, but the elderly aunt as well as the father took responsibility for both children for hours at a time so that the mother had ample chance to rest.

The baby thrived, well-baby check-ups were reassuring, and long before the 7-month visit the entire family felt comfortably able to take care of things. Betty's crib was decorated with all manner of play equipment, and she spent a good deal of time careening about the apartment in her walker. The mother felt that the baby had been spoiled while in the ICU and was anxious to undo this. So, amid much discussion of how much she could understand, Betty was scolded and lightly spanked if she touched forbidden objects. This did not interfere with everyone's desire to treat the baby lovingly and—in spite of themselves—indulgently. The mother wanted to hold the baby on her lap and decided that it was all right to do so if she remembered to put a blanket across her lap. In that way the baby would not become accustomed to the mother's body warmth and therefore would not be spoiled. The father routinely helpd the baby go to sleep by holding her in his arms while he lay down on the bed. (These details are given in order to make it clear that Betty's atypical social responsiveness later on did not arise from a lack of affectionate attention during the early months.)

Brought to the office at the age of 7 months, Betty was a responsive, moderately alert baby whose MDI proved to be 111. Like most 7-month-olds, she functioned on stage three with respect to object permanence and to prehension (sensorimotor intelligence scales). Also like many 7-month-olds, she had recently begun to show aversion to the approach of strangers, which turned to screaming if they did not withdraw, but she responded pleasantly to the research staff when they made their usual, very gradual approach.

At 15 months she was very shy initially but with time became a lively and responsive toddler who babbled and smiled at the examiner quite as much as at her mother. Her MDI was 95 and would have been higher had she not lagged in the area of vocalization and earliest speech patterns. With respect to object permanence she was precocious, functioning at the stage six level by finding invisibly hidden objects. Her comprehension of spatial relationships was age-appropriate at the stage five level (sensorimotor intelligence scales). During the play session she initially clung to mother. She then proceeded to make several excursions to the toy area, yet most of the time she played in the close vicinity of her mother. At no time did she become oblivious to her mother or the examiner. She looked at them, smiled, vocalized, and quite often held out a toy for their inspection (this was the only conventional communication gesture she employed). In the open space situation she behaved in a manner more typical of somewhat older toddlers. She took a few steps, turned to look back at her mother, ventured further into the hallway, returned to her mother only to set out again—never losing contact with her mother. We were struck by the correspondence between an accelerated performance on the object permanence scale and this indication of some acceleration in the development of the "object relationship" in the psychoanalytic sense.

The mother was entirely satisfied with Betty's development if not with all aspects of her behavior. Both parents strongly felt that discipline must be enforced early, in part to prevent Betty from becoming as spoiled as her older sister was thought to be. This intention translated itself into the construction of what seemed to us an excessive number of strictly enforced taboos and rules. The number of easily reached household objects she was not allowed to touch was bewildering; normal toddler-like protests at being bathed and dressed were treated as punishable sins. Thus the child spent a considerable portion of each day in tears or in apprehension of the belt, which was used with her only as a threat but which she dreaded, having witnessed its use on her sister many times. She hated to go to bed, and if often took a spanking to get her to remain there. When discipline was not at issue, on the other hand, she received affectionate and indulgent care. Mother, father, aunt, and sister enjoyed playing with her. She was kissed and hugged often, she was dressed up in loving pride before the daily outing to the park, and she had more toys than she could possibly have used.

When she returned at the age of 28 months Betty proved to be so timid, so resolute in avoiding any contact with us, and so unwilling to respond even to her mother that testing and other procedures could not be carried out at all. We decided to spend some time talking to the mother and paying no overt attention to the child for whom intriguing toys were provided. Her behavior under these circumstances was revealing. She was fascinated by the toys and would stretch out her arm as if to touch them, but invariably she would withdraw her hand before making contact. The impulse to reach was clearly strong, but so was her sense that she should not do so. In hopes that during this long visit the strangeness had worn off to some extent, we scheduled another visit three days later. On this second occasion extraordinary caution on our part, as well as tactful assistance from the mother, did enable Betty to overcome her shyness to some extent. After 60 minutes (!) during which no demands were made on her, she began to say an occasional word and even to involve the examiner in some of her play activity. All was well as long as no one sought to direct her attention to a particular object or to engage her in an activity. When this was attempted, by either her mother or the examiner, she, in the words of the examiner, "presented the most extreme example of stubborn passive resistance I have ever seen." The mother was asked to administer some of the test items and did so in a highly skillful and friendly manner, but to no avail. The child froze into total immobility—clearly determined not to give in. She won this battle, and a valid test score could not be obtained, nor was it possible to perform the pediatric neurological examination.

During the play session, on the other hand, she seemed pleased to use the toys. She freely traversed the room to get the toys she wanted, though she played with them in mother's corner of the room. Nor did she avoid contact with the examiner, smiling at her when their glances met. In order not to jeopardize procedures yet to come, the separation procedure was omitted. In the open space situation she moved out into the hallway, stayed within six feet of her mother, but did not need to turn around to make sure of her continued presence.

The mother was not at all surprised. She said that what we observed during the second visit was typical of how Betty often behaved at home. Moreover, we were told that with us the child had been a "great deal better" than she usually was away from home. The mother had not expected her to make friends with us as, in her opinion, she had done. We, in turn, were surprised by the mother's attitude. Except for the stubbornness she was wholly pleased with the child's development. At long last Betty had learned *not* to do what she knew to be forbidden. To her mother this meant that a major goal had been achieved. She welcomed the child's timidity in contrast to the sister's venturesome disposition and enjoyed the many portions of the day when Betty was sociable and affectionate. Yet she told us that Betty had to be spanked or threatened before she would stay in bed; that she could not entertain herself and always needed someone to play *with* her; that she became very angry when something she wanted was not forthcoming; that she would not obey requests; and, that she was angry and irritable very often. In her mother's eyes these unpleasant episodes were overshadowed by her enjoyment of the child at other times and by the fact that Betty did not get into mischief.

The 34-month visit was dramatic. As before, Betty sat on the sofa close to her mother, mute and unresponsive while the examiner did all in her power to elicit the child's interest in test materials, in toys that she had enjoyed the last time, in refreshments or any other thing. Betty ignored the staff member's antics altogether, although after thirty-five minutes we saw a fleeting smile. When the mother was asked to administer some of the test items she fared no better. Betty showed neither annoyance nor interest, and her face was so inexpressive that she seemed somehow lifeless. This pattern, however, was interspersed with remarkable episodes during which mother and child turned to each other and hugged, kissed full on the lips, spoke and cooed to each other lovingly, and seemed entirely oblivious to the examiner in the room or the staff behind the one-way mirror. These interchanges were so intense that the staff felt embarrassed to be witnessing something very private. Another kind of behavior was also unique in our experience. The mirror was to the side of the child and in full view if she turned her head. As Betty caught sight of her reflection in the mirror she cried,

"No, Mommy, no!" and buried her face in her mother's chest. She caught sight of herself a few more times and each time said *no* in acute discomfort, although she did not again show agitation. It seemed that she felt fascination as well as distress with her image, since she could easily have avoided looking at it altogether.

As a last resort we decided that the examiner should equip the mother with test material and instructions and then leave the room entirely. What we then witnessed through the one-way mirror struck us as an almost miraculous transformation. The moment the door closed behind the examiner Betty became a lively, alert, and cooperative little girl. She eagerly worked at all the tasks that her mother gave her, was willing to name pictures and objects upon request, spoke in full though brief sentences, and danced around the room exploring everything. In other words, her behavior and responsiveness were entirely normal and age-appropriate. An IQ could not be calculated, but her performance on most items that were administered was in keeping with normal expectation. The exception was the verbal area, where her responses corresponded to norms for children between 24 and 28 months of age.

The mother went through the body awareness procedure, and Betty had no difficulty pointing to body parts on herself, dolls, and pictures. Yet even when she was alone with her mother, the mirror image caused uneasy self-consciousness, and her mother wisely did not insist on that part of the test. Peculiarly, the examiner was tolerated as she presented the Achievement Motivation tasks after a break, undoubtedly because Betty could remain on her mother's lap throughout and interesting materials were presented that she could use or not as she chose. In this situation Betty was subdued and would not speak, but she was responsive and answered some questions by shaking her head to indicate yes or no. With her mother's encouragement she could persist in the face of difficulty; she accepted help whenever it was offered, but success yielded no pleasure. In other words, achievement motivation as we defined the term was not yet present.

In the play session Betty seemed tense and perhaps anxious throughout, though she did use the toys in fairly simple play, inviting her mother's participation. She surprised us once again by not protesting when her mother—after due explanation—left the room (separation). She continued simple listless play with minimal interruption. We could not interest her in the Level of Aspiration experiment or the concept formation scale; the latter would almost certainly have been too difficult for her in any case.

The mother's detailed report confirmed that Betty never spoke when she was away from home; in fact, she did not speak even within the home while visitors were present. She continued to be a child who "wants what she wants when she wants it" and became very upset when this condition was not met. The major developmental change of which mother was aware was that in recent months Betty had become much more closely attached to her than she had been before. We were told that throughout the day she trailed her mother as she went about her work. When prevented from doing this—for instance, when the mother went to the bathroom—she would scream or at least whine. Also, she no longer allowed the aunt to bathe or feed her, which had always been acceptable before. Betty was described as very jealous of anyone to whom her mother paid attention. In addition, and this pleased the mother a good deal, many times each day Betty asked her mother, "How much do you love me?" and she needed to be told that she was loved more than any other member of the family. In addition, the mother told us, once a day at least, "She has to be close to me, and I mean *real* close," clearly referring to the kind of smooching we had observed.

The mother saw the child's closeness to her as positive, although she did worry about the youngster's fearfulness. For instance, Betty feared the hole in the toilet seat. She understood what was expected of her, ran to the bathroom—and relieved herself on the floor, for which she was never punished. Other misdeeds, such as unwillingness to eat or to go to bed, failure to come when called, or breaking her sister's toys, led to threats with the belt (which usually worked) or a spanking by hand. At the same time, the mother's description left no doubt that appreciable portions of each day were peaceful and enjoyable for all concerned—helping her father in the workshop, playing with family members, outdoor play, watching her mother cook and clean, long playful conversations with the aunt, and much more.

In view of Betty's overly close tie to her mother, it may well be relevant that the mother's health was again precarious. She felt drained and unable to meet the needs of two demanding children, not to speak of her own compulsive need to maintain a spotlessly clean house. She considered that her difficulty was primarily emotional whereas her physicians maintained that the causes were purely physical. She even arranged to seek psychiatric help but canceled her appointment at the last moment.

It was a relief to find that things had much improved by the time of the 40-month visit. Betty would still not speak to us but she allowed the examiner to administer all but the verbal test items. These were given by the mother while the examiner left the room. She obtained an IQ of 71, and this seemed to be a reasonable index of her current abilities. Vocabulary and verbally mediated concepts were again her weakest areas in that she performed as would be expected of a two-year-old. The Achievement Motivation tasks aroused her interest, but she needed encouragement to persist and was only too glad to accept help. She seemed to prefer someone else to do what was needed to achieve the goal (such as dressing a doll or fastening a decal on paper). We never learned whether or not she understood the matching task (concept formation), because as she approached the material she caught sight of her mirror image, and this was sufficiently disturbing to prevent her from returning to try again. The Level of Aspiration experiment was not attempted. In the play session her behavior was similar to what it was at 34 months, but her play with toys was somewhat more complex. Once again, separation as her mother briefly left the room was tolerated without distress.

The mother looked better than she had for a long time and reported that her symptoms had diminished and that she felt able to cope with things as they came along. Objectively there was more for her to do because on weekdays she took in the young infant of a relative. Everyone in the home enjoyed the baby, who received most of his care from the elderly aunt, and the mother now did a larger share of the caretaking for Betty and her sister than she had. Although Betty remained nearly mute with outsiders and barely whispered a word or two in the presence of visitors whom she knew quite well, she was said to have formed much closer ties to her father and aunt. She still could not play by herself and still asked several times a day how much mother loved her, but her demands on her mother were less intense. The description of their daily life suggested to us that all adult members of the family were more relaxed than they had been, perhaps in part because Betty's outbursts when things went wrong occurred more rarely, although they were as dramatic as before ("she can go on for hours"). There is no way of knowing the sequence in which several changes occurred, but the fact that the mother no longer hit or threatened Betty may explain some of them. The mother now punished the child by sending her to bed, at which she cried bitterly, but, the mother said contentedly, "she does go when I tell her to."

Had we seen Betty for the first time at 40 months we would have viewed her inability to speak to us and to be at all relaxed, her failure to enjoy any part of the visit, her clinging to her mother, and her cognitive immaturity as unusual and worrisome. As it was, we were impressed with the progress she had made and wondered once again about the degree to which Betty's (relative) well being fluctuated with the ups and downs in mother's physical health and basic moods.

Discussion

Betty was seen again at six years and also at nine years of age. On both occasions she had been placed in a class for slow learners and, in academic terms, barely held her own. The parents not only helped with homework but drilled her in weak subjects. Teachers and parents recognized that without such help she could not have met the minimal standards for promotion from grade to grade. Her IQ remained in the low 70s. The pattern of her cognitive development was somewhat different from what might have been expected. She now did poorly on performance items, especially visual-motor integration, and functioned in the dull normal range on verbal tasks. Arithmetic was poor, and at age 9 her reading fell well below standards for her age and grade. At the time of the 9-year medical examination a mild dysplasia was diagnosed, and she was classified as neurologically suspicious.

Behaviorally she had remained true to pattern: it took five months of full-time attendance before she spoke her first word in the schoolroom. She was said to have remained aloof from her classmates and did not play with children in the neighborhood. In our offices she was extremely shy during the 6-year visit, although she cooperated to the best of her ability. During the physical examination, however, in her mother's presence, she relapsed into the mute and entirely uncooperative state we knew so well, so that a valid examination could not be carried out. At home she still screamed and stamped when hurt or angry, and she was still reluctant to acknowledge persons other than members of the household. At 9 years she had learned how to cope with the testing situation. She was friendly and cooperative though neither curious nor the least bit assertive. The teacher's evaluation described her as submissive to authority, easily led by other children, sensitive to criticism, and given to daydreaming. At home her behavior must have been somewhat different. The mother described her as a child who cried often and easily and was excitable and impulsive. The parents and the school authorities regarded her as a child with special learning difficulties but not as a behavior problem.

Whatever the underlying causes may have been, Betty's developmental difficulties lend themselves to description in terms of Erikson's understanding of the central developmental processes during the toddler and early preschool years. Even during the first year of life Betty had been subjected to more stringent prohibitions than most babies are. Her experience must have given her the feeling that independent actions, such as touching objects, were often punished. Yet the lively interactions with her mother and other members of the household, and the warmth and affection by which she was surrounded, also nourished a sense of self as lovable and important. During the second year the inevitable urge to test her powers, the desire to resist coercion, and the wish to engage in activity at her own initiative all seemed to become more intense the more her mother sought to prevent their expression. Erikson defined the polarity of what he termed the autonomy phase as consisting of a sense of the self as a powerful agent at one extreme and a sense of helplessness and dependence at the other. In his view healthy development during the toddler years requires experience at both extremes before a more realistic sense of self can emerge. Betty's experience was one-sided in that it overemphasized helpless dependency. She had much less occasion than most other toddlers to experience the other extreme—that is, to sense herself as strong and self-determining. Precisely because the bond to her mother and other members of the family was strong and yielded so much pleasure, she did not lose the impetus toward autonomy but instead had to confine its realization to a narrow sphere of action.

During the 28-month visit she presented a textbook example of a child nearly paralyzed by the conflict inherent in the autonomy phase. At that time her behavior at home was as passively resistant as we saw it in the office. Temper tantrums were rare though when they occurred they were massive. She had now learned not to carry out actions that she knew were disapproved. One way of describing what we thought had happened is to say that she had been taught *not* to do what was (or might be) forbidden but had also learned *not* to do as she was bid. Her sense of power found expression and fulfillment in her ability to withstand social pressure. Under the best of circumstances, ambivalence is highly typical of this developmental phase and during the abortive developmental test at 28 months we saw this enacted as she would tentatively move her arm as if to touch the proffered toy only to withdraw it, not once or twice but again and again for well over an hour. She clearly vacillated between wanting the toy(s) and not wanting to comply—exhibiting all the tension and discomfort that unresolved ambivalence arouses. Erikson specified that one necessary component of the autonomy phase is a heightened awareness of body boundaries, an awareness that one is visible to others, with the result that shyness and self-consciousness typically occur at this age. Betty's extreme reaction to her mirror image, and yet her fascination with it, can serve as an exclamation mark for our understanding of her condition at the time.

Subsequently her willfulness expressed itself at home in severe and long-lasting tantrums, although she still did not attempt forbidden actions. Away from home, and even in the presence of strangers in the home, she remained mute and almost entirely inactive. To construct a cohesive picture of these more complex developments would require more detailed knowledge of the mother-child relationship, and also of her relationship with father, than we possess. She dichotomized her behavior organization in terms of within and outside the home and later in terms of interaction with mother in contrast to her dealings with anybody else. Certainly, major issues related to autonomy remained important: the overly intense, symbiotic-like bond to her mother can be seen as an emergency solution made possible by the mother's not-so-subtle encouragement of it, and although Betty finally came to deal more effectively with other persons and with broader segments of the environment, this was a slow and anxious process. While we knew her, Betty never achieved the degree of spontaneity and independence one observes in most other children.

Whether or not she was exceptionally vulnerable because of an undetected weakness or deficit in the CNS remains an open question. Her slow and uneven cognitive development may well have been due to the presence of an inherent deficit, and if so, such a deficit might have lessened her resiliency to stressful experience. In its own right speculation of this sort is futile; it is mentioned nonetheless for two reasons. One is that Betty's unusual behavior patterns are intelligible only in light of her individual experience within the family, whether or not CNS pathology was present. The other reason is that extreme though comprehensible reactions to environmentally induced stress and strain were seen more often in this group of prematures than the literature and past experience would lead one to expect in a comparable full-term population. It is conceivable that the immaturity and hence the lability of the CNS that necessarily exist in prematures entail a risk for stress-induced developmental irregularities even in the absence of specific abnormality.

Georgia: An Unlikely and Partial Triumph

Background

Georgia was reared in a family that set unusually high standards of behavior and enforced them with unusual severity. Both of the parents had been raised by sternly religious and moralistic families, and they carried this tradition into their own home. The father earned a steady but marginal income, and they lived in constant dread of having to apply for welfare. Life was made difficult for the young couple by the fact that the mother suffered greatly from the neurological and emotional sequelae of a freak accident (a car went out of control and hit her on the sidewalk). We never met the father. The mother presented herself as a harsh, scornful person and spoke as though she felt no tenderness or affection for her child or anybody else. A kind of grim satisfaction at the result of her childrearing efforts was the most positive sentiment that we heard her express. At the same time she was an extremely conscientious and responsible person who took excellent care of her family. The more we saw of this mother, and the more we saw of the child's responsiveness to her, the more certain we became that her harsh manner masked a good deal of warmth and affectionate concern, however unacknowledged. Mother took exclusive care of her baby, with an occasional assist from a grandmother or an aunt.

Ratings at 40 Months

Impulse control. As was so often true of our deviant children, the level of ego control was difficult to assess. Throughout the relevant age span Georgia showed good to excellent control in some situations but in other circumstances lacked appropriate controls. She was able to sit still in church for long periods of time and also for shorter periods during Bible reading sessions in the home. She learned at an early age to refrain from actions that were considered destructive or aggressive by the parents. At the slightest provocation, however, she cried inconsolably and for long periods of time, often willing her body to become limp. Weeping and loud crying were her response to prohibitions, to scolding, and to any situation in which things did not go her way. Thus it seemed that the impulse to protest was limited to crying and that she was unable to suppress it to the degree expected of children at ages two and three. As she was neither overcontrolled nor lacking controls, an IC score of 3 was reluctantly assigned.

Structure. All previous ratings for this pattern had been medium (2), largely because the mother's many commitments to the church as well as her medical appointments caused basic routines to be somewhat irregular, though otherwise family life was well organized. The same rating at 40 months refers to a different situation. Because of the mother's pregnancy at this time, outings were reduced to an absolute minimum, so elements of Georgia's experience that had been regularly present had dropped out. These included play with other children and expeditions to the park, to stores, and to the church. What we called ministructure nevertheless remained intact. Georgia was supervised every minute of her waking time and made to toe the line by being punished at any sign of wildness, selfishness, poor manners, or failure to obey. But both mother and father also spent some time in pleasant interaction with their daughter, the latter playfully and the former during grooming, at mealtimes, and by sharing household tasks. What interfered with a well-structured, day-by-day existence were the constant clashes with the mother over discipline, which led to abandoned crying on the child's part and, while they lasted, disrupted behavior organization and alertness to her surroundings. The EP rating for structure was 2 (present, not prominent).

Accommodation. Georgia's mother was explicit in her conviction that it is wrong for a parent to accommodate a child; it is the youngster who must conform in all respects. Insofar as it is possible to combine such a view with conscientious care, Georgia's mother did just that. She disregarded even trivial preferences on the child's part, such as using one utensil rather than another or wanting a different toy, because one should not give in to whims. In a few situations mother did in fact accommodate: for instance, she could empathize with her daughter's fears (of darkness, of loud noises) and did her best to ease them. But, on the whole, Georgia experienced a minimum of accommodation as we defined the term. Supportive practices, such as providing toys, play with other children, and outdoor activity, were based on what the mother believed was good for children in general, not on behavior clues emanating from the child. The EP rating for accommodation was 1 (minimal).

Focused attention. The mother's vigilance in seeing to it that Georgia was well behaved guaranteed a fair amount of attention concentrated on the child. Much of this took the form of scolding, punishing, and coercing. The mother, however, valued her daughter's appearance, and there were daily leisurely episodes during which hair brushing and general prettifying took place. Briefly but regularly the mother taught the child such things as numbers and letters. The father's custom of playing with the child also added to the total time during which Georgia received undivided attention. The EP rating for focused attention was 2 (present, not prominent).

Didacticism. In addition to teaching Georgia some cognitive skills, her mother also encouraged her to watch educational television programs and faithfully bought each book related to the best known series ("Sesame Street"). In comparison to that of our other three-year-olds, Georgia's exposure to cognition-related activities fell at the lower end of the medium range. The EP rating for didacticism was 2 (present, not prominent).

Frequency of conflict. If the mother's account were taken at face value this experience pattern would have to be rated as high. However, we came to know that from her perspective *any* open conflict was too much. A frequency much like that observed in many mother-child pairs would surely be excessive in her eyes. The mother told us of a good many recurring situations that were conflict-free and confirmed what we had occasion to observe; namely, that Georgia was able to ignore her mother's scolding.

We thus felt justified in assigning an EP rating of 2 (present, not prominent) for frequency of conflict.

Selected pattern of discipline. The mother described herself as "strict, strict, strict," and that was the simple truth. From infancy onward and surely at 40 months, the number of things Georgia was not permitted seemed endless, and punishment followed swiftly. Typically, the mother began by forbidding or requesting something in a harsh manner, proceeded to show the belt, and if the child cried instead of obeying right away, used the belt. The mother said that her child must understand that if she says something she means it and that the only way of convincing the child is to use the belt promptly after the threat. Punishments were not brutal but they were sharp and swift and administered in full conviction of utter righteousness. What made severity in this home so pervasive was that it was not so much the offense that was punished as the fact that transgression had occurred at all. In a manner we did not see in any other family, the mother seemed to feel distress rather than anger at the child. The firmness that she deemed necessary existed side by side with interest in the child, with some pride, and—we thought—with concealed affection. Unlike other punitive mothers in the sample, Georgia's mother gave no sign of feeling guilty, of apprehension at the intensity of her own affect, or of considering that the necessity for so much punishment might indicate a degree of parental failure. On the contrary, observing that most other children were undisciplined and "savage," she blamed their parents, feeling that they got their just desserts for neglecting discipline. The EP rating for discipline was 4 (overall severity).

Intensity of maternal involvement. Clearly this mother was committed to providing the best possible care for her child. Nonetheless, the primary focus of her emotional and intellectual life was her religion. Church activities, including missionary work, were exceedingly important to her. Additionally and of necessity, much of her concern focused on her own poor health. Thus persons and activities outside the home and concerns other than childcare loomed large, contrary to our definition of overly intense involvement. It is intriguing to note the difference between Georgia's mother and Caroline's. The latter lived her religion with equal fervor but used her intense beliefs as a crutch to support her precarious personal integrity. For Georgia's mother, on the other hand, family life and its obligations were given a broader meaning through religion, and this circumstance probably prevented her personal relationships from becoming overly intense. The EP rating for intensity of involvement was 2 (present, not prominent).

Developmental Course

Georgia was born about two months before term. She was and remained a healthy infant although her growth curve was peculiar. At the beginning, measures of length and weight placed her near the bottom of the normal distribution. She gained weight and grew well during the first year so that by 15 months both measures had moved closer to the midrange of the distribution (35th and 40th percentile, respectively). Things went awry during the third year and by the age of 34 months height and weight measures dropped off the curve entirely. She recouped again thereafter but remained a "tiny sparrow of a child," as one record put it; her weight never went above the 7th percentile. Also, from birth through six years of age her head circumference was unusually large (80th percentile). Yet, in medical and neurological examinations she was found to be healthy and normal at all times.

During the first four months the baby was said to cry nearly all the time, and neither the family nor the doctor could find a remedy. The condition, which sounded like a colic syndrome, disappeared spontaneously, and thereafter she functioned and developed normally. The mother told us that once she learned that there was nothing she could do to stop it, she left the crying baby in the crib for hours, checking on her from time to time. The mother made a point of saying that from the beginning, and also after the crying stopped, Georgia was "a loner" and a baby who "doesn't like anybody." Further, we learned that Georgia was exceptionally sensitive to sound. Even a rustling paper bag or a doorbell caused her to startle and cry.

Having told us all this and more at the time of the 7-month visit, the mother predicted that her baby's response to the research staff would be negative. Actually, Georgia proved to be an engaging and alert baby who kept a weather eye on the examiner but showed no aversion. On the contrary, she responded eagerly to the material, vocalized expressively, and enjoyed reciprocal social play of the peek-a-boo variety. Her MDI was 102. She functioned at the stage three level with respect to prehension and had gone slightly beyond this with respect to object permanence (sensorimotor intelligence scales).

When she returned at 15 months Georgia was described as a well-functioning and happy toddler. She was allowed to move freely throughout the apartment and spent most of her waking day moving about as she picked up and discarded various toys. She was content provided that either her mother or father was nearby, as they always were. She cried when punished by scolding or light slaps, had no tantrums, showed a good deal of demonstrative affection for both parents ("she likes to kiss"), and was not especially distressed at the approach of strangers. During the weeks preceding this visit the mother's symptoms had become more severe, and it was necessary for her to rest for large portions of each day. Her usual frequent church attendance was replaced by services within the home. We were struck by the mother's blandness as she described disturbing symptoms and reported her physician's grave concern.

In our quarters Georgia was friendly, cooperative, and at ease. She achieved an MDI of 87. All aspects of her behavior, motoric competence, communication skills, and vocalizations were congruent with low-normal developmental status. During the play session she used most of the toys in typical short-lived toddler fashion and maintained contact with both the mother and the examiner, mostly by showing or offering them toys (the only conventional communication signal she employed). Confronted with the large expanse of hallway space (open space procedure) she hesitated for a bit, moved away from her mother, and kept on going, though at least once she turned around for a sight of her mother. Nothing we saw or were told prepared us for the stormy and stressful times ahead.

The mother was unable to bring Georgia for the 28-month visit, largely because it was so difficult to take the child out of the home. A good many telephone conversations between the mother and ourselves, as well as an extensive interview later on, provided a picture of what was happening at the time. After Georgia had reached the age of two and had begun to speak in sentences, her mother judged that she was old enough to learn obedience. Up to that time this had not been an issue, perhaps because no unusual demands were made. Now, however, Georgia was expected to be tidy, to share her toys, to eat and go to bed when told to do so, to be quiet in church or in waiting rooms, and in general to be instantly obedient. The little girl could not live up to these high standards; the mother tried to enforce her dictates by various means, yet remained baffled by the child's response. When she was sent to stand inside a closet or off to bed this proved to be no punishment at all. As her mother said, "She'd prefer to stay there all day long." Ordinary scolding was apt to be ignored, but when it was followed by being shown or hit by the belt, Georgia began to cry bitterly and kept this up for long periods of time. In other words, she neither conformed to what was asked of her nor calmed down after a reasonable time. The mother perceived the act of crying as yet another misdeed and punished it as such, which led to more intense sobbing during which Georgia allowed her body to go limp. There was nothing anyone could do to stop her. By all accounts (we spoke to a close relative as well) this became *the* issue between the two. The child cried for hours each day and behaved in the same manner while away from home, with the result that neither the mother nor other relatives ventured to take her out at all. Things reached the point where the mother could no longer meet her obligations to the church, the father or others had to do the shopping, and the entire household was in turmoil.

The mother understood the crying as an act of rebellion if it occurred in response to unwelcome requests. What she could not understand, and what caused us to label Georgia as showing behavioral deviancy at this time, was that very often the child cried just as bitterly for no reason that anyone could discern. For instance, when Georgia's mother awakened her with a cheery "Good morning" (hoping to get the day off to a good start), the child would look at her as her eyes filled with tears and she would then begin to cry. Inexplicable crying would also occur in the park or on the street; it could happen while she was playing by herself or at any other time. The mother sought help from a child guidance clinic. However, in part because of the mother's rigidity and in part because of ineptness on the part of the clinic staff, no serious counseling took place. It should be mentioned that during this period Georgia's appetite was very poor, so that by the time of the 34-month visit she was alarmingly underweight.

By then all that has been described above was still present though the intensity and severity of the crying spells had diminished so that outings to church and other places had become possible again. Also, the still frequent clashes between child and mother were not interspersed with pleasant or at least neutral periods. The mother still worried about the episodes of inexplicable crying but spoke of them as though they were essentially a problem of proper management. Not once did she verbalize feeling sorry for the child or angry at her, though distress and annoyance at her inability to solve the problem found free expression. On the more positive side, the mother spoke of the fact that Georgia was much better behaved than many other children of her age in that she was neither destructive nor aggressive; "she won't go that way" was said in satisfaction. The one soft note was introduced when we were told of Georgia's fearfulness (of the dark, for instance). "I know what it is to be afraid," the mother said (referring to the aftermath of her accident), and she made clear that she tried to be reassuring. In passing, as though it were unimportant, the mother also told us that with other people, including strangers, Georgia was always sociable and friendly.

And so we found her to be during the research sessions at 34-months. Using a playful and encouraging approach, we were easily able to motivate the child to undertake even those tasks that initially did not attract her. Yet she looked physically unwell, there was a fluttery, restless quality to her behavior, and she spoke in a very low tone of voice. Her articulation was so poor that quite often we could not understand her. In addition, all aspects of her behavior were distinctly immature, and the IQ of 71 struck us as descriptive of her competence at this time. In response to the Achievement Motivation tasks she showed little persistence, needed a great deal of encouragement, and derived no visible pleasure from the end product. It was therefore not surprising that the Level of Aspiration experiment did not challenge her. During the play session Georgia kept busy with the toys and maintained social contact with both her mother and the examiner. Throughout this and the other sessions the mother frequently intruded by admonishing the child, by making disparaging remarks about what she was doing, and by outright scolding. Georgia paid little attention to this and nevertheless approached her mother in a friendly manner, most often to call her attention to a toy. The staff members, however, were so troubled by mother's attitude that the separation procedure was not attempted. One play episode is worth mentioning for its possible relevance to Georgia's lagging cognitive development. While handling a tiny toy bathtub Georgia tried to turn the faucet and seemed genuinely puzzled when it released no water. She tried repeatedly, inspected the underside, and tried again. For the time being she lost sight of the make-believe nature of the object. We have often seen precisely this kind of behavior with toy objects in toddlers between the ages of 12 and 15 months when objects are recognized but the capacity for symbolic functioning has not yet emerged (concept formation assessment).

Taking all these things together, Georgia at 34 months impressed us as an unhappy child, a child whose cognitive development was slow and in addition showed an atypical unevenness. We wondered whether her apparent friendliness to one and all might be a façade concealing impoverished and/or conflictual interpersonal relationships. And of course we wondered whether or not the mother always remained as scathing and remote as she claimed and as she demonstrated during this visit.

By the time of the 40-month visit marked changes had again occurred. The mother was pregnant and had been advised to reduce her activity as much as possible. She looked unwell and spoke of many physical discomforts. She rather dreaded the idea of having to train another child just when the worst was over with the first one. She was able to let us know that she felt deprived, isolated, and somehow resentful about her life at present. Most of the time the family remained at home. She told us that Georgia now had no opportunities to play with other children and in fact was hardly ever out of doors. Georgia was said to cry almost as much as she did before but to have matured in other ways. The youngster now liked to help with household chores, she ate well, and she seldom needed assistance with such things as bathing or dressing herself. Except for the crying, the mother said that she was a good girl.

In her contacts with research staff Georgia was as friendly but also as tense as she had been before. She spoke a great deal, in longer sentences, but with poor articulation (the mother's speech was exceptionally clear). Fine motor coordination had improved but gross coordination remained poor. Cognitive development had taken a leap forward. Perceptual acumen and memory had markedly improved, and categorical thinking and low-level abstraction were now within her repertoire. As before, cognitive functioning was uneven. She failed one item (vocabulary) at the two-year level, yet on another verbal test (response to picture) her response met normative expectation for six-year-olds. Her IQ was 87.

The assessments dealing with Achievement Motivation and with response to success and failure (Level of Aspiration) reflected next to no change in these dimensions. She took little pleasure in successful outcome, showed minimal self-confidence, and was compliant rather than assertive. With the World Test materials she was able to build a structure that was decorative rather than representational in nature.

Discussion

Results obtained at the time of the six-year follow-up examination clarified some aspects of Georgia's development that had puzzled us, but not all of them. She had made substantial cognitive progress in that her IQ had risen to 102, in spite of the fact that she proved to have a severe but circumscribed deficit in the area of visual-motor integration. When it came to such tasks as block design, which requires the child to reproduce with colored blocks a design presented in picture form, her performance was dismal. Yet she was alert to perceptual detail and did well on all verbal items. In retrospect it seems to us that the peculiar unevenness in her earlier test performance can be accounted for by the presence of a minor CNS deficit which could not clearly manifest itself until the requisite maturational level had been reached.

There remained the issue of how it was possible for this young child to adapt to nearly unremitting severity and frequent unfriendliness on the part of a mother who was an all-important person to her. We thought that Georgia was overly (and synthetically) friendly and downright loquacious with us. The mother told us that Georgia had now become what she ought to be: she did an appreciable share of the housework, she was so devoted to her baby sibling as to "mother her more than I do," she was "into religion" very deeply, and she frequently surprised her parents by performing chores that had not been assigned to her. The teacher was pleased with her in school. The mother regularly taught school subjects to her daughter because, as she said in her old scathing manner, in kindergarten all they do is play. The impression was inescapable that Georgia was being too good altogether and too eager to please. A small hint at what it may have cost her to live up to parental expectation came from her drawing of a human figure. She drew a very large grinning face from which there dangled a small shapeless appendage which she designated as the remainder of the body. It had no arms or hands, no legs or feet to stand on, and nothing with which harm could possibly be done.

Caroline: A Born Survivor

Background

Caroline was the fourth child born to a family whose existence might be described as an unending series of crises. The mother, her children, and many other members of the immediate family lived on welfare. They moved from one overcrowded apartment to another, always in close proximity to their relatives. The mother and others in the group had severe health problems so that hospitalizations, surgery, clinic visits, and the like took up much of their time.

The mother was a volatile, nervous person who had sought psychiatric help for what appeared to be periodic agitated depressions. During some of our contacts with her she was full of energy, good will, and hopefulness. At other times she was deeply troubled, angry, resentful, and afraid of a complete breakdown (an apprehension shared by her physician). Fortunately the bond between the family and several relatives was very close. In fact the households often merged. Most members of this large tribe had a share in raising the children, especially Caroline, who was regarded as special in both the positive and negative connotations of that word.

In order to understand Caroline's EP ratings and the descriptions of what happened to her, it is necessary to convey a sense of the ambience in which this family lived. All of them took violence for granted, both in themselves and in general. Thus the children, beginning for Caroline at a very early age, were allowed to beat each other up (for example, one sibling might beat another with a broomstick). They bit, scratched, and pulled hair to the point of inflicting real injury on each other, and adults very seldom interfered. Similarly, the fact that some men abuse and beat their women was accepted as part of life and did not necessarily prevent a positive appreciation of men who did so. Also, the mother knew that her own anger at the children could become uncontrollable. At such times she used a variety of means to separate herself from the children because she seriously believed that inadvertently she might kill. At less extreme moments, no one doubted that hitting and other physical punishments were natural responses to misbehaving children. When the mother said of her small daughter, "She likes violence," it was not said with regret or alarm. She rather appreciated the child's toughness as she added that this applied not only to her actions but to Caroline's response to mayhem on the television screen ("She sits there and laughs"). In a manner we had not seen before, these attitudes and actions existed in a kind of harmony with strong affection for the children and for one another; with a readiness to give pleasure, material goods, and loyalty to each other; and, last but not least, with genuine enjoyment in shared pleasures such as outings, family celebrations, or simply a good time at home. Another essential ingredient of this mix was that the mother was an articulate, thoughtful, and imaginative person who could describe an event or the quality of a relationship so vividly that the listener became a vicarious participant. Insofar as we could learn, there was only one thing this subculture held in contempt and that was weakness. It was made explicit that those who do not fight and scheme for what they want simply get what they deserve and are not to be pitied. From all this it will be understood that our ratings of experience patterns failed to capture much that was essential in the experience of this child.

Ratings at 40 Months

Impulse Control. At 40 months Caroline presented an unusual combination of behavior characteristics. The mother was accurate when she said that the child's temper was very bad but that she was now able to control it as she had not before. She meant that Caroline could refrain from overt action for long periods and release unbridled anger at a time when it was most effective. One example is that recently she had become angry at a sibling and let this be known by speaking to her furiously but quietly. She then hid a stick and late at night, when everybody was in bed, severely beat her sister with this weapon. It was common for her to request a particular kind of food while no one else was eating. The family complied, but if it took a while for the food to be prepared she became so angry that when it came she threw the plate at whoever brought it. She was relentless in demanding particular things that she wanted. Neither repeated refusals nor punishment stopped her clamor, and if her mother finally gave in Caroline had worked up so much anger that she no longer wanted it and threw a tantrum. Yet when engaged in an activity or task that interested her, her quiet concentration and prolonged perseverance were impressive. When harshly punished she typically neither moved nor spoke, but her mother thought she looked frightened. Thus in some ways her self-control was extreme, but she was a child so active and so given to unrestrained aggressive outbursts that an IC score of 4 would have been inappropriate. The impulse control score was 5 (both over- and undercontrolled).

Structure. During the previous several months Caroline's life had been more irregular and unpredictable than usual. While mother was once again in the hospital, Caroline and her siblings lived with their grandmother, where the mother had joined them upon her release. As Caroline rarely wanted to eat when meals were served and insisted upon bathing and dressing herself when it suited her to do so, the family had come to terms with the necessity of allowing the child to determine not only what she did, but also when and where. Other recurrent events, such as trips to the park or to stores or lunch at McDonalds, depended entirely upon the presence and the inclination of various relatives—there was no regularity to such outings. Caroline was described as spending an inordinate amount of her time in battles with her siblings and tempestuous altercations with her mother, grandmother, and other relatives. But she had also taken to solitary play and to watching television for prolonged periods of time.

The relative lack of structure in Caroline's life was not due to indifference on the part of the adults in the home, though their customary way of doing things—primarily the fact that the children were allowed to run wild and that punishments were frequent but haphazard—was an important factor. The only routine in Caroline's life was that, after others had gone to bed, she and her grandmother habitually spent an hour or two at the television and conversing. To some degree Caroline provided ministructure for herself during solitary play, much of which centered on rather rousing fantasy themes such as monsters or violent catastrophes. The EP rating for structure was 1 (minimally present).

Accommodation. This child was deferred to and sometimes indulged rather than accommodated. The mother and grandmother were aware of Caroline's sensitivities and difficulties but their response was chiefly to accept her as she was. Beyond that, both perceived her as an exceptionally strong (their word) personality whom nothing and nobody could sway ("The king of Jehova could not even move her," her mother said in something like admiration). An example may clarify why this family's way of dealing with the child could not be considered accommodative. All the adults knew and often said that with Caroline no punishment was effective—yet all of them hit and punished her when she "deserved it" (many times each day). One instance of attempted accommodation in this area reveals something of what was amiss. When Caroline could not be controlled, her mother tried to gain the child's cooperation by pretending to cry. Sometimes this led Caroline to be good, but only if her mother and grandmother went through a ritual during which the grandmother pretended to beat mother (for crying), at which act Caroline was said to show delight. It goes without saying that some things that would have been helpful to Caroline did not happen, not because no one thought of them, but because they were impossible to provide. The mother knew, for instance, that Caroline suffered from their frequent changes in living quarters and the abrupt loss of close relationships this entailed, but she had no control over these events. The EP rating for accommodation was 1 (minimally present).

Focused attention. Although she did play by herself and watch television, Caroline was the kind of child who compelled concentrated attention from other people, in part because her demanding, provocative behavior and stubbornness led to efforts at persuasion and to punishment very often, but also because whatever it was about this child that the family felt to be exceptional also caused her mother, grandmother, and other relatives to vie for her acceptance. They went out of their way to give her pleasure or to improve her mood, and this usually entailed giving exclusive attention to the child. By comparison to most children in our research group, Caroline received an amount of focused attention that falls near the lower end of the high range. The EP rating for focused attention was 3 (very prominent).

Didacticism. As in a good many of the other low SES families, but not in the research group as a whole, direct teaching of anything related to cognition was rare indeed in Caroline's life. We were told that one aunt occasionally taught her the numbers. There were magazines and picture books in the home, but it was claimed that she refused to look at them with someone else even though she was observed to study the pictures while mumbling to herself. Her television viewing was limited to the more highly dramatic among the horror and adventure stories (this is one of only two families that never once mentioned educational television or educational toys). The EP rating for didacticism was 1 (minimally present).

Frequency of conflict. This variable by definition referred only to conflict with significant adults, which, at 40 months, meant mother and grandmother. Caroline had had more than her share of such experience in the past, and, of course, still did. However, both of these adults tried to avoid open confrontations. The mother, because she was afraid of the intensity of her own anger, tended to send the child to the grandmother for what she called chastisement. On occasions when she had not been involved directly, the grandmother did not necessarily follow through. Open conflict with persons other than primary caretakers was very frequent indeed in Caroline's experience, but her opponents were primarily her siblings and secondarily some of the less tolerant of her relatives. The EP rating for frequency of conflict was 2 (present, not prominent).

Intensity of maternal involvement. Through good times and bad this mother was deeply involved with Caroline, clearly more so than with her other children. In part this came about because mother saw her own "bad" characteristics in the child and in part because the admixture of admiration, distress, intense anger, and maternal concern trapped the mother in a state of ambivalent feelings. At the time of the 40-month visit, which followed her prolonged hospitalization as well as profound upheavals in her personal life, the mother's thoughts and feelings centered on Caroline. She recognized that her daughter's current behavior difficulties were the result of distressing events in recent months, and she felt fiercely protective of the child. At this time, as throughout the baby's life, the quality of the mother's feelings for her child could not be described as chiefly affectionate concern, though this was also present. To her, Caroline represented much that she was afraid of in herself and much in the child's father that had caused her pain (she spoke of the possibility of reincarnation). Even as an infant Caroline was perceived not only as mean and evil but also as a child who, unlike her siblings, "doesn't want to be loved." The mother was greatly troubled by this.

When the child became old enough to show defiance, her mother had to deal with her own tendency to become enraged. Various phases of trying to cope with these feelings included unsuccessful efforts to withdraw and also periods when she gave reign to her feelings and dealt with the child in a harsh and punitive manner (reported and observed). She had now reached the point of safeguarding both the youngster and herself by removing Caroline from her presence as soon as she felt her anger rise. None of this interfered with her determination to cherish and protect the child. Caroline and her siblings received meticulous medical care. At considerable sacrifice, the mother saw to it that the children received excellent food and in general were provided with what was "good for them." In this respect too she may have overdone it. For instance, Caroline's Christmas wishes were extravagant by any standard, yet, during the 40-month interview, the mother declared her firm intention to fulfill them all ("Christmas is for them," meaning the children). Thus both her inner and her outer life revolved around Caroline to a higher degree than was true for the other children. The EP rating for intensity of maternal involvement was 3 (very prominent).

Developmental Course

Caroline was only slightly premature but required care in the ICU because of initial apnea. She responded well to respiratory assistance and, upon discharge two weeks later, she was considered to be a healthy infant. Up to the time the study ended there was only one unresolved medical problem. Several times each year she developed brief episodes of high fever (without seizures) for which extensive diagnostic studies failed to find the cause.

At the 7-month visit Caroline was a well-developed and well-functioning infant who received an MDI of 99. She demonstrated greater sensitivity to perceptual stimuli of low intensity than most and became excited in response to moderately intense visual, auditory, and tactile stimulation. She was highly responsive to social approaches, and she smiled, cooed, and babbled at a great rate when she was on her mother's lap but not otherwise. With respect to prehension and object permanence (sensorimotor scales) she functioned at stage three.

Largely because the mother was concerned about the baby (while we were concerned about the mother), Caroline was seen again when she was 12 months old. At that time her MDI was 89, which was thought to be an underestimate. Testing was made difficult by the fact that Caroline was friendly with the examiner only as long as she kept her distance; when the examiner came close enough to touch her, the child became distressed and unresponsive. Speech development had progressed to the point where Caroline uttered random syllables with an intonation so closely resembling ordinary speech that one felt one ought to know what she was saying (what the books call jargoning). She could also repeat short phrases and appeared to comprehend simple verbal directions of the *give me* and *don't touch* variety. During the play session she remained seated at her mother's knee, never approaching the toys, which is not uncommon at this early age. In other words, her behavior was fairly typical of that of alert 12-month old babies.

When the family returned for the 15-month visit the mother reported somewhat atypical behavioral developments, some of which could be confirmed by observation. For the first time we were told in some detail about the family's living conditions and Caroline's everyday experience. Elaborating on the theme that Caroline was mean and evil, the mother described not only severe temper tantrums but also strong combative tendencies. In interaction with her preschool-age siblings, the baby had learned to bite hard enough to draw blood, to pull hair so forcefully that it took adult strength to unclasp her hand, to hit, and to throw objects. It turned out that the siblings treated her in the same manner, so that Caroline, who was perceived as provocative, merely gave as good as she got. The mother and grandmother, who shared caretaking, responded to her tantrums by hitting and threatening. The mother felt it necessary to "get the badness out of her" before it was too late. Curiously, the mother was more concerned with the effect these scenes had upon the child than with their occurrence. She described how the baby first became stiff with tension and then began to "shake all over" and sometimes also to vomit. She took less seriously what concerned us most—the fact that Caroline had begun to bite and scratch her own body hard enough to leave marks. What worried the mother most of all was that the child was not cuddly: "She doesn't want you to bother her, even look at her," she said. Throughout this visit the mother was harsh and punitive toward the child and volunteered that she was too annoyed to act in any other way.

Caroline's cognitive development had not been hindered by all of this as she attained an MDI of 92. Like many other toddlers, she had become active and distractable, and her favorite activity was to throw objects, not in anger but as a game. Unlike most toddlers, she managed to ignore the examiner completely, avoiding any contact or acknowledgment of her as a person. She was intrigued by the test materials and responded to *them,* but not to the person who offered them. We also noted that when she was playing by herself and not interfered with she would nod her head in the gesture usually meant to express agreement. Her mother explained that after punishment she, the mother, usually bent over the child telling her that she was a bad girl. While doing this she habitually nodded her own head and when finally Caroline also began to nod this was taken to mean that the child admitted to being bad. We thought that the out-of-context nodding gesture might have its roots in the same mechanism that underlay the biting and scratching of her own body. Both can be understood as a primitive way of turning a passive experience—that which was meted out to her—into an active experience, by administering it to herself.

During the play session she again tended to cling to her mother but was also attracted to the toys. She occasionally walked away from her mother to manipulate the toys only soon to return. Unlike the majority of toddlers she did not show a single conventional communication signal. When confronted with the open space situation Caroline moved a few steps into the hallway, turned and glanced at her mother, and then walked past her back into the playroom.

By the time Caroline had reached the age of 22 months things had gone from bad to worse. The mother felt herself on the verge of a nervous breakdown, was seeing a psychiatrist, and felt that the tranquilizing medication did not help. She attributed her condition to the stress and strain of living with three children in a tiny "hellhole" of an apartment as well as to financial pressures. For the time being the grandmother was not able to help as much as she usually did, and Caroline's troublesome disposition was felt to be the last straw. Part-time placement with a sitter came to an end after a few days because Caroline was ungovernable and hurt both the sitter and her belongings. Her tantrums were described as terrible, and the constant fighting among the siblings remained unabated. When things got unbearable the mother said she often locked Caroline in the bedroom. There the child would take her revenge by putting the room in shambles. Caroline continued to hurt herself and also to reject affectionate attention. The mother believed that the only creature Caroline felt close to was the family cat.

The mother's account may well have been exaggerated, but the angry tension between the two was evident to observers. The research staff noted in some astonishment that Caroline was guardedly friendly with all of us but distinctly negativistic, and it seemed actively hostile, toward her mother. The latter, on her part, made no attempt at friendliness. Even when not scolding or threatening, her voice and manner toward the child were harsh even as she extended friendly warmth to the research staff.

During developmental testing Caroline was somewhat ill at ease but responded positively to the examiner, who was very careful neither to thwart the child nor to invade her privacy. Caroline obtained an MDI of 80. The symbolization experiment proved that the child's capacity for representation (in this case, imaginative play), was more advanced than that of most peers. She was able to point to two body parts on herself and on the doll though not the mirror, which is in keeping with normative expectation (body awareness procedure). In the play session her behavior differed from what we had seen before. She at once left her mother to use the toys and showed no observable reaction to separation. She did exhibit a few of the conventional communication signals, but these were addressed to the examiner, not the mother. In the open space experiment she behaved as is usually seen in somewhat younger toddlers in that she roamed the hallway, never looked back, and had to be retrieved.

Twenty-eight months is the age at which many of our research children reached their nadir with respect to behavior integration. Not so Caroline, but neither had she overcome her difficulties. The major change was a great improvement in the mother's state. Although the family still lived in the same small apartment, the mother's application for housing in a better building had been approved. Also, the grandmother was again available as a companion and part-time caretaker. We had an object lesson in what hope alone can do. The objective situation was exactly as before: Caroline was as difficult, all the children as unruly, overcrowding and lack of funds as severe, mother still on tranquilizers—but she was so buoyed up by the prospect of a better state of affairs as to be a different person. Among other things, this meant that friendly and companionable interchanges could take place between Caroline and her mother, side by side with the fighting and the punishments that, according to report, were not much diminished.

The mother's description of Caroline's behavior was so detailed and incisive that it would take pages to do it justice. She considered Caroline to be as self-willed and evil-tempered as before. Simply said, the child would brook no interference and when frustrated bit, kicked, broke things, and screamed. With siblings and other children it was often Caroline who provoked the fights. Yet at other times she listened to television programs with interest or played with her dolls, and her mother noted that the theme of a bad girl who was punished was often reenacted. The mother expressed genuine admiration for the child's strength of will, her excellent memory, her resourcefulness, and her ability to teach herself skills (such as independent dressing, using the play equipment in the park, etc.). The only developmental changes mentioned were that Caroline now spoke in words and short sentences and had begun to protest separation from the mother.

In the office we saw a distinctly active, somewhat tense, and rather self-willed little girl. On the Stanford-Binet she attained an IQ of 75. She refused a number of items of which we thought her capable, and we believed her to be a normally endowed and developed child. She was not yet able to match objects by category (concept formation scale), and in other ways as well the more abstract and objective modes of dealing with words and objects as yet had no meaning for her. Comprehension of pictures and nonverbal problems was fully adequate for her age. In response to the body awareness procedure she could now point to four body parts except on the mirror image (where posturing and clowning had more appeal). In the play session she was intrigued by the toys and used them, but she seemed tense and perhaps mildly anxious during most of this session. Throughout the play period she maintained contact with her mother and occasionally left the toy area to hug her briefly or spoke to her across a distance. Separation troubled her; she showed mild distress and ceased playing altogether. Her response to the open space situation was equivocal in that although she moved freely in the large hallway, she frequently looked back as if to see if mother was still there. The assessment of impulse control revealed her tendency to behave impulsively but also her capacity to maintain control over herself. However, her inability to wait even briefly before touching the toys, her near-tantrums when something she asked for was not given or done, and her restlessness were so striking as to overshadow the episodes of good control. Overall, she was rated as very excitable and as showing relatively little modulation or inhibition. There was every indication that at the age of two years Caroline had moved into the realm of symbolic mental functioning and that her relationship with her mother had several (but not all) features characteristic of what Mahler calls the rapprochement phase.

The interval between 28 and 34 months brought greater changes and upheavals than Caroline could cope with. The move into the new apartment entailed the loss of the family cat, to which Caroline was greatly attached. More important, soon after the move the mother became very ill and was in and out of the hospital for months. For several brief spells the children lived with their natural father, whom Caroline barely knew and in whose home she had never been before. For several other periods they were with the grandmother, and between times they lived with their largely incapacitated mother. The latter still looked and felt unwell and once again worried lest she might collapse.

Caroline's response to this sequence of events was dramatic. A few weeks before the research visit, when the mother was back home again, Caroline awoke in a strange state. At first she acted as though she did not recognize her family and within hours began to behave like a small baby. She used baby talk, wet and soiled herself, refused food except by bottle, and clung to her mother. At first she was punished, but then the mother noted that the child became timid and afraid and vomited with each upset. Thereupon the family gave in and "let her be." By the time we saw Caroline again she had returned to a nearly normal state though she was still in diapers and used baby talk much of the time. We were told that temper tantrums and fights with siblings continued to be frequent and that she was often seen to hit her dolls in what was described as a state of fury. For the first time since we had known her Caroline was shy in our presence and looked unhappy.

Although she was less defiant than before, she managed to evade many test items, chiefly by sitting there looking so unhappy that the examiner could find no way of coaxing her into a better mood. Yet when the materials and activities were attractive to her she did become involved and mildly pleased. Her IQ was now 73, and we felt that in some areas, especially the comprehension and use of verbally mediated concepts, she was truly deficient. As before, however, there was evidence of complex symbolic activity and good reasoning in relation to more concrete problems. When the miniature toys used in the scale for concept formation were presented she played with them in various ways but clearly failed to understand what matching meant, even with many demonstrations. The tasks used in the Achievement Motivation procedure were comprehensible and congenial to her. She worked with interest and persistence, showed pleasure when difficult items were achieved, but throughout conveyed a sense of low self-confidence and needed a great deal of encouragement. Similarly, in response to the Level of Aspiration experiment she chose to throw the ball from the very easiest position and stayed there after several successes. After a single failure she broke the rules by dropping the ball into the basket from immediately above. She used the toys throughout the play session, but in a listless manner. In response to separation she grew tense, fussed briefly, but then returned to handling the toys.

During the interval between the 34- and 40-month visits more serious upheavals and frightening events had taken place. Soon after the family had moved into their new apartment the mother's male friend joined them—with disastrous results. Suffice it to say that on numerous occasions he became abusive with the children and also with the mother when she tried to protect them. All the children were afraid of him and Caroline especially so. When he came home she went to bed and pretended to be asleep; she got to the point where she would neither eat nor speak in his presence. What made things worse for her and everybody else was that, whether his mood was good or bad, she refused to obey him and therefore bore the brunt of his wrath. On a few occasions she was painfully injured, and she as well as the other children watched as this man beat their mother. At such times Caroline's entire body trembled and she vomited, but, though terrified, she still refused to obey his commands. The mother thought it fortunate that after a few weeks of this she herself became ill and required prolonged hospitalization. This enabled the grandmother to take the children back into her home, where the mother joined them when she was discharged from the hospital.

In spite of the crowding and other hardships, the mother was delighted to be back and appreciated the material and emotional support given by her own mother and other relatives. The description of Caroline's experience patterns at 40 months provides details about the tumultuous home life and the manner in which the entire extended family helped to take care of the children and, beyond that, went out of their way to provide pleasurable experiences for them. They continued to take for granted the constant battles between the children and now as before, Caroline was not expected to obey adult requests. The major changes in Caroline's behavior were described as follows. Her fantasy life had become so intense that her mother wondered whether the child always distinguished between what was real and what was not. For instance, she often believed what she saw on television and could not or would not accept her inability to make the same things happen. When the appropriate movements failed to turn her into a being possessed of magic powers, and also when she found out that, try as she might, she could not fly, she became enraged and kept on trying. After seeing a show in which there was a talking cat she severely punished her own cat for not doing the same. She also awakened crying from bad dreams, apparently about monsters.

On a more realistic level, Caroline had become adept at protecting herself from her siblings and from all intrusions. She seemed really content only in solitary play; if she could not find an empty room, she settled down with her dolls beneath the table. The adults saw the wisdom of this arrangement and did all they could to separate Caroline from her siblings. The mother emphasized again how impossible it was to influence her daughter. No bribes or punishments, no appeals or reasoning affected her resolution. Once she disliked a person this was immutable; once she was determined to do something nothing but force could stop her, and even then she would try again. The mother also said that Caroline's mood "changes with the moon and the stars." One last anecdote highlights some of Caroline's unusual characteristics and symbolizes her desire for greater stability. Shortly before the last research visit she observed a toddler walking in a harness and urgently demanded that mother buy her one. When her astonished mother pointed out how inappropriate this was for a child of her age and asked why she wanted it, Caroline is reported to have said: "I want to know where I am at"!

Observers thought that Caroline was more comfortable with herself and with us than when last we saw her. In response to the test material she showed fine perceptual acumen, considerable imaginative powers, considerable impulsivity, and—as always—unusual determination in the pursuit of goals. Also as before, conceptual labeling and sorting lagged behind. Her IQ was now 81 and was thought to reflect her current abilities but probably not her potential. Especially noteworthy in one so young was the manner in which her relationship to the examiner changed by degrees from initial shyness to friendliness and finally to real warmth and something resembling intimacy. She now understood and carried out the matching task (concept formation) with toys but could not do the same with pictures. The Achievement Motivation assessment reflected somewhat greater self-confidence and much greater pleasure in accomplishment than before, though she still needed a fair amount of encouragement. She avoided confrontation with possible failure in the Level of Aspiration experiment by throwing the ball once and no more. In response to the World Test she became absorbed in building a fairly complex structure (something about half of our three-year-olds were unable to do). Although it did not represent anything in particular, it was more than a design in that animals, vehicles, and houses were grouped in a systematic manner.

Discussion

We were able to see Caroline again at six and also at eight years of age. Her IQ was 87 at age six, and at eight her abilities in school-related subjects (reading, spelling, arithmetic, sentence comprehension) fell well within the average range. She enjoyed school, and the teacher's independent evaluation described her as doing well in all areas and as a child whose feelings were easily hurt and who tended to sulk and hold a grudge. At no time did the school consider that she presented a behavior problem. From the mother's detailed accounts it would seem that her unusual determination and other early characteristics were still present. The fact that school attendance separated the children from one another much of the time, that the family lived in a somewhat larger apartment, and that the adults continued to accept her special ways probably contributed to her better overall adaptation. We were told, however, of unusually intense and lasting reactions to certain painful events such as her grandmother's illness and the death of her beloved cat.

We cannot offer a full discussion of how this unusual child developed under stressful conditions, partly for reasons of confidentiality and partly because for the later ages information is too scanty. We do consider Caroline to be a survivor par excellence and a good example of how reasonable competence can be achieved by very different routes. In her case, the atypical developmental course involved, among other things, the ability to turn initial weaknesses into strengths. Weaknesses may not be a good term since Caroline's unyieldingness, her overly intense fantasies, and her active way of responding to what befell her may also be regarded as unusual capacities. Over and over again Caroline found ways of protecting herself from unbearable conditions, whether by temporary regression, by isolating herself from constant battles with her siblings, by achieving tender closeness with a pet when this was not to be had from her mother, or by the constant working through of difficult experience in play and fantasy.

Chapter 9

Concluding Comments

Our intention was to establish a set of relationships between some stable features in the life experience of young children, some factors that play a major role in determining these life experiences, and some broadly defined aspects of developmental outcome. Having come to the end of our detailed analyses of ratings, test scores, and socioeconomic variations, to what extent have we succeeded? What have we learned that was not known before?

One way of putting it is to say that we specified some concrete values that must be entered into well-known equations, analogous to the particulars of weight and volume required when the law of gravity is to be applied to actual phenomena. The most general of these "equations" is that development is shaped by the interaction of biological and environmental factors. And, of course, it is well known that socioeconomic status is one of several powerful indexes of environmental circumstances. What we did was to specify, for a given locus (a metropolis in the United States), at a given time in history (the late 1970s and early 1980s), and for a group of infants vulnerable because they were premature, what aspects of the childrearing environment tend to vary most as a function of social class, and which of these variations are linked to early cognitive development. By tracing the interrelationships among social class, experience patterns, the development of impulse control, and cognitive development it was also possible to substantiate, and to make concrete and plausible, another well-known fact: that the cognitive and overall development of children from equally low socioeconomic strata runs the gamut from subnormal to distinctly gifted.

Another area in which a general formulation was translated into specifics was the emergence of impulse control and its significance for adaptation and cognitive development during the preschool years. Psychoanalysis and, in one way or another, all developmental theories have postulated that the voluntary inhibition of action impulses (the ability to delay), modulation in the expression of excitation, and in general ego control (especially the ability to forego or postpone immediate satisfaction in order to avoid subsequent displeasure and/or attain more highly valued goals) are essential components of normal development during the preschool years. Just how and when impulse control emerges, what fosters its development and what can hinder it, and how it is first manifested had not previously been studied in detail.[1] For our research population we were able to discern a fairly regular sequence of behavior patterns that mark the progression from a near-absence of intentional control to its establishment to the degree required for coping successfully with expectable dosages of stress and for reasonably harmonious adaptation to the social and physical environment. Beyond this, we described the consequences of more than ordinarily high levels of impulse control; in toddlers and young preschoolers, this tends to suppress spontaneity while, at the same time, cognitive development tends to advance rapidly.

That there is a connection between cognitive development and impulse control (the latter variously referred to as reflectiveness, delay capacity, distancing, and by other terms) is another well-established formulation. What was added by our work is a clearer understanding of the intrinsic cohesiveness between the emergence of symbolization, the basic first steps in formal thinking (abstraction, concept formation), and delay capacity. On the basis of this understanding we found evidence to suggest that the connection between impulse control and intelligence (as reflected in IQ scores) is time-limited. Once ego controls are sufficiently mature to permit thinking on the symbolic level, and hence to permit abstraction, the intellectual development of children whose impulse control was initially delayed does not differ much from that of children who entered the symbolic realm at an earlier age. Thus, while relatively poor impulse control is associated with relatively poor cognitive test scores during the preschool years, there is no reason to believe that this association persists into later childhood.

One topic about which we did *not* acquire new information is prematurity itself, or rather the consequences of low birthweight for subsequent development. We confirmed the well-established fact that neurological and pulmonary abnormalities occur more frequently in this group than in the full-term population. We did gain some impressions and generate some hypotheses in the course of our study. These include: (a) that low birthweight infants are less resilient in the face of stress than are full-term infants; (b) that emotional and behavior difficulties arise more frequently in this group, especially during the early preschool years when so many of the premature infants manifest signs of CNS immaturity; (c) that the presence of so-called soft neurologic signs during the first two years often heralds the emergence of specific learning difficulties and/or diagnosable neuropathology at school age; and, last, (d) that the developmental consequences of CNS abnormalities or deficits can be overcome or minimized if early life experience is growth-supportive, yet comparable handicaps may lead to grave impairment or impoverishment of personality and intellectual development under less favorable environmental circumstances.

To document and confirm such suppositions would require a comparison group

1. The literature on normal child development includes references to many of the behaviors that served us as criteria for assessing impulse control but that were not described in that context. Case histories that focus on the issue of ego control, on the other hand, have described pathological rather than normal developmental sequences.

of full-term infants. Had we been able to study, during the same interval and by the same methods, full-term infants from similar socioeconomic backgrounds, the consequences of prematurity could have been traced with reasonable confidence. Those who planned the study were keenly aware of this requirement, but fiscal and other practical impediments compelled us to accept a more limited research design.

We have bemoaned the fact that there are no good measurement devices for such encompassing variables as impulse control and stable aspects of life experience. Yet, we have also stressed the shortcomings of technically more precise techniques, such as standard tests and measures of socioeconomic status. We regard the numerical results as pseudoprecise in that tests measure limited aspects of overall intelligence, and in reality socioeconomic conditions comprise a great deal more than income, vocation, and education. It is as though the more directly and the more concretely one approaches variables that are patently important in reality, the more crudely they are indexed by the instruments we devise—and it is also as though arithmetical and hence statistical refinement have to be purchased at the price of considerable distance between that-which-is-to-be-measured and that-which-is-reflected by the final score.

Methodological shortcomings of this kind beset all psychological child-development research, but in our view, they are not the major obstacle to the conclusive demonstration of developmental laws. The real difficulty is that the hybrid area of child development does not lend itself to formal research in the classical mode, largely because the psychological and behavioral development of children cannot be dealt with in terms of any one—or even several—of the established scientific disciplines. Genetics, physiology, and other branches of biology play a role, but so do psychology, sociology, ecology, and even history. Rarely if ever is it possible to separate out for study the effects of genetic or biochemical determinants upon development, just as it is impossible to understand developmental changes by studying them only in terms of learning theory or psychodynamic processes or cognitive transformations. Each and every potential and actual determinant of developmental change modifies, and is modified by, all of the coexisting variables. For instance, just as identical geneotypical dispositions lead to widely different phenotypical end states, so will traumatic events in early life have a widely different impact upon personality development depending upon a host of circumstances, including the child's genetic endowment.

In principle, the same state of affairs prevails whenever scientific scrutiny is applied to uncontrolled phenomena in nature. Even physics does not deal with the entire physical universe, nor is the most advanced among the sciences always able to control or predict the consequences of its interventions. Brief mention of a highly developed scientific discipline is made in order to aid in the formulation of reasonable expectations for child development and, in fact, for psychology as a whole. Epistemologically speaking, child development has much in common with an area such as agriculture. There, through careful observation, simple measurements, and the experience of farmers in many regions of the world, a good deal has been learned about the effective cultivation of many plants. Not so different is the way in which the experience of untold generations in rearing and teaching children has yielded much valid information about what children need in order to thrive. Agriculture was transformed primarily by the application of two scientific disciplines: chemistry and genetics. Chemical analyses helped to define and to create the best environments for different plants in different regions. Genetic engineering created especially resistant and productive strains adapted to various environments. Yet even the most scientific farming remains dependent upon uncontrollable forces such as the weather, luck, and the intuition of those who work the land. No one ever thought of agriculture as a branch of science in its own right.

The parallels between agriculture and child development—in some respects, psychology as a whole—are obvious. Close observation of child behavior under different conditions, observation of regular and recurring changes with advancing maturity, and registration of different adult characteristics associated with different antecedents laid the groundwork. Thoughtful speculation about these observations provided hypothetical explanations (which we like to call theories), that in turn can be supported or refuted by more selective and partially controlled observations (which we like to call experiments). It is no accident, I think, that the statistical methods that have proved most useful in psychology were first developed to meet the needs of agricultural research. Psychologists soon recognized the suitability of parametric and nonparametric methods to their own data precisely because of the fundamental similarities between agriculture and empirical psychology.

Most psychological research, including that in the area of child development, employs the language and to some extent the techniques of the so-called hard sciences. There are mathematical models, there are hypotheses presumably testable by the experimental method, and there is a tendency to accept successful prediction for a limited sample as proof of the truth of the hypothesis upon which the prediction had been based. None of these qualms and reservations about the research establishment in the psychological and social sciences is new, though critical discussion of these issues has had little influence upon the mainstream of psychological research. These epistomological considerations are mentioned in support of my contention that—in child-development research, at any rate—we have fallen short because we aimed too high. The investment in developing and validating an overarching theory, be it learning theory, Gestalt, psychoanalytic, or any other, has narrowed the focus of empirical inquiry to items held to be directly relevant (and those that can be readily quantified). In consequence, systematic observation of a wide range of phenomena and of apparent relationships between them, and informed speculation about how these relationships came about, are not sufficiently encouraged. In other areas, including biology and geology, the formal scientific edifice has been likened to a pyramid: it rises from a broad base of factual information about the phenomena it seeks to understand and to explain. In much of psychology, and certainly in child psychology (and, parenthetically, also in present-day sociology and anthropology), the network of abstractions and models is more like an inverted pyramid. A rather narrow field of cumulative and systematic observation supports massive and complex theoretical formulations.

Limited but stringent research enterprises, such as our study of preterm infants and their families, may serve to broaden and to strengthen the empiric underpinnings of whatever theoretical abstractions will make it possible to better understand our children and ourselves.

Appendixes

Appendix A.1: Socioenvironmental Data Background: Scoring Directions and Scoring Blanks

The demographic and other background information for each index baby is coded in a single booklet although information may be obtained at various times in the course of our contacts with the family. The procedure is to code all relevant information on the basis of the summary of the seven-month visit. A list is made of those items still lacking, and this is incorporated into the pink sheet in preparation for the 15-month visit. After that visit the summary is again used to code the additional information that has been obtained. If necessary, a list of missing items is again placed with the pink sheet so that they can be obtained at the 22-month visit. By that time the process should be complete, but it is possible that the same procedure may be followed for an additional time interval. In any case, *information missing* scores (0) will not be entered until after the last interview with the family.

All information on this background coding form refers to events and circumstances prior to the index subject's birth. We have added birthweight and estimated gestational age (EGA) as well as sex to the identifying information only because certain preliminary calculations can then be made without recourse to the computer data stored centrally.

Columns 1 through 18 are self-explanatory. Columns 19–25 provide for seven siblings (a number not likely to be exceeded). When our subject is the first and only child, score NA, for *not applicable*. If any of a mother's other children lived for more than two weeks but died thereafter, score *deceased*. The next few columns are self-explanatory, but note that where we ask for the birth-order position of the mother and father, only one of the two relevant columns can be scored. In other words, if the mother's birth order is from first to eighth, a score will be assigned in column 28; if she is the ninth child or a higher number, it would be coded under column 29. Columns 30 and 31 are scored in the same way. For column 32 please consider our subject's position in relation to all surviving siblings and half-siblings. Column 33 refers to the mother's marital status on the day the infant was born, regardless of whether she is married to the baby's father. Both common-law and legalized marriages are scored as *married*. *Previously married* refers to women who are separated or divorced from their previous husbands as well as to widows. Column 34 refers only to whether or not the mother's parents have remained married to each other. Columns 35 through 38 describe the marital status of each grandparent whenever the score for column 34 was other than married. When a grandparent is deceased, please score *not applicable*. Columns 39 through 44 are self-explanatory. Columns 45 through 50 employ the categories used in the calculation of socioeconomic status as defined in working paper number 15, U.S. Department of Commerce, Bureau of Census, *Methodology and Scores of Socio-economic Status*. Columns 51 through 53 are self-explanatory. Column 54 refers to the period when mother was pregnant, and she is counted as having worked or gone to school even if this was discontinued during the last trimester. Column 55 refers to the presence of familial disease to a marked degree; that is, the same medical disorder must have been experienced by at least three members of the family. These will usually be the families subject to high blood pressure and to asthma, although, of course, other familial diseases may appear.

Everything through column 61 should be self-explanatory. Column 62 scores the mother's plans about who will take care of the infant, either herself or some other person. For mothers who plan on a pattern of shared caretaking, the appropriate scoring on column 62 is *not applicable*. The reverse applies to those who plan on a single caretaking pattern; their score on column 63 will be *not applicable*. The SES status of the mother's and father's families of origin (that is, their parents) is also to be calculated by the method provided in the U.S. Census Paper 15.

Socioenvironmental: Background

Variable		Col.	Code
Card No.		1	1
Code No.	hundreds	2	
	tens	3	
	units	4	
Acc. No.	thousands	5	
	hundreds	6	
	tens	7	
	units	8	
Infant's birthweight in grams	1000 or less = 1; 1001–1500 = 2; 1501–2000 = 3; 2201–2500 = 4; 2501 or more = 5	9	
Infant's gest. age in weeks at birth	tens	10	
	units	11	
Infant's Sex	Male = 1; Female = 2	12	

At Time of Infant's Birth

Age of	12–15	16–19	20–29	30–34	35–40	>40	Don't Know	Dec.	Col.
Mother	1	2	3	4	5	6	9	7	13
Father	1	2	3	4	5	6	9	7	14
Mat. grandmo.	1	2	3	4	5	6	9	7	15
Mat. grandfa.	1	2	3	4	5	6	9	7	16
Pat. grandmo.	1	2	3	4	5	6	9	7	17
Pat. grandfa.	1	2	3	4	5	6	9	7	18

app. continued

Variable											Col.	Code
Age of infant's sibs or half sibs in years		Not Appl.	<2	2–5	6–10	11–16	17–24	25+	Deceased	Don't Know		
	I	1	2	3	4	5	6	7	8	9	19	
	II	1	2	3	4	5	6	7	8	9	20	
	III	1	2	3	4	5	6	7	8	9	21	
	IV	1	2	3	4	5	6	7	8	9	22	
	V	1	2	3	4	5	6	7	8	9	23	
	VI	1	2	3	4	5	6	7	8	9	24	
	VII	1	2	3	4	5	6	7	8	9	25	
No. living siblings		None	One	Two	Three	Four	Five	Six+	Don't Know			
Of mother		1	2	3	4	5	6	7	9		26	
Of father		1	2	3	4	5	6	7	9		27	
Birthorder of Mother		First	Second	Third	Fourth	Fifth	Sixth	Seventh	Not Appl.	Don't Know		
		1	2	3	4	5	6	7	8	9	28[a]	
		Eighth	Ninth	Tenth	Eleventh or more	Don't Know						
		1	2	3	4	9					29	
Birthorder of Father		First	Second	Third	Fourth	Fifth	Sixth	Seventh	Not Appl.			
		1	2	3	4	5	6	7	8		30[a]	
		Eighth	Ninth	Tenth	Eleventh or more	Not Appl.	Don't Know					
		1	2	3	4	5	9				31	
Birthorder of Infant (live sibs only)		First	Second	Third	Fourth	Fifth	Sixth	Seventh	Eighth	Don't Know		
		1	2	3	4	5	6	7	8	9	32	

[a]Score either column 28 or 29, *never* both.

Marital status at infant's birth:	Married[b]	Previously Married	Always single	Not Appl.	Don't Know	
Mother	1	2	3	4	9	33

Mother's biol. parents	Married[b]	Separated	GM dec.	GF dec.	Don't Know	
	1	2	3	4	9	34
If not married to each other or one partner deceased:						
Mat. grandmother	1	2	3	4	9	35
Mat. grandfather	1	2	3	4	9	36
Pat. grandmother	1	2	3	4	9	37
Pat. grandfather	1	2	3	4	9	38

Highest educational level of	<6th grade	7–8 gr.	Some H.Sch. 1–3 yrs.	H.Sch.[c] Dipl.	Some Coll. 1–3 yrs.	BA or BS	Grad.	Don't Know	
Mother	1	2	3	4	5	6	7	9	39
Father	1	2	3	4	5	6	7	9	40
Mat. grandmother	1	2	3	4	5	6	7	9	41
Mat. grandfather	1	2	3	4	5	6	7	9	42
Pat. grandmother	1	2	3	4	5	6	7	9	43
Pat. grandfather	1	2	3	4	5	6	7	9	44

[b]Common law included.
[c]Include equivalence.

app. continued

Variable										Col.	Code
Last or present job	Prof. tech.	Mgr. prop.	Cler. Sales	Craftm. foreman	Operative	Serv. incl. domest.	Labor	None	Don't Know		
Mother	1	2	3	4	5	6	7	8	9	45	
Father	1	2	3	4	5	6	7	8	9	46	
Mat. grandmo.	1	2	3	4	5	6	7	8	9	47	
Mat. grandfa.	1	2	3	4	5	6	7	8	9	48	
Pat. grandmo.	1	2	3	4	5	6	7	8	9	49	
Pat. grandfa.	1	2	3	4	5	6	7	8	9	50	
Ethnicity U.S.	Black	Cauc.	Hispanic	Other	Don't Know						
Mother	1	2	3	4	9					51	
Father	1	2	3	4	9					52	
While pregnant (this infant), Mother lived with	Alone	Husb.	Own parents	Relative	Friends	Institution	Don't Know				
	1	2	3	4	5	6	9			53	
During pregnancy Mother employed	Not	Part-time	Full-time	School	Don't Know						
	1	2	3	4	9					54	
Significant familial disease	Yes	No	Don't Know								
	1	2	9							55	
No. miscarriages (Mother)	None	1	2	3	4 or more	Don't Know					
	1	2	3	4	5	9				56	
Mother's age at first miscarriage	Not Appl.	<16	16–19	20–29	30 or more	Don't Know					
	1	2	3	4	5	9				57	

No. abortions, Mother	None	1	2	3	4 or more	Don't Know	
	1	2	3	4	5	9	58

Mother's age first abortion	Not Appl.	<16	16–19	20–29	30 or more	Don't Know	
	1	2	3	4	5	9	59

No. premature sibs of infant	Not Appl.	None	1	2	3	4 or more	Don't Know	
	1	2	3	4	5	6	9	60

		School		Work				
Mother's plans vocational	No Plan	PT	FT	PT	FT	Stay Home	Don't Know	
	1	2	3	4	5	6	9	61

Mother's plans caretaking	Mo	GM	Relat.	Other	Not Appl.	No Plan	Don't Know	
Single CT	1	2	3	4	5	6	9	62

	Not Appl.	Mo.&Fa.	Mo.&GM	Mo.&Oth.	GM&Oth	2 Rel.	2 Oth	Grp.	Don't Know	
Shared CT	1	2	3	4	5	6	7	8	9	63

Religion	Protestant	Catholic	Pentacost.	Other	None	Don't Know	
Mother	1	2	3	4	5	9	64
Father	1	2	3	4	5	9	65

Importance, religion	None / Minimal	Somewhat	Very Devout	Don't Know	
Mother	1	2	3	9	66

SES, family of origin	Low 25 or less	Middle 26–75	High 76–100	Don't Know	
Maternal	1	2	3	9	67
Paternal	1	2	3	9	68

Appendix A.2: Socioenvironmental Data for Each Visit: Scoring Directions and Blanks

For each heading on the left-hand side of the page, one or several scores are appropriate. These scores will be assigned specific numerical values corresponding to the column on the computer card and to each of the alternatives that may be checked as true. Since the computer operates only vertically, any number of more than one digit is spread over several columns. Thus, the sample first page prepared reads: code number 013, accession number 7511, visit number 2, gestational age 1 year no months or days, chronological age 1 year, 1 month, 14 days. Under face-sheet information we also record who responded in the interview, allowing for two possible respondents. When more than two people are interviewed on any one visit, please choose the two most important ones. Thus, on the sample page (columns 22 and 23) respondent 1 is the grandmother and her role is that of secondary caretaker. The second respondent is some other relative whose role is that of occasional caretaker (columns 24 and 25). If there is only one respondent, score columns 24 and 25 *not applicable*. Once we come to the actual data, beginning with household composition, a number is assigned to each possible score, but the number 9 will be reserved for *don't know* while the number 0 will be used for missing information.

Under household composition, the number of persons includes the baby and everyone else who permanently lives in the same residence. The baby is also included under number of children less than 6 years of age. By sick or aged we understand persons requiring care; so, a younger person with severe handicaps might be counted, while an older person, even one with significant health problems, might not be counted unless he or she was disabled to some degree.

Under income and vocation (column 32), we included a score for "income per person." This would simply be the estimated weekly income (column 31) divided by the number of persons in the household (column 26). For the calculations, use the midpoint of the range indicated in the score. We thought it would be easier for us to do this simple calculation as we scored rather than to wait for the computer to do it for us. We thought that the dollar income per household would tell us nothing on first surveying the data unless it was put in some relationship to the number of persons that the income had to feed. Support from father (column 33) is applicable only where the baby's father is *not* a member of the household. The same rule applies to column 34, support from other individuals. The health and life insurance items (columns 36 and 37) must apply to mother and baby in order to be scored here whereas, if the home in which mother and baby are living is owned by the grandparents (column 38), it receives a score.

For vocational status (columns 39 and 40) we attached a separate memo that assigned a score to each occupational level. This was taken from an SES determination instrument developed by the U.S. Census Bureau. Vocational status to be scored here is only for members of the household; the scores for *don't know* and *missing information* will be entered as appropriate for the various members of the household.

For the income and vocation items as well as some others, the interviewer should determine whether or not there have been any changes in the relevant categories since the previous visit. A statement to the effect that there have been no changes should be included with the summary. When the summary indicates that there has been no change the coder should enter the same scores as were entered the previous time. Otherwise, of course, the newly-appropriate scores should be entered. (The purpose is to determine by machine calculation whether or not changes have occurred in these dimensions.)

In scoring *dwelling type* (column 41), an apartment house is considered small if it contains from two to ten separate apartments. *Project* refers to large apartment-house complexes such as Co-op City or Mitchell Llama. The score for marital relationship (column 48) must be based on things the mother actually said as she described aspects of her life. When a lack of harmony (or its presence) is thought to exist on the basis of clinical inference from what was *not* said, a score of *don't know* is appropriate.

Under caretaking patterns someone is considered the primary caretaker if he or she has responsibility for the baby's safety and well-being at least 80% of the time. By *primary caretaking shared* we mean something close to a 50–50 split between two people who between them have responsibility for the baby at least 80% of the time. Working mothers who take care of the baby after working hours and the entire weekend are considered as sharing the primary caretaking with whoever babysits during the day. By secondary caretaker we mean persons who regularly or often enough for this to be a recurring element in the baby's life assume full responsibility for the baby's well being. The fact that relatives or others may perform caretaking functions such as feeding while the primary caretaker is present does not make them secondary caretakers since they are not really in charge of the baby at those times. *Time spent with father* does not refer to the father's caretaking activities. Fathers who play with the baby every evening would be scored here. Here (column 54) we refer to situations when the father actively devotes himself to the baby; just being in the room but paying only intermittent attention to the baby would not count. This means that a father who does share in the caretaking would be scored in column 52 or 53 and again in 54, while those who do not participate in caretaking may still be scored under 54.

All categories that follow *time spent with father* will be rated by changing criteria according to the baby's age level. Thus, freedom of movement at 7 months would be considered limited only in infants who are rarely placed on the floor, in playpens, on sofas or beds while they are awake, or in babies who are frequently strapped down or habitually wear clothes that interfere with kicking and the like. At later ages this becomes more significant in terms of walking, running, climbing, being taken to the park, etc. Similarly and obviously, what might constitute a limited amount of social play at one age may be considered adequate at another. Here it is not only the amount but the appropriate sociability that enters the rating. For this variable it does not matter whether play takes place primarily with caretaking adults or other persons. Beginning with the second year, social play will be considered to include interaction of a playful nature with other children including peers. By contact with nonhousehold members we mean more than being smiled at by strangers in the store; we refer to occasions when persons not members of the household interact directly with the child. When scoring *exposure to places other than home* we include quite familiar places such as the homes of neighbors or other relatives as well as streets, parks, stores, and visits to unfamiliar homes. Again, the supply of toys and objects that can be used for manipulation and play will be judged in terms of appropriateness and customary standards as these vary from one age to another. By television viewing we refer to those occasions when the baby is held or placed in such a way as to invite him to view the screen *and* there is some evidence that, in the respondent's view, the baby is paying attention. *Comforted when crying* must of course reflect what we are told. We are referring here to the caretaker's reported manner of dealing with the child who cries not from hunger, pain, or other immediate need. When we know what one of the primary caretakers does but she cannot tell us how the other one handles the problem we would have to go either to *variable* or *don't know* depending on how much the respondent can tell us. Peer-group contact will be scored *not applicable* for the 7- and 15-month visits. Thereafter it refers to more than brief and casual encounters—that is, to sharing play or other situations with children of similar age for at least a half hour at a time and usually for a longer period. If the child attends an organized group such as a daycare center or nursery school he receives a rating of not applicable under this heading, which refers to informal association in his own home or the home of friends or relatives. The next variable, group care, refers to organized groups only. It is possible to receive a score for both group care and peer-group contact.

The next section concerns mother's attitudes and characteristics. Some of the variables refer to overt statements made by the mothers while others refer to the interviewer's observations and judgments. By mother we mean any primary caretaker who participates in the interview. Emotional difficulty reported refers only to instances in which mothers spontaneously mention that they have suffered or are suffering from a difficulty that they themselves regard as being emotional or nervous in nature. We shall regard as professional help any contacts mother may have with a professional or paraprofessional person that the mother perceives as taking place for this reason. Thus, a mother who states that she had been helped by talking with a counselor or social worker receives a score as does a mother who says that she turns to her physician for help with her depression. *Emotional difficulty observed* is a judgment on the interviewer's part, incorporated in the summary, to the effect that the mother manifested overt signs of clinical disturbance during the visit. *Mother feels isolated* refers to mother's direct or indirect communication to the interviewer to the effect that she feels cut off from normally close communication with other people. By *isolation* we here mean that she has no one to whom she feels close, whether or not she is in contact with other people. The coding *self report* (1) is limited to instances where mother directly indicates that she is very lonely, etc. The score of 2 refers to the interviewer's considered judgment that the mother in fact lacks access to people with whom she can communicate although the mother failed to make this explicit. The score of 3 is appropriate when the mother reports isolation and the interviewer's judgment concurs with that report; neither applies when the mother does not mention feeling isolated and the interviewer does not consider her isolated. *Don't know* here refers to the interviewer's inability to judge this variable.

Column 71 refers to a tendency to read into the baby's behavior complex motivations and personality characteristics of a nature not appropriate to the child's age. A mother who believes that a 7-month-old baby prefers men because he knows he will be a man someday would be an extreme example. Mothers who attribute entirely normal responses of crying and moving about during grooming procedures to stubbornness or meanness show the same tendency to a lesser degree. To assume that a 7-month-old purposely does something he knows to be forbidden in order to annoy his mother or to describe a child of this age as selfish or generous are other examples. It may be that this variable will become meaningless toward the end of the second year.

By didactic tendencies (column 72) we refer to intentional, deliberate teaching of the baby on the caretaker's part. There may be "lessons" in reaching or walking, there may be practice in learning to say words, there may be systematic efforts to teach the child self-feeding, table manners, or anything else. The coding of mother's view of the child's physical and mental normality refers to mother's opinion at the time of the interview. It may be influenced by what she has been told during the visit though not all mothers accept diagnostic information. This code represents the interviewer's judgment of what mother said on the topic and may or may not include overt expression of her beliefs. Therefore, *don't know* may apply when the interviewer cannot be certain how the mother views the baby.

On card 2 columns 27 and 28 refer to the mother's behavior during the visit in relation to the interviewer and to the infant. The term spontaneity is used in its usual meaning, referring to a sense of ease, freedom, and lack of inhibition. Columns 29 and 30 are both limited to overt verbalization accompanied by appropriate affect on the mother's part. When the interviewer is certain that a mother takes pleasure in the baby, but fails to comment on this or demonstrate it very openly, she would nonetheless receive a score of 3; the same applies to the negative affect. In the latter category we include all indications of negative feeling, whether disappointment, worry, dislike, anger, or anything else.

Card 2, column 31, represents the interviewer's judgment, as expressed in the summary, about mother's tendency to reflect and think about the baby as well as herself and family life. A case in point are mothers who have developed theories about why the baby likes or dislikes certain things, mothers who spontaneously wonder what the baby may be thinking or feeling, mothers who debate with themselves about what might be the most appropriate way of dealing with the baby or a family issue rather than acting on established convictions or spontaneous impulse. In most instances, column 32 refers to a commitment to upward social mobility. However, parents from middle-class backgrounds who place special value on material security and maintaining social status would also demonstrate this characteristic. A code of 1 (actively/seriously) is reserved for mothers whose current activities are very strongly governed by efforts to gain or maintain material security. People who save at a real sacrifice to immediate convenience, people who work in order to make a move to a better neighborhood possible, people who seek out schooling or vocational training in order to improve their lot would fall into this category. A code of 2 applies to the large group of mothers who do indeed resent their limited material security but seem unable or unwilling to do anything about it. A code of 3 does not necessarily mean that a mother does not have motivations of this sort. It may mean that neither directly or indirectly was there any evidence as to how she feels about the matter.

The next section deals with a few aspects of the interval history. Brief and long separations from the primary caretaker (columns 33 and 34) refer to temporary separations that occurred during the time interval since the last visit. If there has been a permanent change in caretakers this will have been scored in one of the preceeding sections. We refer here to such events as mother's having to leave home for a few days and then returning, or to any other circumstance that for a limited period of time has created for the baby a separation from a primary caretaker. Brief is defined as three to five consecutive days; long is defined as anything more than five days. Serious illness of household member is meant to refer to disruption of the usual routine due to an accident to or illness of a permanent member of the household, causing anxiety or other strong feeling. The death of a household member, if preceeded by an illness, would be included here. Column 36 is a catch-all for any event that causes major disruption and concern in the household. It is impossible to be specific, but such things as sudden death of a significant person, fire, robberies, major fights and/or confrontations with the police, and the like would be included.

Financial improvement refers to an easing of the financial situation during the interval since the last visit. For instance, a debt may have been paid off or a cheaper apartment may have been obtained or expenses related to an illness may have dropped out. Similarly, a reported decrement refers to a worsening of the financial situation whether it be due to a rent raise, unexpected expenses, or whatever. The coder will have to judge whether the change is sufficiently substantial to make a real difference to the family. A rough guideline is that the added or subtracted amount should correspond to no less than 20% of weekly income.

For technical reasons it seemed necessary to include items relevant to each of the hypotheses on each coding sheet. Thus, at any given visit a great many of the variables will be scored as not applicable. For visit 1 *not applicable* applies from columns 39 through 65. Walking ability refers to the state of affairs on the day of the visit. Column 40 refers to mother's report as to when the child began to walk easily and freely. The score is applicable only when column 39 receives a code of 1—all other visits receive a *not applicable* for column 39. The same applies to column 41, which refers to the frequency with which the child is allowed free walking, and column 42, which describes the spatial areas within which the child is allowed to roam.

Column 43 refers to mother's report as to whether any of the conventional communication signals have been observed at home and, if so, how long they have been in the baby's behavior repertoire. Column 44 is based on the scores recorded on the intentional communication blank. A *yes* is appropriate if the child was scored for at least two instances of any kind of conventional communication behavior. Column 45 assumes a developmental sequence running from *show/points* to such behaviors as uttering the word "bye-bye" clearly as a request to terminate.

For hypothesis II, column 46 refers to the mother's report as to the child's behavior when a primary caretaker leaves the room. It does *not* refer to behavior when the child leaves the caretaker or to outdoor situations, but only to instances when the caretaker leaves a room in which the child remains; other familiar persons may or may not remain with the child. Column 47 refers to the history of protest or distress at separation. A child who has not shown this behavior would receive a score of *not applicable*. Column 48 is based on mother's account of the degree to which the child is inclined to follow the caretaker actively as the latter moves from one place to another. Column 49 deals with the history of this behavior, provided that there has been a tendency to follow. *Demonstrative hugging and caressing* refers to mother's report of a tendency on the child's part to approach his primary caretaker spontaneously with demonstrations of affection. In order to qualify for a score here the child must be said to direct such behavior either only to primary caretakers or very noticeably more often to primary caretakers. Column 51 is a catch-all since many other behaviors may be reported which the interviewer understands to reflect the presence of strong attachment. We record merely whether or not such other unequivocal signs of strong attachment have been reported in addition to the specific ones mentioned in the other variables.

Column 52, speech performance, is to be based on whatever the mother reports the child's present vocabulary to be. Clear-cut and convincing idiosyncratic words may be included, but call sounds are excluded. The next variable (53) refers to the reported history of the ability to use any conventional words understandably. The last column (54) is based on credible reports of particular two- (or more) word-phrases that the child may have uttered at some time before the visit. (Since we shall have scores of taped speech samples I did not include mother's account of the child's present performance in this respect as a separate variable.)

The variables under hypothesis III, beginning with column 55, attempt to specify behaviors that would reflect the absence or presence of a degree of impulse control.

Beginning with column 61, interview content relevant to achievement motivation is specified. The first variable refers to the child's tendency to ask for help in accomplishing his goals while the second scores mother's response to our questions of how the child behaves when offered or given help for which he did not ask. The remaining variables are self-explanatory. (An effort was made to make this last group of variables correspond to those that can be observed during testing and the play session. Whether or not mother's report and our observation yield the same picture remains to be seen.)

Summary Coding: Each Visit

Variable			Col.	Code*
Card No.			1	1
Code No.		hundreds	2	0
		tens	3	1
		units	4	3
Acc. No.		thousands	5	7
		hundreds	6	5
		tens	7	1
		units	8	1
Visit No.			9	2
Gest. Age	years		10	1
	months	tens	11	0
		units	12	0
	days	tens	13	0
		units	14	0
Chron. Age	years		15	1
	months	tens	16	0
		units	17	1
	days	tens	18	1
		units	19	4

Item								Column	Code
Baby's Sex	Male 1	Female 2						20	
Birthweight	1000 or less 1	1001–1500 2	1501–2000 3	2001–2500 4	2501 + 5			21	
Respondent I	Mo 1	Fa 2	GM 3	Rel 4	Other 5			22	3
Caretaking role	Prim 1	Sec 2	Occ 3	None 4				23	2
Respondent II	Mo 1	Fa 2	GM 3	Rel 4	Other 5	Not Appl. 6		24	4
Caretaking role	Prim 1	Sec 2	Occ 3	None 4	Inappl. 5			25	3
	Household Composition								
No. persons	2 1	3–4 2	5–7 3	8–10 4	10+ 5	Don't Know 9		26	
No. children < 6 years	1 1	2–3 2	4–5 3	6+ 4	Don't Know 9			27	
No. children 7–16 yrs.	1 1	2–3 2	4–5 3	6–7 4	8+ 5	Don't Know 9	None 6	28	
No. sick or aged	0 1	1 2	2 3	3+ 4	Don't Know 9			29	
Head of Household	Fa 1	Mo 2	GF 3	GM 4	Other 5	Don't Know 9		30	

*Code numbers in columns 1 through 25 were entered as examples only.

app. continued

Variable	Categories (code)	Col.	Code
	Income, Vocation: Baby's Household		
Est. Weekly Income, dollars	<85 = 1; 85–115 = 2; 116–155 = 3; 156–200 = 4; 201–300 = 5; 300+ = 6; Don't Know = 9	31	
Income per person	Col. 26 / Col. 31; <15 = 1; 16–20 = 2; 21–30 = 3; 31–50 = 4; 51–99 = 5; 100+ = 6; Don't Know = 9	32	
Support from father (not in household)	Not Appl. = 1; Major: reg. = 2, occ. = 3; Minor: reg. = 4, occ. = 5; None = 6; Don't Know = 9	33	
Support from others	Not Appl. = 1; Major: reg. = 2, occ. = 3; Minor: reg. = 4, occ. = 5; None = 6; Don't Know = 9	34	
Public Assistance (in household)	Yes = 1; No = 2; Don't Know = 9	35	
Health Insurance	Yes = 1; No = 2; Don't Know = 9	36	
Life Insurance	Yes = 1; No = 2; Don't Know = 9	37	
Own their home	Yes = 1; No = 2; Don't Know = 9	38	
Vocational status,[a] family	Fa; Mo; GF; GM; GF; GM; Sib 1; Not Appl. = 8	39	
Vocat. status, others[a]	Sib 2 = 1; Sib 3 = 2; Other = 3; persons = 4; In Appl. = 5	40	

Physical Setting

Item								Column
Type Dwelling	One Family House	Apt. small house	Apart. house	Project	Instit.	Rented Room	Don't Know	
	1	2	3	4	5	6	9	41
Density: No rooms / No persons	<.99	1.0–1.5	1.6–2.0	2.+				
	1	2	3	4				42
Baby's sleep location	Own crib own room	Own crib parents	Own crib others	Share Mo's bed	Share Other's bed	No perm. place		
	1	2	3	4	5	6		43
Neighborhood perceived	Good acceptable	Undesirable	Bad	Unbearable	Don't Know			
	1	2	3	4	9			44

Family

Item							Column
Mother's marital status	Married	Previously married	Single	Don't Know			
	1	2	3	9			45
Contact w. extend. family	Share home	Frequent regular	Occasional	Rare	None	Don't Know	
maternal	1	2	3	4	5	9	46
paternal	1	2	3	4	5	9	47
	Not appl.	Good, no conflict	Some Strife	Chronic Strife	Don't Know		
Marital Relationship	1	2	3	4	9		48
Relationship ext. family maternal	1	2	3	4	9		49
Relationship ext. family paternal	1	2	3	4	9		50

[a]See separate memo, attached to scoring instructions. Enter appropriate vocational status for each member of household. However column 39 or 40 should contain score for *head of household*. Either 39 or 40 (whichever does not list head of household) must be scored "Not appl."

app. continued

Variables										Col.	Code
	Caretaking Patterns										
Single prim. CT.	Mo. 1	GM 2	Rel. 3	Other 4	Not appl. 5					51	
Prim. CTing shared	Not appl. 1	Mo/Fa 2	Mo/GM 3	Mo/Oth 4	GM/oth 5	2 Relat 6	2 Oth 7	Don't Know 9	Group 8	52	
Second CT present	None 1	1–2 alw. 2	1–2 occ. 3	3 or more alw. 4	3 or more occ. 5	Don't Know 9				53	
Time spent with father	Daily br. 1	Daily prol. 2	2 Week br. 3	2 Week prol. 4	Weekends br. 5	Weekends prol. 6	<Weekly 7	None 8	Don't Know 9	54	
Freedom of movement	High 1	Medium 2	Low 3	Don't Know 9						55	
Social Play	High 1	Medium 2	Low 3	Don't Know 9						55	
Contact non-HH members	None/rare 1	Moder. frequ. 2	Daily 3	Don't Know 9						57	
Exposure places not home	None/rare 1	Moder. frequ. 2	Daily 3	Don't Know 9						58	
Lingual environment	Predominantly English 1	Predominantly Other 2	About equal 3	Solely English 4	Solely Other 5	Don't Know 9				59	

Item	Categories (codes)	
Objects & Toys	Plentiful 1; Moderate N 2; limited 3; None 4; Don't Know 9	60
Basic Routines	Regular 1; Variable 2; Unpredictable 3; Don't Know 9	61
TV viewing (baby's)	Daily 1; Often 2; Rarely 3; None 4; Don't Know 9	62
Comforted when crying (not hunger etc.)	Seldom 1; Variable 2; Usually 3; Almost alw. 4; Don't Know 9	63
Peer group contacts	Above 15 months only: Not appl. 1; Daily 2; >Once weekly: reg. 3, irreg. 4; <Once weekly: reg. 5, irreg. 6; Don't Know 9	64
Group Care	None 1; Daily: PT 2, FT 3; >Twice weekly: PT 4, FT 5; Occasion. 6; Not appl. 7; Don't Know 9	65
	Mother's attitudes characteristics	
Emotion, difficulty reported	Yes 1; No 2	66
If yes, received prof. help	Not Appl. 1; Yes 2; No 3; Don't Know 9	67
If yes, reported as	Not Appl. 1; Chronic 2; Recurrent 3; Recent / now 4	68
Emotion. diffic. observed	Yes 1; No 2	69

app. continued

Variable									Col.	Code
Mother feels isolated	Self report 1	Interviewer's judgement 2	Both 3	Neither 4	Don't Know 9				70	
Mother attributes too mature beh. char.	Very much 1	Somewhat 2	Very little 3	Don't Know 9					71	
Mother didactic	Very much 1	Somewhat 2	Very little 3	Don't Know 9					72	
Mother judges baby to be (at time of interview)	phys. 1	Abnormal ment 2	both 3	phys. 4	Slow ment. 5	both 6	No opinion expressed 7	Don't Know 9	26	2[b]
Mo. spontan. with interviewer	Very 1	Somewhat 2	Not 3						27	
Mo. spont. with baby (during visit)	Very 1	Somewhat 2	Not 3						28	
Mo. expresses delight re baby	Often/strong 1	Medium 2	Barely/none 3						29	
Mo. expresses concern, neg. affect	Often/strong 1	Medium 2	Barely/none 3						30	
Mother reflect thoughtful	Very 1	Somewhat 2	Minimal 3	Don't Know 9					31	

	Actively/seriously	More wish than deed	Not manifestly	Don't Know		
Mother strives social. material gains	1	2	3	9		32
			Interval History			
	None	1–2	3–4	5+	Don't Know	
Brief separations from prim. CT	1	2	3	4	9	33
	None	1–2	3–4	5+	Don't Know	
Long separations from prim. CT	1	2	3	4	9	34
	Yes	No	Don't Know			
Serious illness household member	1	2	9			35
	None	1–2	3+	Don't Know		
Upsetting events (fire/robbery, etc.)	1	2	3	9		36
	Yes	No				
Financial improv. reported	1	2				37
	Yes	No				
Financial decrement reported	1	2				38

[b]Columns 1–25 on second punch card contained identifying data.

app. continued

Variable								Col.	Code
			Relevant to Hypothesis I						
Walking ability	Walks freely 1	Walks with hesitation, brief 2	Walks Supported 3	Does not Walk 4	Not appl. 5			39	
Effortless walking began	Not appl. 1	Within last week 2	1–3 weeks ago 3	4–6 weeks ago 4	>6 wks. ago 5	Don't Know 9		40	
Exercises walking ability	Not appl. 1	Rare/brief 2	Daily brief 3	Daily loads 4	Don't Know 5	Not appl. 6		41	
Locations, walking only	Not appl. 1	1 room 2	thru apt. 3	thru house 4	outdoors 5	Don't Know 9		42	
Convention com. occ. reported	Not appl. 1	Within last week 2	1–3 wks. ago 3	4–6 wks. ago 4	Don't Know 9			43	
Conv. commun. observed	Yes 1	No 2	Not appl. 3					44	
Conventional Commun. highest level	Not appl. 1	Show/point 2	Call/pull persons 3	Recipr. game 4	Bye-bye on request 5	Only score "Other" 6	Don't Know 9	45	
				Hypothesis II					
Separation from prim CT at present	No marked response 1	May cry briefly 2	Usually mild protest 3	Usually strong protest 4	Not appl. 5	Don't Know 9		46	

Item	Noted within last 14 dys.: remained	Noted within last 14 dys.: disappeared	Noted 1–2 mo. ago: remained	Noted 1–2 mo. ago: intermittent	disapp.	Don't Know	Not appl.	
Separation protest, history	1	2	3	4	5	9	6	47

Item	Not noted	Occ.	Frequent	Nearly always	Don't Know	Not appl.	
Following CT present	1	2	3	4	9	5	48

Item	Within last wks.: remained	Within last wks.: stopped	Noted 1–2 mos. ago: remained	Noted 1–2 mos. ago: intermittent	Noted 1–2 mos. ago: stopped	Don't Know	Not appl.	
Following CT, history	1	2	3	4	5	9	6	49

Item	Not noted	Occasional	Frequent	Don't Know	Not appl.	
Demonstrative, only CT	1	2	3	9	4	50

Item	Yes	No	Not appl.	
Other attachment signs reported	1	2	3	51

Item	None	1–5 words	6–10 words	2 word phrases	>2 word phrases	Don't Know	Not appl.	
Vocabulary, reported (present)	1	2	3	4	5	9	6	52

Item	Within 14 days: remained	Within 14 days: stopped	1–2 months ago: remained	1–2 months ago: stopped	Not appl.	Don't Know	
Speech history (any words)	1	2	3	4	5	9	53

Item	within 14 dys.	3–6 wks. ago	>6 wks. ago	Not appl.	Don't Know	
2 or more word phrases history, first heard	1	2	3	4	9	54

Hypothesis III

Item	No patience	Some control	Often controlled	Very patient	Don't Know	Not appl.	
Ability to wait, reported	1	2	3	4	9	5	55

app. continued

Variable								Col.	Code
	None	Rare	Occ.	Often	Very frequent	Don't Know	Not appl.		
Anger: tantrums, screaming	1	2	3	4	5	9	6	56	
	None	Rare	Occ.	Often	Very frequent	Don't Know	Not appl.		
Anger: vocal only, little motoric expression	1	2	3	4	5	9	6	57	
	None	Rare	Occas.	Often	Very frequent	Don't Know	Not appl.		
Anger: looks mad, stiffens, quiet	1	2	3	4	5	9	6	58	
	Never	Rarely	Occas.	Often	Not appl.	Don't Know			
Joy or excitement: jump, shriek, active	1	2	3	4	5	9		59	
	Quiets droopy	Restless fussy	keyed up/ active	Very active	Don't Know	Not appl.			
With fatigue	1	2	3	4	9	5		60	

Hypothesis IV

Item								Col.
Ask for help	Easily/often	Variable	Seldom	Not appl.	Don't Know			
	1	2	3	4	9			61
When offered/ given help	content/ accepts	Sometimes demurs	Protest sometimes	Protest often	Angry sometimes	Not appl.	Don't Know	
	1	2	3	4	5	6	9	62
With difficult tasks perseveres long time	Never	occ.	quite often	typically	variable	not appl.	don't know	
	1	2	3	4	5	6	9	63
Tries for a while gives up	Sometimes	Usually	Rarely	Variable	Not appl.	Don't Know		
	1	2	3	4	5	9		64
Gives up or asks help at once	Sometimes	Usually	Rarely	Variable	Not appl.	Don't Know		
	1	2	3	4	5	9		65
Attempts, diff. ambitious	Not typical	Occ.	Highly characteristic	Not appl.	Don't know			
	1	2	3	4	9			66
Baby's HH SES Index	25 or less	26–75	76–100	Don't know				
	1	2	3	9				67

Appendix B: Global Assessment of Impulse Control: Manual and Guidelines (28, 34, and 40 Months)

Definition and Implicit Developmental Assumptions. The term impulse control refers to overt behavioral manifestations of what is generally understood by the words self-control and patience—that is, the ability to inhibit, suppress, and modulate the expression of excitement and strong affect. Conceptually, impulse control rests on the capacity to delay the overt bodily response to an excitatory—internal or external—stimulus condition. Note that, as defined for scoring purposes, impulse control must be generated from within the child. Inhibition externally induced does not necessarily bespeak the presence of impulse control. For instance, a child who freezes in his tracks while and only while seriously threatened with a belt may be incapable of modulating movement or other impulses by means of self-generated mechanisms at times when he/she is not under immediate external compulsion.

Developmentally, delay capacity and impulse control first emerge well before the age of two years. It is during the third and fourth years, however, that impulse control becomes a central and critically important aspect of ego development. During the time span for which ratings are made (28 through 40 months) impulse control develops in a gradual fashion. It is not a matter of the presence or absence of such control but a matter of degree. In addition, normal adaptation and development may occur in the presence of *relatively* low and *relatively* high impulse control. Similarly, maladjustment can at times be characterized by a pattern of either over- or undercontrol. Whether or not normal cognitive and personality development can occur in the presence of extremely low or extremely high impulse control is unknown at this time. At any rate, inhibition and suppression of impulse can be so rigid and pervasive that spontaneity and age-appropriate responsiveness to rousing stimuli are diminished or—in extreme cases—seriously impaired.

The development of impulse control is known to depend on familial and cultural conditions to the degree that these factors influence or shape the childrearing milieu. It also depends on individual differences in temperament. (One of several purposes to which the ratings will be put is to learn more about the sociofamilial conditions that facilitate or counteract the development of impulse control.) In evaluating how far a child has progressed with respect to impulse control the sociofamilial context will be disregarded almost entirely. That is, a child who is extremely impatient by comparison to the majority of agemates will be evaluated as low in this respect even if childrearing conditions amply account for this behavior characteristic. There is one exception: Among the things to be examined is the child's behavior with respect to certain routines such as going to bed at a fixed time or remaining seated during a meal. Marked inability to conform with bedtime routines without major upset, or leaving the dinner table to roam and having to be retrieved can contribute to a relatively low rating of impulse control in households that maintain fairly stable routines in such matters. A few of our families do not maintain stable sleeping or eating locations or times. If and when the child's behavior conforms to what is expected and accepted in the home these particular situations are *not relevant* to the rating. However, if caretakers attempt to make the child comply with requests or commands in situations such as these the child's typical response is scorable. This applies only to routines of daily life.

An impatient child reared by an impatient mother will nonetheless be considered and rated as impatient.

All ratings of impulse control are based on judgment of the degree of control, across a wide range of situations, shown by this child as compared to the majority of children at the same age. Normative expectations with respect to impulse control are based on prevailing and culturally determined standards; that is, they are those characteristic of the dominant middle-class American customs. There are no norms in the precise meaning of that term. The closest approximation to normative data on impulse control is provided by certain items on the Vineland Scale of Social Maturity (Sparrow and Cichetti 1984). The criteria to be used in our ratings are derived from research and clinical experience with this age group. In considering a behavior characteristic for which we do not know the average expected pattern for age, raters will compare the behavior in question to what is most typical *in our sample*. If insufficient data are contained in our files, that is, if the situation in question is rare or unique, the particular uninterpretable behavior datum will be disregarded.

The Rating Procedure. Ratings will refer to the level of impulse control shown by the child in many different situations and will reflect his predominant pattern. Considerable variability over time and across situations is expected, especially at 28 months, and this is specified in the rating guidelines. In some cases a rating of fairly low (2) or good balance between control and spontaneity (3) can be documented, but in one or two specific situations the child consistently shows unusually high or even overly rigid control, out of keeping with his or her typical behavior. In such instances, a separate rating reflecting maximal capacity is added. For example, a child may typically show a fairly low order of impulse control, but when physically hurt the child nearly always fails to cry and makes visible efforts to suppress sobs. Such a child might receive a predominant rating of 2 and a capacity rating of 4. The capacity rating may be based on only one kind of situation, but not on a single or a very few behavior episodes.[1] (In the example above the child suppresses crying whenever he or she is hurt.)

Ratings are based primarily on the caretaker's report of the child's everyday behavior. Ratings of impulse control and behavior observations made during the office visit provide supplementary information. Caretakers' reports must be specific and fairly extensive. Further, if the report is considered to be unreliable (intrinsically inconsistent or deliberately misleading) it cannot be used and a rating of unknown (7) will result.

Caretakers' reports serve to provide concrete instances of behavior relevant to impulse control. Judgments such as "he is very impatient" or "she does not have a temper" are irrelevant. The reported behavior in context is to be evaluated by the rater in light of the criteria specified in the guideline section.

In instances where behavior observed during the research visit differs sharply from credible reports of typical behavior in the home environment, ratings of predominant level of impulse control are to be based on the caretaker's report. This constraint is necessary because young children can be so overwhelmed (or overstimulated) by the novelty of the research situation as to show grossly atypical behavior. If, however, behavior while under observation shows significantly greater impulse control than is said to occur at home, a

1. As it turned out, capacity ratings were almost never made. Therefore they have not been used in the analysis of data.

capacity rating should be made on the basis of observed behavior (again, provided that behavior observed at the laboratory furnishes a good many instances of relatively good control so that the *pattern* we observe is different from the pattern reported for the home).

Documentation. This is to follow the procedure outlined in detail in the manual for the rating of experience patterns. In short, a written statement is to refer to the relevant portions of the summary or other source in order to furnish an adequate basis for a review of the rating if raters disagree.

Rating Categories. The general definition of each score is provided below.

1. Very low.	By comparison to others of the same chronological age, child shows an extreme lack of delay capacity and impulse control. S(he) will necessarily be judged to be immature in this respect. It is expected that a child receiving this rating will show severe difficulty or disruption in adapting to socialization procedures, to caretaking routines, to interpersonal transactions, and to standard testing procedures. The rating will be applied even if cognitive retardation explains the lack of impulse control, as comparison is made to expectations for chronological, and not mental, age.
2. Fairly low.	The degree of impulse control shown by the child falls below that observed in the majority of agemates. A degree of immaturity is present in this respect. It may be that efforts at control and modulation are present but are less effective than for peers, or that such efforts are infrequent and/or immature in kind. Often (not always) such children are perceived as turbulent, labile, or difficult to take care of, yet socialization procedures and everyday routines, as well as developmental testing using the standard techniques, are not seriously impeded or disrupted.
3. Good balance between spontaneity and control.	Child demonstrates age-appropriate capacity for modulation and control. However, s(he) is fully capable of expressing affect freely and displaying all degrees of excitement in motoric and other ways and is subject to loss of impulse control on occasion. There are no signs of generalized inhibition or significant constriction.
4. Rather high.	By comparison to agemates the child is more rigidly or extensively controlled than most. Lack of age-appropriate controls is a departure from typical behavior and infrequent. Affect expression and general responsiveness to stimulating situations are often subdued or slow to emerge; zest and spontaneity may be somewhat diminished although not absent.
5. Very high.[2]	By comparison to peers and even within the most familiar home environment, the child shows extraordinarily rigid and extensive controls. A generally inhibited, constricted

2. When we came to survey the impulse rating data it appeared that a rating of 5 was never assigned in the intact group and very rarely in the deviant groups. Therefore in our tables, ''(5)'' came to designate simultaneous over- and undercontrol.

child who lacks zest, spontaneity, and the unrestrained display of affect to a significant degree. Strong passive resistance and a precocious independence and determination are compatible with this rating, as are excessive timidity, shyness, and lack of assertiveness.

6. Both under- and overcontrolled. Child characteristically shows behaviors reflecting significantly immature (1 or 2) impulse control as well as rigid overcontrol (4 or 5). Both are prominent; neither can be said to be atypical. (In all probability these children will show more than ordinary adjustment difficulties.)

7. Unknown. Caretaker's report is insufficiently detailed or judged to be unreliable.

Rating Guidelines. The relative degree of impulse control shown by a child can manifest itself in a great many different ways and in almost any situation—namely, whenever tension, excitement, and strong affect are aroused. The particular behaviors and situations upon which ratings are based will vary from one case to the next. Prototypical situations and behavioral responses enumerated below are guidelines, based on universally recurring situations. They serve to orient the rater to the range of behaviors observable between 28 and 40 months, and to normative expectation at each age level, extending upward and downward from the optimal score of 3 (good balance between control and spontaneity). The degrees of control and modulation described below need to be applied to such other behaviors and situations as are contained in the data. Impulse control is expected to increase with age, and ratings are to be made relative to each age level.

Prototypical Situation	*Behavior*	*Age*	*Rating*
A delay occurs between expression of demand (e.g., calling for mother, asking for a drink, wanting an object) and the response	Screams, cries, protests immediately. Through gross motor action attempts to get desired response. Or tantrum. This is the typical, expected response.	28 34 40	1 1 1
	If desire urgent, behaves as above. If not urgent, vocalizes or verbalizes insistently but no loss of control. Can tolerate short delay, but typically loses all control if delay lasts more than a minute or so.	28 34 40	2 2 1
	Will ask or vocalize repeatedly if desire is urgent. Tolerates brief delay without upset, usually. Sometimes able to accept prolonged delay. Variable.	28 34 40	3 3 2
	Most of the time accepts delay though may ask, or repeat demand at intervals. Good about waiting on most occasions. Restlessness, mild fussiness may occur.	28 34 40	4 3 3
	Overt affective expression and/or motoric response to delay very rare. May wait contentedly, may look sulky and annoyed, may softly whimper, may arrest other activity (that is, become passively tense).	28 34 40	4 (or 5) 4 3
Being told firmly not to touch something or to stop activity already begun	Completely disregards even very forceful prohibition. Proceeds as though he had not heard or, more typically, as though unable/unwilling to stop. Temper tantrum frequent if child attends the prohibition.	28 28 34 40	1, if always 2, if often 1, if typcial 2, if occasional

Prototypical Situation	*Behavior*	*Age*	*Rating*
	Either disregards or stops briefly in his tracks but resumes at once, the latter frequent. Occasionally obeys.	28 34 40	2 2 1
	Usually stops. May resume after an interval, when adult no longer pays attention. May verbally protest.	28 34 40	3 3 3
	Usually stops at once, often becomes inactive, carries out incomplete token reaching action without touching.	28 34 40	4 (or 5) 4 4
Frustrated, as when object removed from grasp, denied a strong request, etc.	Temper tantrum full blown is the most frequent typical occurrence. Many such each day. Sometimes throws self to floor, diffuse gross motoric and affect outburst. Less frequently, more coordinated aggressive action as in hitting, kicking, throwing objects. Usually with screaming or yelling.	28 34 40	1 or 2 1 or 2 1 or 2
	Temper tantrums as described above occur but are no longer the only or most typical response. Angry explosive vocalizations and verbalizations occur with restrained or modulated motoric component. Deliberate but not extensive aggressive action, such as throwing an object or hitting out can occur, or crying only. Occasional effort to control crying or vigorous motion.	28 34 40	3 2 2
	Full-blown tantrum very rare. Verbal or vocal	28 34	4 (or 5) 3

Prototypical Situation	*Behavior*	*Age*	*Rating*
	protest (crying, "back talk") occurs but not on all occasions. Sadness (crying, complaintive soft vocalizations) may occur, as may token gestures or movements of defiance. Arguing, attempts to negotiate by "being good," efforts to divert or manipulate adult may occur. Withdrawing, not responding to friendly advances may occur at times.	40	3
	No temper tantrums or explosive affect outbursts ever. Withdrawing, becoming unresponsive, "holding a grudge" are typical, and/or a marked reduction in activity. Stubborn refusal of what was previously desired (sour grapes) may occur. Also calm but persistent nagging, or negotiating, provided behavior very contained and modulated.	28 34 40	4 (or 5) 4 (or 5) 4
Upset in response to a physical hurt, afraid of something (a dog, thunder, whatever)	Cries or screams immediately, accompanied by diffuse body motions. Runs to adult for comfort / protection. This is the typical response, uncontrolled.	28 34 40	2 2 (or 1) 1
	If sudden or intense, behaves as above. However, efforts at suppressing, modulating loud crying occur quite often. If not intense, verbal though affectively very expressive statements can replace or greatly reduce diffuse body motion. Self-soothing such as bringing hand or object to mouth, rocking or bouncing motions,	28 34 40	3 2 (or 3) 2 (or 3)

Prototypical Situation	*Behavior*	*Age*	*Rating*
	or getting hold of transitional objects can occur.		
	Looks frightened, may pale, reduces or ceases activity (freezing). May weep (not cry loudly) or visibly suppress sobs. In extreme cases breath-holding may occur.	28 34 40	5 4 (or 5) 4 (or 5)
Engaged in task requiring fine motor coordination, such as bead stringing, buttoning, lacing shoes, building a tower of small blocks. The task must be difficult for child so that obstacles to smooth performance are encountered.	As soon as difficulties are encountered the quality of coordination is impaired. There may be tremors, overflow motions that disrupt performance, and overly forceful motions. Child does not persevere, abandons task showing annoyance, discouragement, or resolute refusal to try again.	28 34 40	2 2 2 (or 1)
	Fine coordination is visibly impaired as above, and on some tasks or occasions child gives up, as above. However, efforts to compensate and to control excess motions are also seen on occasions when child perseveres despite difficulty. Annoyance or discomfort may be shown, both when task is soon rejected and when efforts at containment are made.	28 34 40	3 3 2
	When motivation is very strong, some impairment of fine coordination occurs. More often than not, child makes strong effort to control and compensate, perseveres for quite some time. Numerous fine coordination tasks, which do offer difficulty, are performed without real	28 34 40	3 (or 4) 3 3

Prototypical Situation	*Behavior*	*Age*	*Rating*
	impairment of coordination.		
	Typically delicate manual tasks are pursued in a calm, deliberate manner. Difficulties do not lead to impairment of coordination, though affective responses of annoyance, or at least comments about difficulties ("oops," "fall down") may be present. When motivated, attention span and perseverance are excellent for age.	28 34 40	4 3 (or 4) 3 (or 4)

Appendix C: Rating of Experience Patterns: Manual (All Ages)

The summaries contain a wealth of information about the child's behavior in a great many different situations. They also contain information about childrearing practices and attitudes as well as about family life style. Much of this material does not lend itself to coding and therefore cannot be embodied in computer printouts. This rating instrument deals with relatively stable aspects of the child's experience that are likely to exert an influence on cognitive and personality development, singly or in cluster combinations.

Rating Procedures. Ratings are based exclusively on summaries, supplemented by tape recordings of the interviews with caretakers when necessary. For each variable the entire body of material is to be scanned, and relevant statements are to be indexed or flagged. The relevant aggregate of information bits is then judged for best fit against criteria for each score. This is done largely by comparing information on the child to be rated against information obtained about all other children in the research population at the same age.

Documentation. The next step is to summarize the basis for each rating judgment in written form. This is done in part because in the case of complex, essentially qualitative variables such as these, specific documentation will be useful for the interpretation of quantitative results, especially as the same rating can be appropriate to a variety of different circumstances. For instance, a rating of medium (2) may be assigned because primary caretaking is shared by persons who differ sharply from each other in their caretaking style. Yet a score of 2 may also be assigned when a child's experience with a single caretaker best fits the medium score. In addition written documentation is required when disagreement between raters needs to be resolved.

For some variables at some ages the necessary information will be lacking—for instance, when interviews had to be brief, when caretakers were unwilling or unable to discuss some topics, or when reports were internally inconsistent or thought unreliable for some other reason. Raters are instructed to assign a score of "unknown" whenever convincing documentation is not available. A lesser number of valid ratings is preferable to a more complete but inaccurate data pool.

Definition of Experience Variables

Physical closeness between mother (as always, "mother" refers to whoever is the primary caretaker) and baby [applicable at 7 and 15 months only]. This variable refers literally to the amount of skin contacts—such as holding, rocking, or touching. A 3-point scale in which (1) means low. Mother(s) have physical contact as required for caretaking routines but little beyond that. Diapering and the like are performed with dispatch; bottle is propped for at least some feedings. In general, a physical distance is typically maintained at times when the baby appears content, not in need or acute discomfort. Departures from this pattern at times when the baby is unwell or irritable are compatible with this score, but such times must be limited in frequency and duration. Thus an infant who is irritable or unwell much of the time and is therefore held a great deal would *not* receive a (1) even if mother tries to minimize touching the baby.

A score of 3 means high. During baby's waking time (and possibly even when baby sleeps) mother rarely loses physical contact with the baby for more than a short time. Thus, times when baby is awake and mother is not touching are markedly less frequent than the reverse. Mother's attitude is irrelevant. She may constantly hold the baby, much against her wishes, in order to keep the infant quiet or because she is overly anxious. Or she may enjoy the physical closeness. All that matters in this rating is that body contact between infant and primary caretaker(s) is provided more amply than in most other research families.

2 refers to a wide range between the extremes. The experience of being awake and not in bodily contact must be regularly present for more than short periods of time (except when ill health *temporarily* disrupts this pattern). The score of 2 is also applicable when there are two primary caretakers one of whom merits a score of 3 although the other does not.

An additional score (4) refers to a pattern in which the baby is in body contact with an adult (aged 12 years or older) but the holding, rocking. etc., is provided by a person(s) other than the primary caretaker. This pattern is like (3) except that the massive body contact and caretaking functions are performed by different individuals.

Intensity of maternal involvement with the child (applicable at all ages). Refers to the intensity and pervasiveness of the mother's (or caretaker's) emotional investment in the child. It is very much like the dimension sometimes referred to as emotional closeness (versus distance). It refers to mother's feelings and the degree to which her inner life as well as her behavior revolves around the baby.

The low score (1) applies when mother's self-report concerning her behavior, as well as what is observed, has a distant, remote quality. Mothers at times verbalize a lack of closeness or warmth which will be scored if it is in harmony with observed behavior. The rare mothers who are truly withdrawn and demonstrate outright disinterest (perhaps not only in relation to the baby) would of course receive this score. It is also possible to justify a score of 1 when a mother is reasonably effective in caring for her child but does so in such a way that it is not the baby that is important but the general obligation to maintain family life. In such instances there appears to be no more grief or joy or importance connected with the baby than with other practical tasks such as keeping the kitchen clean. A (1) may be assigned for shared primary caretaking situations only if both caretakers are relatively uninvolved; it is not appropriate if one of them merits a (2) or (3).

A score of 3 means high. It applies to situations where the baby, his care, and his well being, are focal points in the caretaker's life. Strong affect exists in relation to the baby, but it need not be verbalized as such. The pattern of the mother's life is to a large extent determined by the importance of the baby, as compared to other considerations. She tends to react strongly to whatever baby does or does not do. In this context the nature of the involvement—whether primarily positive, ambivalent, or negative—is not relevant. In addition to reported behavior and feelings, clues are provided by mother's general demeanor with the baby, her tone of voice in speaking of him, her response to whatever happens during the office visit. As described in the summaries, all of these must convey the existence of an exceptionally strong feeling of close connectedness with the baby. There are some mothers who are closely involved with the baby but are equally close to other persons (siblings, parents). The score of 3 applies to them as well, provided that the baby is perceived as an individual, not a component of the "kids" or the family as a whole. A score of 3 often implies that interests and commitments other than the baby are limited or excluded, in effect crowded out by the overwhelming importance of the child. If caretaking is shared, both caretakers must be described as deeply involved with the baby; otherwise a compromise score (2) becomes appropriate.

The score of 2 again refers to a fairly wide in-between range. A real sense of closeness, whether enjoyment or concern and apprehension, may be demonstrated, yet the caretaker's emotional life and everyday behavior are not dominated by the baby more than is implicit in an appropriate investment in the baby and his care. The score also applies if only one of two primary caretakers merits a score of either (1) or (3).

A score of 4 may be applied beginning at age 15 months. It is appropriate when someone in the household has a deep and persistent emotional investment in the child but is not a primary caretaker. For instance, a father may focus intense or overly intense feelings upon the child and act accordingly, yet seldom assume caretaking responsibility. In order for this score to apply it is required that the noncaretaking adult have frequent and regular contact with the child. A score of 4 may be assigned in addition to scores appropriate for the primary caretakers.

Frequency of overt conflict between child and caretaking adults (applicable beginning at age 15 months). This variable deals with the frequency, not the intensity, of overtly antagonistic encounters between child and adult. As usual, a score of 1 means relatively rare. The frequency of conflict needs to be considered in light of what is typically seen at different ages (at least among our research families). In a 15-month-old, situations in which the child resists and is coerced or is in some other way opposed by the adult occur repeatedly on most days in a great many families. At this age a score of (1) might apply even when such confrontations regularly occur in a few situations, such as hair combing or being removed from the bath. The score applies if, by comparison to agemates in the sample, such head-on collisions are in no way a dominant pattern in the daily child-adult interactions. Relative infrequency of open conflict may be due to relative inactivity or lack of initiative on the child's part, or to skillful caretaking techniques. It is the relative prominence of conflict—not the probable reason for it—that is rated. At 28 months, the frequency of conflict tends to be greater than either before and after. By 34 months, and certainly by 40 months, overt conflict is usually less frequent and ratings must be adjusted accordingly.

A score of 3 means unusually frequent. Open conflicts between the child and caretakers must be so frequent as to be highly characteristic of the form that social interactions take for this pair at this time. A fairly frequent occurrence of affectionate and harmonious caretaker-child interactions can also be compatible with this score (especially in families where fighting followed by appeasement or reconciliation is a stable pattern). Again, whether undue frequency of collisions is attributable to overly severe demands on the adult's part or to excessively resistant tendencies on the child's part does not affect the rating.

The rating of 2 covers the wide range of moderately or fairly frequent conflicts between child and adult. It applies when head-on collisions are a phasic phenomenon (that is, when weeks of constant collision alternate with fairly tranquil periods), and also if conflict is either rare or frequent with one of two primary caretakers but not with the other.

A score of 4 designates situations in which, regardless of what happens with primary caretakers, the child's waking day involves very frequent conflict with persons who are not primary caretakers. Frequent fights with *young* siblings (less than 9 or 10 years old) are so common as to be disregarded; however, constant conflict with an older sibling, father, or anyone else who spends a fair amount of time with the child on an almost daily basis is scored here. A rating of (4) may be assigned in addition to whatever rating is appropriate concerning interaction patterns with primary caretakers.

Freedom of movement (applicable up to the age of 28 months, but not beyond). Here we assess the degree to which caretaking practices provide scope for the age-appropriate exercise of motility. Criteria will therefore vary with age.

A low score (1) applies when movement restraints are typically present during significant portions of the baby's waking day. For example, (1) applies if at 7 months the child remains strapped in an infant seat much of the time and is seldom or never placed on a bed, the floor, or other surface that permits free movement; at 15 months, if the child is given minimal opportunity to cruise, walk, or creep (use of a playpen does not in itself constitute restraint). If all waking time is spent in a walker it merits a low score because the range of possible movement is so narrow. At 28 months, movement restraint is very rare; the rating of (1) would apply if the child spent a very large proportion of his waking day in a crib or playpen and were seldom permitted to walk, climb, or run about.

A score of 3 is high and refers to the absence of movement restraint except as required for caretaking routines and for very brief periods at other times.

The rating of 2 covers a wide range and applies whenever movement restraint occurs with some regularity, but side by side with sufficient or even ample time spent in the absence of restraint.

Degree of structure in the caretaking environment and child's behavior organization. Criteria for the presence of structure include a fairly regular rhythm of daily life such as regular meal- and bedtimes, a specific place to sit for meals, a relative sameness in the sequence of events from one day to the next. Also, beginning at 15 months, reasonable consistency in the adult response to various situations contributes structure. For instance, certain actions on the child's part consistently bring disapproval, demands made at one time are maintained over longer time periods, etc. In short, a cohesive and fairly stable relationship exists between the child's behavior (or certain child behaviors) and the adult's response. Structure is also produced by physical arrangements in the environment, by suggestions, and, in general, by some direction of the child's activity. One mother of several young children assigned a color to the belongings of each so that our subject knew that the yellow plate, towel, toothbrush, etc., were for her to use. Placing a child on the toilet at certain times is structuring, and so is having a toy box, or suggesting dolls, blocks, the tricycle, or any other plaything or activity when the child is bored or restless. A large number of prohibitions, if they are enforced, may, but need not, lend structure depending on the child's response. With this variable, the intention is to distinguish between a highly structured and a fluid or even chaotic lifestyle for the child. Whether the degree and kind of structuring are appropriate and constructive in their consequences or are deemed unfortunate should be disregarded in arriving at a rating judgment.

The low score (1) indicates an extremely fluid, seemingly haphazard sequence of behavioral events. Children are left to their own devices until and unless they get into mischief or danger. Children go to bed at various times and in various places and are fed either whenever they wish or at the (variable) convenience of the adult. The same misdemeanor sometimes leads to punishment, sometimes is appreciated for its entertainment value, and sometimes is ignored. The children have little or no opportunity to focus on an activity that requires adult participation (such as sharing household tasks, looking at picture books, etc.). In all cases so far reviewed, low structuring was characteristic of family life as a whole and easily identified.

A score of 3 means that the household and the child function in terms of well-defined rules and customs. Consistent and usually enforced prohibitions are only one component. If evening is the habitual playtime with one or the other parent; if there are bedtime rituals (such as reading a story, being sung to, having toys placed in the crib and being said good night to); if being dressed always precedes breakfast or vice versa; if breakfast goes with "Sesame Street" and the cartoons are turned on at 5 P.M., putting an end to the afternoon; if things are planned with and for the child and usually carried out; if the child is diverted and his activity is channelled before he gets into trouble—all these can be structuring elements. So, of course, are group daycare attendance, regular outings, consistent rewards and punishments, and the like.

The rating of 2 is in between. Structure and regularity exist but do not pervade the day. The score is also applicable if there is reason to believe that at the babysitter's or grandmother's home there is next to no structure while at home life is highly structured, provided that the child regularly spends considerable time in the nonhome setting (shared primary caretaking).

Degree of accommodation to the child. By accommodation we refer to alterations in the behavior of adults, and especially in the demands made of the child, in response to behavior characteristics noted in the child. By contrast to indulgence, accommodation is limited to flexibility in childcaring practices judged to be appropriate to the child's developmental level. Thus, a mother who modulates her voice when scolding the child after noting that when she yells the child is unable to listen is accommodating. Arranging a night light once the child has shown fear of darkness is accommodating in our age range, as is cutting a child's hair shorter to avoid regular distress during combing. Other examples are providing toys in keeping with the child's preferences and changing meal- or naptimes in accordance with the child's apparent biological rhythm. If the adult behavior reduces stress without sacrificing appropriate immediate or long-range goals, if it increases time spent in focused, age-appropriate activity, or if it is a change in the means used to achieve unaltered goals, it will usually meet criteria for accommodation.

Clearly, the same behaviors that may be accommodating at age 15 months (such as feeding a child who does not want to use the spoon) can be infantalizing at age 34 months. Another frequent though not invariant criterion for what we mean by accommodation is that what the adult does is designed not to achieve greater convenience for herself but to make things easier or more effectively didactic for the child (though both can be achieved at the same time). Thus, a mother who removes all *don't touch* objects from the reach of a 15-month-old is sensibly accommodating. If she follows the same practice late in the child's third year it is simply because it spares her trouble but at the expense of socialization training for the child. We score not merely the intention to be accommodating but its effectiveness in developmental and adaptive terms.

The score of 1 is low and refers to homes in which how the adult proceeds is dictated by conviction, belief, tradition, requirements of other members of the household, or convenience, without regard to the child's response. Whether by necessity (as might be true of movement restrictions in a crowded home) or by choice, the child is expected to conform (accommodate) to the social and physical environment.

The high rating (3) is appropriate when caretaking adults are able and willing to plan and modify their way of dealing with the child in the light of what works best with this youngster and often (always would be impossible) are successful in so doing. Examples are given in the introductory definition. The score applies when there is evidence that the child is seldom if ever faced with demands or expected to cope with situations that lead to prolonged upset, to behavior disruption, or to malfunctioning in such areas as eating, sleeping, and learning. Note that high degrees of accommodation can be associated with what we might regard as either unduly high standards of behavior and/or more didactic cognitive ambition than is appropriate. As always, (2) refers to the midrange. A score of 2 can occur in association with the entire range of scores on other variables. It may also result from a compromise in a shared caretaking situation where the two milieus yield sharply different experience sequences in this respect.

Patterns reflecting a generally indulgent or harshly disciplinary childrearing atmosphere or a combination of these. Because disciplinary patterns are endlessly varied among our families, and similar patterns can yield very different behavioral and affective consequences, we make no effort to assess this aspect of the child's life across the board. Instead we decided to select only three patterns which represent extremes and which are rare among our families. It is probable that where these patterns exist they color the child's experience in such a way as to affect some or all aspects of development. Again, we define our terms before a statement of rating criteria.

Indulgence refers to what is ordinarily called spoiling, but judged by the developmental and behavioral criteria that prevail in middle-class culture. Thus, a family whose subculture sees nothing wrong with a three-year-old who still insists on his bottle, is not toilet-trained, and is unable to tolerate delay would still receive a score of (1) if they were generally indulgent, provided only that the child gives evidence of developmental readiness to function in more mature ways. Therefore, what constitutes indulgence for a healthy, normal child at a given age might be accommodation when applied to a handicapped peer. In general, by indulgence we refer to modes of behavior on the adults' part that, in our judgment, tend to support and encourage immature, relatively infantile modes of functioning in the child. Another way of approximating a definition is to say that indulgent caretakers demonstrate weakness and indiscriminate compliance vis-à-vis the child. They subordinate their actions to the child's demands, and it is the child who determines the course of events to an unusual degree. Examples are children who are allowed to eat only what they want and when they want it, or children who are not taken out of doors "because he doesn't want to go."

(1) This is a difficult rating to make. It refers to consistent and pervasive indulgence in all respects where it is practically feasible. A score of (1) is appropriate when indulgence is practiced in a variety of important behavioral domains over an appreciable period of time (months, not weeks). The overall climate must be indulgent though some instances of accommodation or (rarely) of severity may be reported. These must be viewed as atypical—that is, as departures from what ordinarily occurs.

The score of 2 refers to marked and pervasive severity, judged in the light of developmental norms and standards prevailing in the dominant culture. Severity refers to the *means* used to enforce compliance, not to the frequency or nature of prohibitions and demands. Depending upon the child's age, spanking or using "the belt" may be more severe than administering slaps by hand; merely threatening with the belt can be less severe than using it, but the threat remains severe if it is regularly followed by application of the belt. Loud, impatient screaming is severe in comparison to stern but modulated admonition. Another aspect of severity is a lack of flexibility. A home in which every transgression, however trivial, is punished harshly is more severe than one in which lesser misdemeanors lead to comparatively milder punishment than serious misbehavior. A score of 2 is appropriate to a child-rearing environment that overall is a good deal more severe than the great majority in our research population. Accommodations or indulgences must be very rare and atypical.

A score of 3 identifies a childrearing environment in which marked harshness exists side by side with marked and conspicuous indulgence. Almost always, severity is found in relation to social and moral issues (defiance of adults, behaviors viewed as bad). Indulgence, on the other hand, is likely to be practiced in areas that are held to be unrelated to the good-bad polarity (sleeping, eating, patience, clinging to caretaker, etc.). Quite often the adults expect more control of behavior than can reasonably be expected at that age and tend to punish failures the child is unable to correct. Indulgence tends to be practiced in behavioral realms where maturational and developmental readiness for more mature behavior is demonstrated by the child.

The score of 4 is assigned to children to whom the above scores do not apply. In other words, it means inapplicable or "none of the above."

Didacticism. We define as didactic all activities with and for the child that teach and support developmental advance in the—broadly speaking—cognitive sphere. This includes language, numbers, letters, writing, etc. Encouraging the child to watch "Sesame Street" when it is viewed as educational in contrast to other television programs that are considered amusement is relevant, as is purchasing educational toys. (Didacticism with regard to socialization and moral issues is dealt with elsewhere.) As one element in rating the degree to which the family atmosphere is didactic, we include an assessment of how important learning and intellectual ability are in their scale of values. That is, in some families children are given educational toys, yet new skills are not noted and appreciated as they arise; slow progress may not cause concern. In other families new accomplishments or demonstrations of being bright may be responded to as important events. It is important that didactic input must be *experienced.* When children are read to but pay no attention, no didactic input has taken place. Also, if what is taught is incomprehensible to the child he is not being given a learning opportunity. (For instance, one mother of a retarded 2-year-old who was barely able to produce a scribble tried to teach her child to write his name. To him this was no more than a game in which mother moved his hand.)

A low score (1) means that the child is taught very little or nothing at all as far as cognition-related skills are concerned. Whether this is due to ignorance, preoccupation with character training, lack of time, or any other cause is irrelevant. Also, next to no steps are taken to provide the child with other learning opportunities (toys, etc.), and many developmental advances are not acknowledged. In order to receive this score in a shared caretaking situation, neither of the two settings may be more than minimally didactic.

A score of 3 means high and is self-explanatory in view of the foregoing.

A score of 2 designates caretaking environments in which some didactic experiences are provided but they are not a pervasive or dominant feature of the child's life. Children who attend a group daycare center while the home environment is not at all didactic receive this score as do children in whose lives only one regularly seen person (sometimes the father) teaches the child. This score is also applied to the appreciable number of families that are somewhat or moderately didactic but in which teaching the child is but one of many interests, neither more nor less important than others.

Amount of focused social attention. Here we rate the frequency with which the child is the recipient of concentrated attention from an adult (anyone above 12 years). Often this occurs during caretaking routines. Play with the child can take place in this mode, as can teaching him something or letting him share a household task. During disciplinary encounters adults may also give undivided attention to the child. Situations and events to be considered for this rating are such that the child has reason to perceive himself to be at the center of the adult's attention, which ordinarily leads to full reciprocity and to especially vivid social interactions.

A low score (1) refers to a family milieu in which the child is responded to and is a participant in many social situations. However, except on comparatively rare occasions (as against the majority of peers in our group), adult behavior and attention are not exclusively focused on the child. For instance, while feeding a child or dressing him mother may also keep an eye on other children or watch a television program intermittently. In many social situations the child is somewhat at the periphery of things. A rating of (1) does *not* imply a relative lack of intense and individualized interactions with adults.

A score of (3) is high and describes homes in which almost everything the child does elicits a direct response. Often focused attention will receive a (3) rating in families where adults engage in prolonged episodes of reciprocal play as well as other varieties of non-caretaking, one-to-one social interactions with the child. Caretakers in such homes typically devote themselves totally to such tasks as feeding, dressing, or bathing the child in the form of playful rituals or in order to manage the task efficiently. If we think that the child behaves in such a manner as to compel attention and succeeds in focusing social attention upon himself for large portions of time, a score of 3 is appropriate. Note that certain varieties of social attention are not relevant—for instance, being held on the lap but not spoken to or played with actively. Also, the adult's willingness to comply with the child's requests (for snacks, toys, or whatever) does not count here.

The score of 2 is the usual in-between range where the child receives his full share of focused attention from adults but typically there are also prolonged episodes during which he is at the periphery of ongoing events or plays by himself.

Appendix D: Assessment of Behavioral Deviancy (15, 28, 34, and 40 Months)

The original research plan anticipated the need for a separate and parallel analysis of results for an abnormal and a normal group. It was not until data collection had moved into the third year that we recognized the need for a third group that also required separate analysis. A much larger proportion of our prematures than we had expected manifested maladaptive and distressing behaviors. In many instances these were sufficiently severe to disrupt family life patterns and also to impede the child's developmental progress. A few of these children suffered from the kinds of emotional difficulty that come to the attention of clinics and child psychiatrists. Many more showed behaviors typical of the stormy toddler age, but atypical in their intensity and especially in duration. Daily severe temper tantrums, or an intense fear of the dark, or debilitating shyness, for example, are transiently observed in a great many children between the ages of two and four years and tend to disappear within a reasonable period of time. When these same behaviors persist over months and even years, however, so that temper tantrums or fearfulness are as conspicuous at four years as they were at two, both families and professionals consider that something has gone amiss. A second characteristic of behavioral deviancy as we defined it is that the atypical behaviors represent extremes. For instance, head banging forceful enough to cause bleeding or defiance so extreme that everyday routines (such as dressing or bathing) could not be carried out at all were included if they persisted over an appreciable period of time.

Behavior difficulties of this kind are not attributes of the child; they always result from the relationships and feelings, and the concrete circumstances, that make up the child's life situation. In the illustrative vignettes of individual children we tried to show that the behavior difficulties of these children were often accounted for by parental ineptness, by hostile tensions within the home, or by unreasonable demands placed on the child. Not infrequently, children whom we defined as deviant could and did function normally when they found themselves in more congenial and supportive circumstances than those that prevailed at home. It is for this reason that we have emphasized throughout this study that when a child was judged to show deviant behavior this did not imply a diagnosis of psychopathology. Our behaviorally deviant children *were* maladjusted, nevertheless, even if the emotional and physical conditions in which they lived were such that no child could have adjusted to them. Whether we were dealing with basically healthy responses to inappropriate situations or with a psychological disturbance already internalized, the fact remains that the deviant children lived troubled lives, were the objects of worry and disappointment to their parents, and, most importantly, did not have the opportunity to function and develop in an undisrupted fashion. As it was our aim to explore the interrelationships between stable patterns of experience, cognitive and personality development, and the sociocultural environment, it was necessary to identify the children who fell into this third group.

In order to convey a picture of the variety of deviant behaviors encountered in our research group, we provide a condensed summary of maladaptive patterns seen in those children who were *not* discussed in the vignettes.

1. By the age of 22 months, and reportedly before then, this child was hyperactive and distractable, to the degree that it was impossible to take him into stores or anywhere except

the street or the park or other outdoor areas, where he could run freely. Throughout the period of our study he depended on his security blanket and dragged it about even within the home. Late in the second year he showed echolalia, which was still present at age 40 months, although in milder form. He developed and maintained an extreme fear of doctors, nurses, and all things medical.

2. Even as an infant this child seemed odd and somehow unrelated to the world about her, especially to people. Late in the second year she seldom responded to anything said to her; nor would she comply with requests or return affectionate or playful gestures. For reasons no one could discern, she left the living room for her bedroom, only to return after a while. Speech development was severely delayed but when she began to understand and utter words, by the end of the third year, she often addressed her parents in peculiarly intoned nonsense syllables and cried bitterly when told that they could not understand her. She did not seem to know how to play except that, at 40 months, she liked to throw a ball—in no particular direction. The autistic-like features of her behavior persisted into the fifth year. Thereafter she remained retarded and very peculiar but in better contact with other persons.

3. Up to the age of two-and-one-half-years, this girl's wildness and demandingness were perceived as age-appropriate and cute by the family. By the time we saw her, at 28 months, she had reached the point of more or less automatically refusing any suggestions or requests. Also, she made constant demands and went into severe tantrums if they were not met instantly. Thus it is no exaggeration to say that she spent most of her waking time in tantrums involving screaming, hitting, throwing herself to the floor, and kicking people and objects. For many months, friends and relatives would neither visit nor allow the child into their homes because she never failed to create havoc. Her mother was resigned to the fact that if it was not stringently constrained, her play consisted of upending flowerpots, emptying drawers, climbing dangerously on top of cabinets, or applying crayons to walls. Yet, she also required her security blanket near to hand and, peculiarly, showed a consistent fear of dolls. Last, there were few nights during which she did not wake up crying at least once. By 40 months she was still a stubborn and defiant child, difficult to live with but containable, and hence no longer considered to be deviant.

4. This had been a tense, fearful, and yet resistant little girl since early toddlerhood. When we saw her at 34 months she had become alarmingly unhappy and constricted. Even at home she almost never played with toys; she seemed to be afraid to touch or manipulate anything. She looked unhappy and cried a great deal, even when given something she had asked for. Although she was afraid of many things, her fear of water approached panic levels, so that a bath had not been attempted for many months. At 40 months her behavior had changed, but was just as deviant. She was still afraid of "almost anything" but cried less and could participate in routine activities. Even though she showed no actively directed resistance, it had become usual for her to show anger by lying face down on the floor and remaining thus mute and immobile for fairly long times. She still needed her security blanket close by. Most important from our point of view, the child was deeply involved with fantasies much of the time and became angry when interrupted. Even the developmental test could be administered only when the examiner thought of using a doll that, in relation to test materials, had all sorts of adventures.

5. This child's difficulty might well be described as seemingly unprovoked unhappiness. At 28 months of age he screamed in response to any delay or frustration. In addition, several times each day he threw himself to the floor and cried bitterly for no discernible reason. When upset but not frustrated in situations that the family could not understand as disappointing or disagreeable to him, he quite often went into a clothes closet and remained there in the dark for a long time. At age 34 months the family was at its wit's end and seriously considered him to be deranged. The inexplicable crying spells had become more frequent and lasted two hours or more. He had taken to chewing at the finger of one hand continuously, even while doing something with the other hand. He tended to break down and cry at transition points and in response to novelty. For instance, he cried and became unhappily resistant at the first bite of a meal only to eat normally after a while; he became upset when the first garment was put on in preparation for an outing though he wanted to go; and his first response to a new toy was to throw it into the trashcan though later he liked it well enough. When this child was 40 months old these behavior characteristics had not disappeared but had abated. He was still a troubled child whom it was most difficult to satisfy, but he was no longer deviant by our definition.

6. For this little girl, who shared many behavior characteristics with several other deviant children, the course of events was rather different. At the time of the 28-month visit she was notable for the split-second changes in her mood. She could go from high glee to extreme anger and back again in seconds. Her negativism was so extreme that her inept mother usually lost the battle, with the result that the child might be outdoors in her pajamas covered by a coat, or might remain unwashed for days. In addition, she was inseparable from her transitional object. By 34 months she was still an extremely resistant child, now old enough to be vengeful. To annoy her mother she might dump freshly cooked food onto the floor or take and hide her mother's wallet. Yet, half a year later things had improved so that family life patterns could be maintained. When we saw her again at 40 months she had developed numerous rather serious difficulties, including extreme behavioral regression after the birth of a sibling. It was necessary to bottle feed, burp, hold, and diaper her at the time. Also, she now showed a pronounced fear of darkness, thunder, and—most of all—monsters, which seemed to lurk in every corner. She also seemed to have disturbing dreams; at least she awoke crying and slightly confused quite often during the night. What especially impressed us was her intolerance of large and stimulating settings, which evoked sudden outbursts of uncontrolled destructiveness. In the supermarket she went "berserk," sweeping articles off the shelves while screaming. Sitting on her mother's lap in the movies she suddenly took her mother's heavy purse and hit the head of the person seated in front of her. Surprisingly, her physical health and her cognitive development remained rather better than average.

7. A combination of intense aggressiveness and marked fearfulness was also seen in what struck us as a quite different context. The boy in question hit or bit his mother (or any other person who offended him, including staff members) whenever he felt thwarted or insulted. He also threw objects across the room and screamed. But this same child became anxious and generally upset at the sight of any broken object, especially a toy. During the developmental session he became still and inactive as he found a broken truck, only to resume his animated play when the examiner made a ritual of fixing it (at home family

members had become adept at spotting and hiding broken things). He also feared that he might fall off steps or other high places and seemed terrified of darkness. All this would be regarded as regrettable but not necessarily deviant in a two-year-old. However, this child's behavior did not change at all over the next year and a half. By the time he was 40 months old the family considered him to be unmanageable, and he met all criteria for deviancy.

8. Finally we want to mention an exceedingly bright child whose desire to do everything well and whose intolerance of irregularity and disorder were at first welcomed by his family, who described themselves as perfectionists. They largely overlooked his constant finger sucking and his fear of noises. Before he had reached his third birthday, however, and from then onward, his difficulties had become conspicuous. Finger sucking had turned into severe nail biting and any unexpected noise (even if familiar, such as traffic sounds) upset him greatly. He could not be comforted at such times and often crawled beneath a table. At all times he lacked spontaneity and zest; the parents commented that even in sleep he did not look entirely relaxed. Further, he "went to pieces" at any change in routine. The only thing that was said to fascinate him were superheroes on television programs. His unwillingness to risk failure is exemplified in one of many anecdotes. He had been hammering away at pegs happily enough when he observed his father driving a nail with a single stroke; thereafter he did not touch his hammer again.

These accounts do not describe each and every deviant syndrome that we observed. Some of the problems were quite frequent—for instance, negativism and high levels of activity. Some were rare—for instance, overly deep involvement in fantasy and autistic tendencies. We hope that these summaries substantiate our report that the children in the *behavior-deviant* group were unlike those we regarded as intact.

Appendix E.1: The Play Session Procedure (15, 28, 34 Months)

Of all situations in which toddlers and preschoolers can be observed, free play with an array of toys is potentially the most revealing. The choice of toys, the complexity of play, the thematic content, the degree of concentration and the duration of play bouts, the motoric skills displayed, the affective tone and its variability are only some of the features of behavior organization during play that can provide information about the child's cognitive level and style, his temperamental disposition, his interests and preoccupations, and—with luck—his imaginative powers. The play session can also tell a good deal about the nature of mother-child interactions. From the researcher's point of view, the disadvantages are that play behavior is so variable as to defy rigid classifications and that a child cannot be coaxed to play—he will become involved in active play if he so desires and not otherwise.

When play behavior of young children has been used as an experimental variable, the procedure has most often been to ask the mother to remain in the playroom but to refrain from interacting with him unless her intervention becomes necessary. To young preschoolers this is an unprecedented and puzzling situation. They are used to playing while mother is otherwise engaged yet ready to respond or intervene intermittently. To have her sit there closely watching yet unresponsive causes tension and discomfort to both mother and child. We therefore arranged the play session to resemble more closely what the child might experience when visiting the home of friends. Throughout the session the mother and the staff member shared a sofa and conversed with each other. If the child addressed either of the adults, a brief acknowledgment was made (such as "I see" or "thank you"). If he asked one of the adults to join his play or to do something for him, he was told "in a little while, we have to talk right now" or some such thing.

Procedure and Scoring. The play session lasted for ten minutes, beginning at the moment when the adults were seated and the child had been told, "These are for you to play with; Mommy and I will sit right here and talk." An assortment of toys, a different set for each age level, had been placed in a predetermined spatial distribution on the floor, at a distance of five feet from the sofa. Two or more observers watched through the one-way vision screen. They tallied, timed, and scored ongoing behavior and also recorded nonscorable but relevant events. Below we reproduce the scoring blanks for each age level. For the most part they are self-explanatory. When they are not, abbreviated definitions are provided.

Appendix E.2: The Play Session Procedure: Scoring Definitions and Blank for 15 Months[1]

Initial Behavior (First 45 Seconds)

Plays with toys alone—no mother contact.
Plays with toys—has mother contacts.
Inactive (except looking), may be immobile.
Clings/turns to mother actively.

Behaviors[2]

Self-initiated contact with mother across distance.
Evokes mother's interest in toys (show, point, etc.).
Turns to mother, loses interest in play, clings, etc.
Mother shows or offers toy; baby accepts, turns toward.
Mother shows or offers toy; baby disregards, rejects.
Leaves mother to approach toys.
Plays oblivious to people for at least one minute.
Seeks or maintains contact with staff member.

Pattern Ratings[3]

Plays actively; no mother contact.
Plays in mother's orbit.

Mother-Baby Contact over Time (Check One Box Only)

Most during first few minutes.
Most in last third.
U curve, most first and last.

1. On the scoring blank, the frequency of behaviors was scored as *noted, absent, low, medium,* or *high;* the pattern ratings were scored as *none, occasional, 50%,* or *dominant.*

2. For behaviors at 15 months, low frequency = 3 times or less; medium = 4 to 8 times; high = 9 times or more.

3. For pattern ratings at 15 months, in mother's orbit = within 5 feet and within visual range; mother-baby contact over time = child-initiated, direct contact with the mother. For a 15-month-old, ten minutes of play is a long time. A tendency to approach the mother more often during the last few minutes usually reflects fatigue or satiation on the toddler's part.

Appendix E.3: The Play Session Procedure: Scoring Definitions and Blank for 28 Months

Initial Behavior (First 45 Seconds)

Child does not play (may look at toys), stays close to mother (mother or examiner).
Child approaches toys, has contact with adult(s) (mother or examiner).
Child approaches toys, no contact with adults.
Child self-conscious, shy, inhibited.
Child spontaneous, pleased.
Child spontaneous, distressed.

Child Behaviors

Plays with toys most of the time (80%).
Pays little attention to mother (80%).
While playing typically maintained contact with mother.
While playing typically maintained contact with examiner.
Predominantly played in close vicinity of adults.
Transported toys to mother (at least 3 times).[1]
Transported toys to examiner (at least 3 times).[1]
Stopped play for refueling 4 or more times.[2]
Stopped play for refueling 3 times or less.[2]
More interested in social interaction than self-generated play.
Addressed questions or requests to mother 5 times or more.
Addressed questions or requests to examiner 5 times or more.
Interested in play only if started and supported by mother.
Mostly at ease and involved in activity.
Seemed tense, anxious, restlessly bored, or uncomfortable.
Showed strong displeasure often.
Showed strong displeasure seldom.
Showed intense pleasure often.
Showed intense pleasure seldom.

Mother Behaviors

Usually responded to child's addresses, seldom intruded.
Within letter of instructions, tended to maintain control.
Despite instructions, intruded with suggestions, prohibitions, etc.

1. For *transporting toys,* The score applies if the child, playing at some distance from the adults, picks up several toys and deposits them on the lap or by the feet of one of the adults. Immediately thereafter he is as likely as not to move to another play area. Sometimes transporting toys becomes a primary activity.

2. The term *refueling* is applied to the following sequence of events. The child plays contentedly at some distance from the mother and suddenly interrupts, goes to mother and hugs or cuddles for a moment, only to return to his previous play almost at once. This frequently observed behavior pattern was named refuelling because it is as though brief physical contact with the mother served to re-energize the child.

Conveyed warm, friendly interest in what child was about.
Often or typically scolding, aloof, scornful, disinterested.
Tense, ill at ease, or at a loss how to behave.
Whatever her style, self-assured, unruffled.

Appendix E.4: The Play Session Procedure: Scoring Definitions and Blank for 34 Months

Mood State Judgments[1]

Child tense, anxious, restless or bored.
Child spontaneous and on the whole pleased.
Child spontaneous but on the whole displeased.

Child Behaviors

Plays with toys most of the time (80%).
Pays little attention to adults most of the time (80%).
While playing typically maintained contact with mother.
While playing typically maintained contact with examiner.
Predominantly played in close vicinity of adults.
More interested in social interaction than self-generated play.
Addressed questions or requests to mother 8 times or more.
Addressed questions or requests to examiner 8 times or more.
Matching categories, thematic.[2]
Matching categories, pure sorting.[2]
Complex imaginative play, macrospace.[3]
Complex imaginative play, microspace.[3]

Mother Behaviors

Usually responded to child's addresses, seldom intruded.
Within letter of instructions tended to maintain control.
Despite instructions intruded with suggestions, prohibitions, etc.
Conveyed warm, friendly interest in what child was about.
Often or typically scolded, was aloof, scornful, disinterested.
Tense, ill at ease or at a loss how to behave.
Whatever her style, self-assured, unruffled.

1. *Mood states:* Rating judgments refer to the entire session.

2. *Matching categories* refers to spontaneous sorting, as when a child collects all the toy cars. Matching was scored as thematic when it was subordinated to a play idea—for instance, if all toy cups were grouped together in preparation for a make-believe serving of tea.

3. *Complex imaginative play:* In order to qualify as complex, imaginative play had to consist of three or more separate play actions, all in the service of the same plan or play idea. For instance, if small cars were loaded onto a toy truck, the truck was then moved to an area called a garage, and was unloaded and "parked" there. The terms *macro* and *micro* play were borrowed from Erikson. Play takes place in macrospace if the child himself is the central actor, as in the example of a make-believe tea party. Play is scored as taking place in microspace if a delimited spatial area serves as the arena for imaginative play of the kind that animates toy objects, making them the actors (as in the above example of a toy truck transporting toy cars).

Appendix F: The Open Space Procedure (15 and 28 Months)

This procedure, which is not intended as a measurement device, is based on the following set of observations. In waiting rooms, hallways, and other fairly large open spaces one often sees young toddlers roam the area, apparently at random and oblivious to their mothers. Typically, it is necessary for an adult to retrieve the youngster, who gives the impression of being entirely absorbed by the activity of unhindered locomotion. Such behavior is not observed among somewhat older children (approximately 20 months and beyond). Under the same circumstances older toddlers may or may not leave their mothers. If they do, their locomotion is not random. They do not forget where mother is and tend to become alarmed if they lose sight of her. In a psychoanalytic frame of reference this observation can be understood as signifying a developmental progression in the mother-child relationship. Mahler's description of the individuation/separation process offers a convenient terminology for this purpose. During what Mahler calls the *hatching* stage, young toddlers still feel themselves to be inextricably connected with the mother-person and thus do not experience *psychological* distance from the mother even when physically they move away from her. Indeed, they can sometimes be observed to become distressed when they suddenly notice her absence, and then show much the same kind of displeasure as when it is the mother who leaves them. (Our scoring system refers to this phenomenon as a *double take*.) Once toddlers have become sharply aware of their separateness from the mother, physical distance comes to imply that, for the time being, mother is inaccessible. During this developmental stage toddlers feel their dependency upon their mothers; they feel comfortable and secure in her presence, and physical distance from the mother arouses anxiety, especially in surroundings that are unfamiliar to the child.

The *open space* procedure rests on the expectation that children who at 15 months walked about in the large area, apparently oblivious to mother, will no longer do so at the age of 28 months. It is assumed that this behavior change indicates a developmental advance in the mother-child relationship. In Mahler's terminology, the child who carefully gauges his behavior to his mother's whereabouts has left behind the hatching phase and entered the stage of ambivalent dependency referred to as *rapprochement*.

Procedure. The open space procedure takes place as mother, child, and examiner leave the playroom after the developmental evaluation. Some time before the procedure was explained to the mother and she was asked to remain standing at the threshold and to pay no particular attention to the child unless he or she demanded it. The mother understood that we wished to see whether or not the youngster would move into the hall without her. Incidentally, many mothers spontaneously predicted what the child would do, and almost always did so correctly.

At least two scorers assumed strategic positions in or near the hallway. They scored and timed the child's behavior and, in addition, recorded unscorable but relevant occurrences such as loud noises or other distractions.

Scoring[1]

Initial Responses: This section refers to the child's behavior from the moment the child and mother stand in the doorway, with the child free to move (that is, hand not held, nothing

1. All possible scores are enumerated in the text. Therefore we have not included a copy of the scoring form.

blocks him) until *either* (1) he comes to a full stop once he has moved *or* (2) 45 seconds have elapsed and the child has not moved. Behavior is scorable in four dimensions: (I) Locomotion, (II) Contact with Mother, (III) Mood, and (IV) Goal-Directedness.

Subsequent Responses: This section is applicable only if the child has moved away from the mother. It refers to the time interval between the first few steps and any of the following events: (a) child returns to mother, (b) child is retrieved by mother, (c) mother joins child, or (d) child begins an activity such as exploring a typewriter, socializing with a stranger, or whatever. Behavior is scorable in three dimensions: (I) Locomotion, (II) Contact with Mother, (III) Mood. Note that under (II) it may be necessary to check more than one score. For instance, a child may turn a corner so that mother is out of his visual range and then do a double take.

Appendix G: Inventory of Conventional Communication Signals (15 Months)

This assessment procedure was designed to determine whether or not our 15-month-olds had reached that point in their development at which commonly used signals serve to convey messages to another person. On the basis of ideas contained in Werner and Kaplan (*Symbol Formation* 1963), and congruent with Piaget's conceptualizations, we think of conventional communications as a wayside station on the road from purely expressive behavior to truly symbolic communication in the form of semantic language. The hallmark of intentional communication signals is that the goal-related and expressive action is still somewhat merged with the signal, but there is evidence to show that the signal (or means) is distinct from the content of the message or the goal. This always involves behavior dictated by comprehension of the mother or any other social partner as a causal agent who can be motivated, utilized, or induced and manipulated in behalf of one's own goals. It also presupposes awareness of the social partner's need to be told or shown what is wanted. Earlier behavior is shaped as though the child expected the social partner to understand or know, as though the adult were sharing the child's experience.

Procedure and Scoring. The assessment of intentional communication signals took place during the play session. Through the one-way vision screen observers tallied each scorable instance and narrated behavior episodes not enumerated on the scoring blank but reflecting the same type of behavior organization. Below we combine a list of scorable behaviors with the definitions as provided in scoring manual.

1. Child points, says "that," etc. This category refers to all instances when the child performs an action designed to call another person's attention to an object or event by using a gesture, a word, or both, that serves as a signal. Expressive behavior which in fact draws attention to an object or event is not scored. There must be a difference between the means (action designed to draw attention) and the direct response to the object or event in question. Thus, a child who points at a picture or toy and, while so doing, looks at the other person receives a score. So does the child who, while pointing, alternates his gaze between the referent and the addressee. A child who merely regards the object, pats it, and vocalizes does not receive a score. In this context pointing alone may suffice for a score; however, saying "that" or the equivalent without pointing may not. The child must not only display what Werner and Kaplan called the "deistic" attitude but must do something specific in order to involve a social partner in the contemplation of the object.

2. Child shows object or offers it. This is a somewhat more mature mode of intentionally involving the social partner with an object that is of interest to the child. A classical scorable situation is when the child is at some distance from the social partner and holds up an object in a showing gesture. This may involve turning the body so as to bring the object into the social partner's view. The child may but need not vocalize "see" or "this." Another common situation is for a child to extend a toy held in his hand toward another person without touching the social partner, in the clear expectation that the person will reach out and grasp it. Depositing the object on someone's lap or placing it in the person's hand is not scorable as the child is not sending a message requesting the person's participation but is carrying out the desired action himself.

3. *Headshake to designate negation, "ok," or "yes."* Any gesture, word, or combination of the two that clearly communicates either negation or approval and affirmation is scored here. When a child says "no" or shakes his head while also actively resisting through body motion, or removing himself in evasion, a score is not appropriate. Although the corresponding affect may be displayed in scorable instances, the conventional gesture or word must replace direct action.

4. *Child pulls the other to the desired location.* This refers to instances when the child engages in sequential action involving movement of the whole body, not for its own sake, but in order to convey a request or desire. For instance, if the child is playing in one area of the room, then walks to the mother and pulls at her hand, clearly attempting to cause her to come with him to the toy location, this is scorable. Another example is when a child brings the mother's purse, places it on her lap, and indicates physiognomically as well as by gesture that he wishes her to remove an object (such as a bottle) from the purse. On the other hand, if the child rummages in the purse and tries to obtain the desired object himself, this is not scorable. The critical element is that the child's actions are designed to communicate a specific content, usually a request, and that the actions do not, in and by themselves, bring him any closer to the desired goal.

5. *Calls mother (to come) from a distance.* The structure of scorable situations is very similar to (4), except that words are used instead of body movements. If a child calls someone by name in a context leaving no doubt that he wishes the person to join him, this is scorable. Such expressions as "gimme" or "fixit" or "again," designed to induce the social partner to perform a specific action, are included in this scoring category.

6. *Spontaneous "bye bye" while moving to the door.* This refers to a somewhat more mature form of the behavior described under (5). It refers to one situation only, namely, when the child wishes to leave the room and utters the desire to go "bye bye" while also moving toward the door as if reinforcing the meaning of his statement. Often the child will approach the door and then return to mother continuing to say "bye bye." The fact that he is asking *her* to take him away is unmistakable. When a child goes to the door, tries to open it by himself, and calls out "bye bye," this is not scored unless he repeatedly turns around and indicates by gesture and/or sound that he is trying to mobilize his mother at the same time. We do not reproduce the scoring form because it adds no information.

Appendix H: Inventory of Body Awareness: Manual and Scoring Blank (28 Months)

Among the things toddlers learn is to recognize and name various parts of the human body. All developmental tests include items requiring the child to point to and/or name body parts on himself, on dolls, and on pictures. The ability to do so with ease presupposes that the child has a mental representation of the configuration that constitutes the human body and also recognizes that all human beings possess the same constellation of legs, arms, trunk, and facial features. Typically, very young children first learn to point to portions of their own anatomy in response to the nearly ubiquitous "Where is your . . .?" question. Doing the same with other persons and with dolls comes a bit later and often overlaps with learning to utter the correct word when someone points at a body part with another ubiquitous question, "What is that . . . what do you call it?"

Psychoanalysis and several other developmental theories have linked these cognitive acquisitions to the process of developing a sense of self as an independent entity and to the emerging body image, which of course encompasses more than anatomy and cannot be demonstrated to exist before school age. This particular developmental sequence culminates in the cognitive and linguistic achievement of the proper use of the personal pronoun.

We thought that these phenomena offered strategic opportunities to study central aspects of personality development by using situations that are familiar and congenial to young children and have the additional advantage of being partially nonverbal. Some of the items that refer to mirror behavior were inspired by the work of Renee Zazzo, who studied the emergence of a sense of self using ingenious experimental situations that involved the response to photographs and to the mirror image.[1]

Procedures and Scoring. The inventory is scored, as usual, by observers, through the one-way vision screen, who note the child's response to a number of situations that are normally part of a developmental evaluation and to a number of mini-experiments. The latter were administered as convenient—sometimes interspersed with test items, sometimes after termination of the play session. There was no need for the items to be administered in a fixed order. In fact, if staff members felt that optimal responses had not been obtained, we tried again at a later time, provided that the procedural ground rules were followed.

Three aspects of what we called body awareness were examined.

1. Awareness of Body Parts. In a playful manner the child was asked to point to ("show me . . .") his feet, his nose, eyes, and ears, his hands or "belly button," and others, if the mother thought we had not asked for the ones the child knew.

The same procedure was followed with a doll, and special attention paid to whether or not the child pointed to the correct portion of his own body before he could locate it on the doll. (This transition stage is common among one-year-olds and was seen quite often in those of our 28-month-olds who were immature in other ways as well.)

While both the child and the examiner stood in front of a very large mirror and the

1. Regrettably, we were unable to locate Zazzo's published work, an article entitled "Images du Corps et Conscience de Soi," which appeared in a journal many years ago. We do know that Zazzo was associated with the Laboratoire de la psycho-biologie de l'Enfant, Ecoles des Hautes Etudes, University of Paris.

examiner pointed to the reflection, the child was asked "who is that?" As toddlers easily become self-conscious in that situation, it was often necessary to initiate a game that involved, among other things, identifying the reflection of the mother, the examiner, pieces of furniture, or toys. Once he was at ease the question was repeated. Either thereafter or some time later, the child was also asked to identify parts of his own body on the reflected image.

2. *Awareness of Own Body As An Object Visible to Others.* A few boxes containing necklaces, fancy belts, hats, and other articles of adornment were placed on the floor. If the child did not spontaneously do so, the examiner tried on several objects, showed them off, commented on her altered appearance, and offered to help the child do likewise—all in a playful and slightly silly manner. As will be apparent from the scoring blank, we noted whether the child displayed his altered appearance before his mother; whether he was curious to watch the visual effects of various adornments in the mirror; and, last, whether he realized that, by turning, he could see rear portions of his body.

3. *Reconstruction of Body Constellation.* We used a fairly large and simple puzzle consisting of the trunk, neck, and head in a single piece, two arms, and two legs. The child was asked to put it together. As it happened, almost none of our two-year-olds could do so. Many named the limbs correctly but placed them in what seemed to be an arbitrary manner on top of the trunk. (At 34 and 40 months the task had become too easy to hold much interest for most of our subjects.)

Scoring Blank[2]

I. *Parts of the body.*
   (a) Own body parts.
      Points to 4 or more parts.
      Points to 1 to 3.
      Points to none.
   (b) Doll.
      Four or more parts.
      1 to 3.
      None.
   (c) Mirror image of own body.
      Four or more parts.
      1 to 3.
      None.
   (d) Body representation.
      Places at least one puzzle part correctly.
      Mends broken doll at least approximately.

II. *Confusions between own body and that of others*
   (a) Doll.
      Points consistently to own body instead of doll's.
      Points to own body as well as doll's.
      Points to parts on self and doll.
      Points to doll parts only

2. The body awareness inventory was scored *present* or *absent* for each category on the scoring blank.

(b) Mirror image.
Points to own body, disregards image.
Points to own body but observes image, or activates body parts asked for while watching image (for example, raises foot so its image is visible).
Points to body parts on mirror reflection but alternates with pointing to own body.
Consistently points only to body part on image.

III. *Mirror play*
(a) Clowns, prances, etc., in order to watch changes in mirror image.
(b) Goes to mirror to observe altered appearance with hat, glasses, necklace, etc.
With urging.
Spontaneously.
(c) Uses mirror to see backside of own body

IV. *Presenting self to others as an object to be looked at*
(a) Prancing, dancing, etc., in front of mother or examiner while looking at audience.
(b) Performing a trick, completing a task, or behaving provocatively, then looking at mother or examiner for reaction.
(c) Goes to mother or examiner to show off altered appearance after putting on glasses (anything).

V. *Recognition of self in mirror*
(a) Refers to self as "baby," "boy," or name of twin.
(b) Refers to image by name used for self (for example, "Mary").
(c) Refers to image as "I" or "me".
(d) Shows embarrassed discomfort at view of self-image.

Appendix I: Separation from Mother Procedure (28 and 34 Months)

The manner in which young children respond when mother leaves the room reflects developmental changes in the mother-child relationship. It also serves as an index of some qualitative aspects of this relationship, at least in 12-month-olds. In part because it is so easy to arrange and not time-consuming, in part because it correlates with other variables, a separation procedure is included in the research protocol of many studies. It has been pointed out that it is easy to overestimate the significance of a child's distress when separation occurs in the laboratory setting; at home, left in the charge of familiar persons, the child might show no distress at mother's departure. Yet behavior seen in the laboratory (and not necessarily elsewhere) can show significant relationships with other developmental variables. Further, an adequate corrective is at hand simply by asking mother about the child's behavior in the home.

We decided that it would not be useful to administer the separation procedure at 15 months, largely because the results would not differentiate among the subjects; nearly all 15-month-olds will cry when mother leaves them with a stranger. At ages 28 and 34 months this is not the case. Even if what we saw was unlike the child's home behavior, the youngsters who tolerated separation with minimal distress had shown the *capacity* to do so. Those who cried and protested had made it clear that, at least under these conditions, mother's leaving them was a threat to their well being.

Procedure and Scoring. Separation took place during the play session at a moment when the child was comfortably settled, usually after about six minutes. The mother had been asked to rise from the sofa, move toward the door, and tell the child, "I have to get something, I'll be *right back.*" She was asked to emphasize and perhaps repeat the assurance of almost immediate return. If the child became extremely upset and clung to mother, we abandoned the attempt, having learned all there was to know. In all but a few instances the mother was able to close the door behind her, only to return after less than a minute.

Observers in the one-way vision room had no difficulty in agreeing which of the five scoring alternatives applied. The possible scores were:

1. Immediate protest, tries to follow, total play disruption.
2. Becomes tense, reduces or stops play, may fuss but makes no strong protest.
3. Dismayed, but accepting, turns to examiner for support.
4. Consents, returns to play, minimal if any disruption.
5. Child was uncomfortable and not playing prior to separation. Distress or tension persists or increases.

Appendix J: Laboratory Assessment of Impulse Control and Scoring Blank (28 Months)

Our interest in impulse control as a major variable was amply discussed in the text. The procedure to assess such control during the 28-month research visit was devised, standardized, and pretested during pilot studies well before we realized that a one-time assessment would be insufficient.

Procedure and Scoring. Impulse control was scored throughout the developmental testing. A number of situations that frequently occur in that situation were preselected. Each time they occurred, observers checked whether or not the child had behaved in a controlled or relatively uncontrolled manner, by criteria specified in a manual and briefly summarized on the scoring blank.

For each incident observers viewing through the one-way-vision screen assigned a score of (a), meaning good control for age; (b), meaning poor control; or (c), meaning inapplicable because the child's behavior did not fit the criteria for either (a) or (b). As most of the criterion situations occurred repeatedly throughout the session and thus yielded several scores, at the end each (a) or (b) response in each situation was scored as either *frequent* or *occasional.* If it occurred more than four times it was held to be frequent. Thus many children received both (a) and (b) scores for a given situation, but as a rule, one pattern of responsiveness was typical and the other relatively rare. The final category, *Overall Behavior Characteristics,* summarizes the frequency distributions across situations as well as the general character of the child's behavior throughout the session.

The manual contains precise definitions of each situation and samples of child behavior meeting criteria for each score in each situation. We do not reproduce it here because the function of these pedantic stipulations was to assure reliability. The scoring blank, reproduced here, is self-explanatory.

Scoring Blank[1]

I. *Refuses unwanted test item or any other request.*
   - (a) Firm but controlled, modulated.
   - (b) Strong overt affect, motor overflow.
   - (c) Inapplicable.

II. *Is refused urgent wish, prohibited, restrained.*
   - (a) Gives up, is resigned or displeased but contained.
   - (b) Persists with increasing intensity, loses control.
   - (c) Inapplicable.

III. *Asked to wait before acting or for fulfillment of wish.*
   - (a) Inhibits action, makes strong effort to comply.
   - (b) Acts at once, restless, unhappy.
   - (c) Inapplicable, turns away or fails to understand.

IV. *Desired object is firmly removed from reach or grasp.*
   - (a) Mild resistance, verbal requests, resigned, gives up.

1. For each category, *frequent, occasional,* or *absent* could be scored.

(b) Protests strongly, resists physically, or tantrum.
(c) Inapplicable.

V. *Startled, frightened, or hurt.*
(a) Brief crying or whimpering, brief disruption, or quickly comforted.
(b) Prolonged disruption, cries, behavioral regression.
(c) Inapplicable, did not seem to mind much.

VI. *Gleeful excitement.*
(a) Looks radiant, smiles or chuckles, no loss of coordination.
(b) Increasing vocal/motor activity, coordination impaired.
(c) Inapplicable, enjoyment without excitement.

VII. *Involved in difficult, frustrating task.*
(a) Patient perseverance, annoyance, no skill impairment.
(b) With obstacles and failure coordination is impaired, angry or distressed, soon gives up.
(c) Inapplicable, not deeply engaged or not distressed.

VIII. *Fatigued, physically uncomfortable.*
(a) Withdraws involvement, becomes quiet, listless, or relatively unaffected.
(b) Increasing activity or restlessness, irritable.
(c) Inapplicable, did not occur.

IX. *Overall behavior characteristics.*
(a) Well-modulated, contained; structures and organizes well; only major provocation leads to loss of control.
(b) Very excitable, motorically active, shows affect strongly, little inhibition or modulation.
(c) Seldom deeply engaged or highly motivated, on placid side, self-control seldom relevant.

Appendix K: The Concept Formation Procedure (28, 34, and 40 Months)

An earlier research project ("The Emergence of Symbolic Functioning") provided us with a ready-made and validated technique to test the comprehension of verbally mediated concepts by nonverbal means. The task of sorting objects into attractive boxes is of intrinsic interest to young children and provided a much needed supplement to the restricted information obtained from the Stanford-Binet test.

The procedure is appropriate only to children who can readily name simple objects upon request. The child's performance on the experimental task reflects the degree to which objects that vary greatly from each other in appearance are nonetheless perceived as members of the same conceptual category. In addition one learns whether or not this ability is generalized to encompass pictures of the same object. (The earlier study taught us that three- and even four-year-olds who are well able to sort real and toy objects flounder when asked to sort *pictures* of these objects. Indeed, with our research subjects it was necessary to instruct them to sort "pictures of chairs," or whatever the objects happened to be.)

On a very low table, or on the floor if necessary, three open, transparent lucite boxes (about twice the size of a shoebox) are aligned, within reach of the child but across an empty space where objects could be placed; the child has to be able to survey the entire table space. During a demonstration trial the examiner piles a mixture of toy and real objects on the table. The objects consist of an equal number of watches, keys, and toy animals. The examiner places one object of each kind in an empty box, telling the child that the game is to "put *all* the watches in this box" and so forth with the other objects. During the demonstration the child may be reminded to put "all the keys in" or asked if he can find another animal. If with all this the child cannot comprehend the task and consistently mismatches, or disregards the sorting aspect altogether, the experiment proper is not administered.

During the experimental trials much the same procedure is repeated. The categories this time are cups, chairs, and shoes. The experimenter, however, never touches any of the objects and names them only once, as he says, "This box is for all the cups, this one for all the chairs, and this one for all the shoes." Thereafter, neither the names of the objects nor the words "more," "another," or "the same" can be used by anyone (the mother is cautioned to this effect). During the last trial simple and colorful 10″ × 12″ pictures of cups, chairs, and shoes are used.

Scoring is simplicity itself. Except for the demonstration, the child receives one point for each category that he correctly and completely sorts. Scores could thus range from 0 to 6.

Appendix L: Achievement Motivation Assessment: Guidelines and Rating Blank (34 and 40 Months)

For purposes of this research *achievement motivation* was defined as that level of cognitive and psychosocial functioning at which self-esteem is enhanced whenever the child can attribute achievement of a goal to his own skillful action, while self-esteem is diminished by failure attributed to his own shortcomings. Once this phase has been reached, children can feel intense pleasure if they succeed on a difficult task whereas effortless success on easy tasks is not nearly as gratifying to them. Another way of describing the same thing is to say that sometime late in the third year or during the fourth, a sense of competence comes to play a larger role in the perception of the self, contingent on the experience of being able to overcome obstacles and to learn. This is distinguishable from earlier phases of development when self-esteem depended primarily on the experience of being praised, valued, scolded, or depreciated by important adults in the environment. At that earlier time the child's sense of success or failure on a specific task depended almost exclusively on the adult's evaluation of the result as good or bad.

Only some of the behavior characteristics that signal the change from mastery striving (pleasure and an enhanced sense of self from exerting muscular energy and effort in overcoming obstacles) to achievement motivation are amenable to formal assessment. These include the child's response to receiving help and a spontaneous tendency to choose challenging tasks or, conversely, to avoid the risk of failure. Specific and quasi-experimental situations were developed to probe these two aspects of behavior. In addition, a more qualitative and global set of ratings dealt with the degree to which the child valued the end product of his efforts (rather than the act of producing it), the relationship between task difficulty and pleasure in success, and various ways of coping with the threat of failure.

The research staff thoroughly enjoyed the pilot work for this assessment. It consisted of inventing, constructing, and pretesting tasks that would intrigue and delight our two- and three-year-olds and that, at the same time, required some skill and perseverance in their execution.

Procedures and Scoring. Achievement motivation was assessed during the developmental evaluation to which five task situations had been added. These were: (1) to activate either a wind-up toy or one that required squeezing a rubber ball in order to cause a toy bear to dance or a rabbit to hop; (2) to dress and/or undress a doll, which required the use of zippers as well as buttons; (3) to flatten play dough and produce small animals with the help of cookie cutters; (4) to cut a piece of paper into pieces; and (5) to make a picture by affixing decals to white paper.

Below we reproduce the scoring guidelines, the scoring blank, and the overall ratings score sheet.

Scoring Guidelines. Certain behavioral events that are relevant to the child's level of maturity, and to preferred behavior styles, in the area of investing interest and energy in tasks that offer at least some difficulty are to be scored for the frequency of their occurrence. Scores are based on behavior throughout the developmental testing as well as during administration of the special procedures. The distribution of scores will reflect response patterns or behavior tendencies even if the absolute number of episodes scored by different observers is unequal.

The scorable responses occur under three different conditions:

1. *Works Alone:* Child is actively engaged in a task and the examiner does not participate (except to show interest in the child's activity). *Works Alone* episodes may be interspersed with any of the other situations. All that is required is that there be an interval of time during which the child is busy with a task while no one offers or gives help, or actively intervenes in any fashion.

2. *Help Offered:* While child is actively working at a task. examiner or mother asks if child wants help but does not provide it except in response to the child's expression (verbal or gestural) of willingness to receive it. It is desirable that the examiner not touch the task material while offering help.

3. *Help Given:* Either immediately after demonstration (if the child seems reluctant to get started) or while the child is working, examiner or mother moves in and provides help without first offering it. Verbal instructions such as "turn it over," "you have to wet it first," and "use your other hand" are examples of help given *if the child heard and understood them.* Evidence that such comments gave help is usually that the child acts in accordance with instructions or asks for clarification ("over here?"; "like that?"). In rare instances he might say something like "don't tell me," showing that help is recognized as such but rejected.

Four different responses are to be scored:

1. *Accepts Help:* Under *Help offered,* score if child verbally agrees (for example, by saying "yes," "help me," or "ok") and accommodates his actions to work cooperatively with the examiner or in accordance with helpful verbal directions. Under *Help Given* the main criterion is that the child's actions conform to directions and suggestions (verbal and/or gestural). In either case, the child continues to work at the task except for brief interruptions needed for the examiner to provide the help and at least briefly resumes work after help is given.

Note that child may verbally accept help but in fact ignore it and continue on his own. Or he may say "no" and then in fact accept help. When there is a discrepancy between what the child says and what he does, *always score the action,* disregarding the verbalization.

2. *Refuses Help:* Score if the child (a) ignores offers of help and continues to work; (b) indicates refusal by word and/or gesture and continues to work; (c) indignantly protests help offered or given and then returns to work on the same task. As above, when verbal and behavioral sequences are in opposite directions score the actual failure to use help, provided only that the child stays with the task. (If the child verbally refuses and immediately abandons the task, turning to something else, this is *not scored.*)

3. *Asks Help:* Scorable only under the condition *Works Alone.* Score when the child spontaneously requests help in words, by gesture, or by both together.

4. *Perseveres:* Scorable only under the condition *Works Alone.* Score any episode during which a child continues to work at a task despite several obstacles, mishaps, or a persistent difficulty. (For example, a child who tries to build a tower and continues to do so although the structure collapses several times and he has to begin over again receives a score. So does a child who has great difficulty threading a bead or getting a button through the buttonhole but continues to try.) The score for perseverance does not depend upon whether or not success is finally achieved.

For each scorable episode a judgment is entered gauging the subjective level of difficulty of the task; for example, an easy task may prove difficult for a child whose fine coordination is impaired. Also, if there is evidence that the child's goal is not as presented by the examiner (for example, a child may not attempt to make cookies with the play dough but strives merely to flatten out the dough), this altered goal may be difficult or easy for him.

It is not always easy to decide whether a time interval during which help is given or offered consists of several episodes or only one. For instance, an offer of help may be repeated but it is not clear whether the child ignored the first offer or failed to comprehend it. *When in doubt, score each instance* as a separate episode unless there is evidence that the child failed to notice the examiner's comment or intrusion.

Overall Ratings. The effort to make a clinical judgment of the degree to which a defined behavior characteristic is represented in the child's behavior organization as a whole, or how much his behavior is shaped or dominated by this tendency, is based on all behavior seen during the period of observation. A rating of zero (to be entered as *0* under the heading *little*) means that not a trace of the behavior tendency was observed. *little* means that one or a few instances of the tendency were noted, but only peripherally, and that they were overshadowed by other modes of responding. *medium* means that the characteristic was displayed, but along with others. It neither dominated nor was it the exception. *high* means that the child showed a very strong, pervasive disposition to behave in this manner; it was an outstanding and dominant pattern. If there was no occasion to display the characteristic because the situation that elicits it did not occur, the phrase *not applicable* is written in.

Values achievement of end product. The child's behavior, including affective responses, indicates that the actions that must be executed in order to achieve a goal are perceived as a means toward an end, and that the result or end product of his efforts is appreciated as such. A child who is deeply invested in, for instance, pushing the cookie cutter on the dough, but then pays no attention to the animal shape that results, would not display this characteristic. One who points at it, names it, calls his mother's attention to as if to convey the sentiment, "Look what I made," displays it to a high degree.

Greater pleasure in more difficult achievement. Affect, verbalizations, or physiognomy indicate that success (or near-success) with items that offered substantial difficulty leads to more intense, more genuine, and more deeply felt satisfaction/pride than success with items that were mastered easily. An end product, such as a dancing bear, may yield great pleasure as a spectacle, but this is not relevant to this variable. The pleasure must clearly relate to the child's sense of accomplishment. Children who clap or exclaim, "I did it" even with failure or equally with easy tasks would fall at the *little* extreme, as do those who do not care much about the end product.

When working alone, tends to become discouraged and to give up in the face of failure and difficulty. To receive a score the child must have begun to work at a task at a time when neither active encouragement nor help is provided. If he then shows the opposite of perseverance and abandons or greatly modifies the task, he shows this characteristic. Note that some children are not observed under this condition (those who require encouragement to work at all, in which case the correct score is *not applicable.)*

When working at a difficult task, tends to persevere provided that active encouragement is given. In the same situation as above, the child tends to continue working with encouragement, and it is judged that without it he would not have done so. Note that it is possible for a child to receive a medium or a high score on this item as well as on the preceeding one, since his behavior may include both responses depending upon his state, the degree of difficulty, or other factors.

Tends to welcome help when it is needed and to refuse it when it is not needed. This judges the degree to which the child's response to help offered or given is determined by how much difficulty he encounters in achieving his goal. Again, it is not the objective difficulty of the task as presented that counts but the experienced difficulty in terms of how the child perceives his goal.

Tends to welcome help even with tasks that do not offer special difficulty. This refers to the child's general attitude toward receiving help. Children who typically dislike accepting help and respond to it as an intrusion would receive a score of *little* or zero. Children who typically welcome or enjoy the attention and social interaction in the situation, and hence are disposed to accept help on most occasions, would receive a score of *high*.

Tends to speak and behave as though success had been obtained though aware that this is not the case. This refers to a tendency in some children to clap their hands, exclaim "I did it," or in other ways go through the rituals signalling accomplishment when observers judge that the child was well aware of failure. This is understood as a defensive or coping maneuver that serves to avoid the discomfort of acknowledging failure.

Tends to speak and otherwise behave as though in need of help and unlikely to succeed when this is not the case. This refers to a tendency in some children (who lack self-esteem) to present themselves as more helpless and incompetent than they are as judged by their performance.

Tends to evade or avoid tasks he believes to be too difficult. The child typically avoids exposing himself to the risk of failure by not entering the task situation. What is being rated is a tendency to avoid tasks that appear difficult while readily attempting easy tasks. A general tendency not to accept suggestions is not relevant here.

Angry and distressed at failure. This relates to the intensity of overt negative affect shown when, in spite of effort, the child is unable to succeed. Note that evidence suggesting that intense distress is felt but *not* given overt expression is not scored here.

Tends to perceive help as intrusion and to show strong resistance and anger in response. A *high* score is merited when the so-called *me do syndrome* is observed. That is, the child so dislikes or resents interventions in his independent activity that they are resisted in general, as a function of autonomy strivings largely unrelated to task requirements. Note that the rating refers to affect-laden vigorous protests (not to quiet or polite refusals).

Self-confidence. A clinical estimate of the degree to which the child approaches tasks with the expectation or confidence that, in all probability, he will succeed. Here we try to gauge how the child really feels. Bravado and blind, unrealistic expressions of confidence most often mask inner doubts and hence do not indicate high self-confidence. Note that this variable is so inferential as to be of doubtful usefulness. Scorers are free to omit it, which is preferable to a forced judgment at low confidence levels.

Achievement motivation limited to narrow area. This is either true or false. A child who receives *little* scores on the first two variables and/or tends not to get involved in or persevere on most tasks, but becomes ambitious and involved only in gross motor tasks (or only on formboards and puzzles, or any other area of activity) would receive a plus. Failure to get involved with a majority of items is not scored, as long as achievement motivation was present for a variety of tasks.

Pattern Rating Blank[1]

Overall Ratings

Values achievement of end product.
Greater pleasure in more difficult success.
Working alone, no encouragement, easily stops.
Working alone, encouraged, perseveres.
Welcomes help when task difficult.
Welcomes help even when task not difficult.
Pretends success, knows better.
Pretends inability though competent.
Tends to avoid tasks thought difficult.
Tends to display anger and distress at failure.
Tends to resent all help (me-do-syndrome).
Self-confidence.
Achievement motivation in narrow area.

1. Each pattern could be scored as *high, medium,* or *little.*

Appendix M: The World Test: Description and Scoring Blank (40 Months)

The World Test is a projective test which in the United States has fallen into disuse. In the mid-1970s test materials and manuals were available only in the French edition (Les Editions du Centre de Psychologie Appliquée). Norms are available for ages 5 years and up.

A small number of modifications had to be made in order to use the test with three-year-olds and in our setting. Several scoring categories were omitted because they referred to behavior of which young preschoolers are not capable. Some toys were removed from the standard kit because they were fragile or else depicted objects not familiar to the children. We also added to the scoring sheet. Further, under *Overall Play Ratings* we described behaviors that prevented children from appropriate participation so that they produced no scorable results.

Procedures and Scoring. Test equipment consists of a very large array of miniature toys representing familiar aspects of the "world." We used a 4′ × 4′ yellow plastic board as the surface on which the child built a construction. Toys were placed on the floor and grouped in the following categories: buildings, wild animals, tame animals, vehicles, trees and fences, and people. The board was placed three feet from the row of toys.

The examiner took the child by the hand and walked him or her past the toys explaining, "Here are all the people; this is where all the cars and airplanes are;" and so forth for each group. The examiner then withdrew from the toy area and enjoined the child to use the toys to "make something," to "make anything you like. You can use any of the toys you want and fix them up on this board the way you want them." Once the child had begun, he or she was also told, "Tell me when you are finished. I will take a picture of what you made, so you can take it home to Daddy [or any appropriate family member]." Except for occasional reminders to limit the structure to the board and brief replies to what the child said, the examiner remained on the sidelines.

Polaroid pictures of the end result were taken to facilitate scoring and to keep our promise. (We were intrigued to find out that almost none of our three-year-olds accepted the idea of a photograph that did not include themselves. Only after they had posed and seen the picture of themselves with their construction would they let us photograph their product.)

Scoring Blank

I. Mood state judgments

Child tense, anxious, or bored.
Child spontaneous, pleased, involved.
Child spontaneous, aggressive play predominates.

II. Object Type	Number handled			Final number		
	1–2	3+	All	1–2	3+	All
(a) People (7)						
(b) Farm Animals (17)						
(c) Wild Animals (5)						
(d) Buildings (12)						
(e) Vehicles (13)						
(f) Fences (13)						
(g) Trees and Benches						

III. Child Behaviors

While playing maintains contact with mother most of the time.
While playing maintains contact with examiner most of the time.

IV. Maternal Behavior

Usually responded to child's addresses, no intrusions.
Intruded once or twice with suggestions, warnings, etc.
Despite instructions, often intruded with suggestions, etc.
Conveyed warm, friendly interest in what child was about.
Often or typically scolding, disinterested, aloof, scornful.
Tense, ill at ease, or at loss how to behave.
Whatever her style, self-assured, unruffled.

V. Spatial Organization

Enter check for all structures and organizational types that occur in *final construction.*

1. Matching:
   3 or more objects of one category in close proximity.
2. Representational:
   Objects of different categories placed together in a logical context (e.g., horse fenced in; building with person). Or objects of same category placed together when verbalizations and arrangement indicated a theme (e.g., several cars for parking lot).
3. Piling:
   Objects are heaped or strewn about with no arrangement, no deliberate placement.
4. Linear alignment:
   Single, unbroken linear arrangements predominate. One of these must extend at least 25% of the length of the board.
5. Discontinuous clusters:
   Unconnected clusters with spaces between them.
6. Continuous clusters:
   Clusters with spaces between them, connected by lines or separate objects that were deliberately placed.

7. Enclosures:
   One or several partial or complete enclosures present.
8. Perimeter placements:
   Placements dictated by shape of board, edges, corners, or both.
9. Interior placements:
   Placements extend to interior—that is, near center—of board.

VI. Structure building versus dramatic play

1. Dramatic play dominant, little or no structure building.
2. Structure building as focused activity for at least one brief episode, not interrupted by dramatic play.
3. Structures predominantly of matching type.
4. Structures predominantly representational.
5. Matching and representational, neither predominant in relation to the other.

VII. Overall Play Ratings

1. Child so inhibited that real play does not occur at all or child fails to engage in play for other reasons.
2. Child unable to sustain play activity because of diffuse excitement or disturbing affect (fear, anger).
3. Play is monothematic (e.g., only car crashes, only eating, etc.).

Bibliography

Bayley, N. *Manual for the Bayley Scales of Infant Development*. New York: Psychological Corporation, 1969.

Beckwith, L. and Cohen, S. E., Interactions of preterm infants with caregivers and test performance at age 2. In M. Field, S. Goldberg, D. Stern, and A. M. Sostek (eds.). *High-risk Infants and Children: Adult and Peer Interactions*. New York: Academic Press, 1980.

Biber, Barbara. *Early Education and Psychological Development*. New Haven and London: Yale University Press, 1984.

Block, J. *Lives Through Time*. California: Bancroft Books, 1971.

Block, J. H. Familial and environmental factors associated with the development of affective disorders in young children. National Institute of Mental Health, *Conference on Mood and Related Affective States*. Washington, D.C., November 1976.

——— and Block, J. The role of ego control and ego resiliency in the organization of behavior. A. Collins (ed.). *Minnesota Symposium of Child Psychology*, volume 13. Hillsdale, New Jersey: Lawrence Erlbaum, 1980.

Broman, S. A., Nichols, P. L., and Kennedy, W. A. *Preschool IQ, Prenatal and Early Developmental Correlates*. Hillsdale, New Jersey: Lawrence Erlbaum, 1975.

Cohen, S. E., Sigman, M., Parmelee, A. M., and Beckwith, L. Perinatal risk and developmental outcome in pre-term infants. Seminars in *Perinatology*, 6, 334–39, 1982.

Drillien, C. M. *The Growth and Development of the Prematurely Born Infant*. Baltimore: Williams and Witkins, 1964.

———, Thomson, A. J. M., and Burgoyne, K. Low birthweight children at early school age: a longitudinal study. *Developmental Medicine and Child Neurology*, 22, 26–47, 1980.

Dubowitz, L. M. S., Dubowitz, V., and Goldberg, C. Clinical assessment of gestational age in the newborn infant. *Journal of Pediatrics*, 77, 1–10, 1970.

Escalona, S. K. *The Roots of Individuality: Normal Patterns of Development in Infancy*. Chicago: Aldine Publishing Company, 1968.

———. Babies at double hazard: early development of infants at biologic and social risk. *Pediatrics*, 70, 670–76, 1982.

——— and Corman, H. Early life experience and the development of competence. *International Review of Psychoanalysis*, 1, 151–68, 1974.

Golden, M. and Birns, B. Social class and cognitive development in infancy. *Merrill-Palmer Quarterly of Behavior and Development*, 14, 139–49, 1968.

Golden, M., Birns, B., Bridger, W., et al. Social class differentiation in cognitive development among black preschool children. *Child Development*, 42, 37, 1971.

Golden, M. and Birns, B. Social class and infant intelligence. In M. Lewis (ed.). *Origins of Intelligence: Infancy and Early Childhood*. New York: Plenum Press, 1976.

Golden, M., Rosenbluth, L., Grossi, T., et al. *The New York City Infant Day Care Study*. New York: Medicine and Health Research Association of New York City, 1978.

Kurtzberg, D., Vaughan, H. G., Jr., Daum, C., et al. Neurobehavioral performance of low-birthweight infants at 40 weeks conceptual age: comparison with normal full-term infants. *Developmental Medicine and Child Neurology,* 21, 590–607, 1979.

Lipper, E., Lee Kwang-sun, Gartner, L. M., and Grellong, B. Determinants of neurobehavioral outcome in low-birth-weight infants. *Pediatrics,* 67, 4, 1981.

Myrianthipoulos, N. C. and French, K. S. The application of the U.S. Bureau of Census SES index to a large diversified patient population. *Social Science and Medicine,* 2, 283–99, 1968.

National Institutes of Health. *Perspectives on Human Deprivation: Biological, Psychological and Sociological.* Washington, D.C.: U.S. Department of Health, Education and Welfare, 1968.

Pavenstedt, E. A comparison of the child rearing environment of upper-lower and very low lower-lower class families. *American Journal of Orthopsychiatry,* 35, 89–98, 1965.

———. *The Drifters.* Toronto: Little Brown, 1976.

Pepper, Stephen C. *World Hypotheses.* Berkeley and Los Angeles: University of California Press, c.1942.

Piaget, J. *The Construction of Reality in the Child.* New York: Basic Books, 1954.

Rose, S. A. and Wallace, I. F. Visual recognition memory: a predictor of later cognitive functioning in preterms. *Child Development,* 56, 843–52, 1985.

Sigel, I. E. The distancing hypothesis revisited: an elaboration of a neo-Piagetian view of the development of representational thought. M. E. Meyers (ed.). *Cognitive Learning.* Bellingham, Washington: Western Washington State College Press, 1972.

Sigman, M., Cohen. S. E., and Forsythe, A. B. The relation of early infant measures to later development. In *Preterm Birth and Psychological Development.* S. L. Friedman and M. Sigman (eds.). New York: Academic Press, 1981.

Sparrow, S. S., Balla, D. A., and Cichetti, D. V. *Vineland Adaptive Behavior Scales.* Circle Pines, Minnesota: American Guidance Service, 1984.

Terman, L. M. and Merrill, M. A. *Stanford-Binet Intelligence Scale: Manual for the Third Revision, Form L–M.* Boston: Houghton-Mifflin, 1973.

Wallace, I. F., Escalona, S. K., McCarton-Daum, C., and Vaughan, H. G., Jr. Neonatal precursors of cognitive development in low birthweight children. *Seminars in Perinatology,* 6, 327–33, 1982.

Werner, E., Bierman, I. M., and French, F. E. *The Children of Kauai.* Honolulu: University of Hawaii Press, 1971.

——— and Smith, R. *Vulnerable but Invincible.* New York: McGraw-Hill, 1982.

Werner, H. and Kaplan, B. *Symbol Formation.* New York: Wiley & Sons, 1963.

Wilson, R. S. Synchronies in mental development: an epigenetic perspective. *Science,* 202, 939, 1978.